Global Hematology

Editors

DAVID J. ROBERTS
SIR DAVID J. WEATHERALL

HEMATOLOGY/ONCOLOGY CLINICS OF NORTH AMERICA

www.hemonc.theclinics.com

Consulting Editors
GEORGE P. CANELLOS
H. FRANKLIN BUNN

April 2016 • Volume 30 • Number 2

ELSEVIER

1600 John F. Kennedy Boulevard • Suite 1800 • Philadelphia, Pennsylvania, 19103-2899

http://www.theclinics.com

HEMATOLOGY/ONCOLOGY CLINICS OF NORTH AMERICA Volume 30, Number 2
April 2016 ISSN 0889-8588, ISBN 13: 978-0-323-41756-3

Editor: Jennifer Flynn-Briggs
Developmental Editor: Kristen Helm

Hematology/Oncology Clinics (ISSN 0889-8588) is published bimonthly by Elsevier Inc., 360 Park Avenue South, New York, NY 10010-1710. Months of issue are February, April, June, August, October, and December. Business and Editorial Offices: 1600 John F. Kennedy Blvd., Ste. 1800, Philadelphia, PA 19103–2899. Customer Service Office: 3251 Riverport Lane, Maryland Heights, MO 63043. Periodicals postage paid at New York, NY and at additional mailing offices. Subscription prices are $385.00 per year (domestic individuals), $707.00 per year (domestic institutions), $100.00 per year (domestic students/residents), $440.00 per year (Canadian individuals), $875.00 per year (Canadian institutions) $520.00 per year (international individuals), $875.00 per year (international institutions), and $255.00 per year (international and Canadian students/residents). International air speed delivery is included in all Clinics subscription prices. All prices are subject to change without notice. **POSTMASTER:** Send address changes to Hematology/Oncology Clinics of North America, Elsevier Health Sciences Division, Subscription Customer Service, 3251 Riverport Lane, Maryland Heights, MO 63043. Customer Service (orders, claims, online, change of address): Elsevier Health Sciences Division, Subscription **Customer Service, 3251 Riverport Lane, Maryland Heights, MO 63043. Tel: 1-800-654-2452 (U.S. and Canada); 314-447-8871 (outside U.S. and Canada). Fax: 314-447-8029. E-mail: journalscustomerservice-usa@elsevier.com (for print support); journalsonlinesupport-usa@elsevier.com (for online support).**

Reprints. For copies of 100 or more, of articles in this publication, please contact the Commercial Reprints Department, Elsevier Inc., 360 Park Avenue South, New York, New York 10010-1710; Tel.: 212-633-3874, Fax: 212-633-3820, E-mail: reprints@elsevier.com.

Hematology/Oncology Clinics of North America is covered in MEDLINE/PubMed (Index Medicus), EMBASE/Excerpta Medica, and BIOSIS.

Contributors

CONSULTING EDITORS

GEORGE P. CANELLOS, MD
William Rosenberg Professor of Medicine, Department of Medical Oncology, Dana-Farber Cancer Institute, Boston, Massachusetts

H. FRANKLIN BUNN, MD
Professor of Medicine, Division of Hematology, Brigham and Women's Hospital, Harvard Medical School, Boston, Massachusetts

EDITORS

DAVID J. ROBERTS, DPhil, MRCP, FRCPath
Professor of Haematology, Radcliffe Department of Medicine, National Blood Transfusion Service; Consultant Hematologist, National Health Service Blood and Transplant, John Radcliffe Hospital, University of Oxford, Oxford, United Kingdom

DAVID J. WEATHERALL, MD, FRCP, FRS
Regius Professor of Medicine Emeritus, University of Oxford; Weatherall Institute of Molecular Medicine, John Radcliffe Hospital, Oxford, United Kingdom

AUTHORS

JASMINA AHLUWALIA, MD
Additional Professor, Department of Hematology, Postgraduate Institute of Medical Education and Research, Chandigarh, India

ANGELA ALLEN, PhD
Research Scientist, Molecular Haematology, Weatherall Institute of Molecular Medicine, John Radcliffe Hospital, Oxford, United Kingdom; Honorary Research Fellow, Department of Clinical Sciences, Liverpool School of Tropical Medicine, Liverpool, United Kingdom

STEPHEN ALLEN, MD
Professor of Pediatrics, Department of Clinical Sciences, Liverpool School of Tropical Medicine, Liverpool, United Kingdom

RONALD D. BARR, MB ChB, MD
Professor of Pediatrics, Pathology and Medicine, Department of Pediatric Oncology, McMaster University, Hamilton, Ontario, Canada

IMELDA BATES, FRCP, FRCPath
International Public Health Department, Liverpool School of Tropical Medicine, Liverpool, United Kingdom

VIVIAN CHAN, PhD, FRCPath
Emeritus Professor, Department of Medicine, Queen Mary Hospital, University of Hong Kong, Hong Kong, China

REENA DAS, MD, DNB
Professor, Department of Hematology, Postgraduate Institute of Medical Education and Research, Chandigarh, India

MEGHAN DELANEY, DO, MPH
Department of Laboratory Medicine, Bloodworks Northwest, University of Washington, Seattle, Washington

HAL DRAKESMITH, BSc, PhD
MRC Human Immunology Unit, Weatherall Institute of Molecular Medicine, John Radcliffe Hospital, University of Oxford, Oxford, United Kingdom

ALAA EL-HADDAD, MD
Professor of Pediatric Hematology/Oncology, Department of Pediatric Oncology, Sayda Zainab, Cairo, Egypt

STEPHEN FIELD, MMed(Path) (SA), FCPath (SA)
Welsh Blood Service, Pontyclun, Wales, United Kingdom

SUTHAT FUCHAROEN, MD
Thalassemia Research Center, Institute of Molecular Biosciences, Mahidol University, Nakornpathom, Thailand

SHAU-YIN HA, FHKAM (Paediatrics)
Consultant, Department of Paediatrics and Adolescent Medicine, Queen Mary Hospital, Hong Kong, China

NICHOLAS J. KASSEBAUM, MD
Institute for Health Metrics and Evaluation, University of Washington; Department of Anesthesiology and Pain Medicine, Seattle Children's Hospital, Seattle, Washington

YOK-LAM KWONG, MD
Professor, Department of Medicine, Queen Mary Hospital, University of Hong Kong, Hong Kong, China

LESLIE LEHMANN, MD
Clinical Director, Pediatric Stem Cell Transplant, Dana-Farber Cancer Institute; Assistant Professor of Pediatrics, Harvard Medical School, Boston, Massachusetts

LUCIO LUZZATTO, MD, FRCP, FRCPath
Istituto Toscano Tumori; University of Florence, Florence, Italy

JULIE MAKANI, MD, PhD, FRCP, FTAAS
Department of Haematology and Blood Transfusion, Muhimbili University of Health and Allied Sciences, Dar-es-Salaam, Tanzania

CATERINA NANNELLI, MSc
Core Research Laboratory, Istituto Toscano Tumori, Azienda Universitaria-Ospedaliera Careggi, Florence, Italy

ROSARIO NOTARO, MD
Core Research Laboratory, Istituto Toscano Tumori; Azienda Universitaria-Ospedaliera Careggi, Florence, Italy

NANCY OLIVIERI, MD, FRCP
Professor, Pediatrics, Medicine and Public Health Sciences; Senior Scientist, Toronto General Hospital, University of Toronto, Toronto, Ontario, Canada; Executive Director, Hemoglobal®, Toronto, Canada

SANT-RAYN PASRICHA, MBBS(Hons), MPH, PhD, FRACP, FRCPA
MRC Human Immunology Unit, Weatherall Institute of Molecular Medicine, John Radcliffe Hospital, University of Oxford, Oxford, United Kingdom

FRÉDÉRIC B. PIEL, PhD
Department of Zoology, University of Oxford, Oxford, United Kingdom

DAVID J. ROBERTS, DPhil, MRCP, FRCPath
Professor of Haematology, Radcliffe Department of Medicine, National Blood Transfusion Service; Consultant Hematologist, National Health Service Blood and Transplant, John Radcliffe Hospital, University of Oxford, Oxford, United Kingdom

MAN UPDESH SINGH SACHDEVA, MD
Associate Professor, Department of Hematology, Postgraduate Institute of Medical Education and Research, Chandigarh, India

DAVID J. WEATHERALL, MD, FRCP, FRS
Regius Professor of Medicine Emeritus, University of Oxford; Weatherall Institute of Molecular Medicine, John Radcliffe Hospital, Oxford, United Kingdom

THOMAS N. WILLIAMS, MBBS, DCH, DTM&H, MRCP, PhD
Professor of Haemoglobinopathy Research, St Mary's Hospital, Imperial College of Science, Technology and Medicine, London, United Kingdom; KEMRI/Wellcome Trust Research Programme, Kilifi, Kenya

Contents

Managing hematologic disorders in developing countries poses problems
not encountered in Western societies. The clinical features of hematologic
conditions may be modified by malnutrition, chronic bacterial infection, or
parasitic illness. Iron deficiency is the major factor in anemia worldwide.
Anemia is more common in the wet season when malaria transmission
peaks. After anemia, eosinophilia is the next most common hematologic
abnormality in children in the tropics. Infection with the human immunodeficiency virus can cause hematologic abnormalities. The pattern of distribution of primary disorders of the blood varies among populations and
some disorders are unique to certain parts of the world.

Anemia is an important cause of health loss. We estimated levels and
trends of nonfatal anemia burden for 23 distinct etiologies in 188 countries,
20 age groups, and both sexes from 1990 to 2013. All available population-
level anemia data were collected and standardized. We estimated mean
hemoglobin, prevalence of anemia by severity, quantitative disability
owing to anemia, and underlying etiology for each population using the
approach of the Global Burden of Disease, Injuries and Risk Factors
2013 Study. Anemia burden is high. Developing countries account for
89% of all anemia-related disability. Iron-deficiency anemia remains the
dominant cause of anemia.

Anemia is common among people living in low- and middle-income countries, and alleviation of the global burden of anemia is an essential global
health target over the next decade. Estimates have attributed about half
the cases of anemia worldwide to iron deficiency; a range of other causes
probably make a similar overall contribution. Individuals living in low-
income settings experience a simultaneous high burden of infection with
inflammation and iron deficiency. At least in children, iron supplementation
exacerbates the risk of infection in both malaria-endemic and nonendemic
low-income countries, whereas iron deficiency is protective against clinical
and severe malaria.

HEMATOLOGY/ONCOLOGY
CLINICS OF NORTH AMERICA

ISSUE OF RELATED INTEREST

Clinics in Laboratory Medicine, March 2015 (Vol. 35, Issue 1)
Automated Hematology Analyzers: State of the Art
Carlo Brugnara and Alexander Kratz, *Editors*
Available at: http://www.labmed.theclinics.com/

THE CLINICS ARE AVAILABLE ONLINE!
Access your subscription at:
www.theclinics.com

Preface
Global Hematology

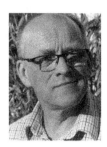 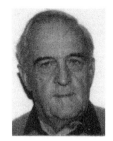

David J. Roberts, DPhil, MRCP, FRCPath   David J. Weatherall, MD, FRCP, FRS
Editors

Many common diseases exhibit marked and complex heterogeneity due to genetic and environmental factors together with variability in their level of management. Hematologic disorders are no exception. In the articles that follow, and which focus particularly on hematologic disease in the developing countries, examples of these problems and the experiences of those who are trying to address them are discussed.

The first article, by Roberts and Weatherall, emphasizes the multifactorial complexity of blood disease in the developing countries, paying particular attention to their modification by nonhematologic disorders, particularly infection. The next article, by Kassebaum, provides a recent updated account of the global burden of anemia based on the Global Burden of Disease program. Pasricha and Drakesmith consider the continuing problems of both the diagnosis and the treatment of iron deficiency, the commonest cause of anemia. The next three articles discuss various aspects of the inherited disorders of hemoglobin, which are the commonest monogenic diseases and which occur at particularly high frequency in many of the developing countries of the tropical belt. The article by Luzzatto and colleagues deals with the problem of another extremely common genetic disease, glucose-6-phosphate dehydrogenase deficiency, particularly in its relationship to severe drug reactions and its role in the pharmacology of *Plasmodium vivax* malaria. Roberts' article deals with the complex hematologic findings related to common infections, particularly those in tropical regions, while the article by Lehmann and colleagues covers the widespread variability in the forms of malignant hematologic disorders. The next two articles provide coverage of the patterns of hematologic disorders in South and Southeast Asia. The article by Makani and Roberts discusses the current complexities and diversity of hematologic practice in sub-Saharan Africa. The article by Roberts and colleagues deals with the problems and approaches for developing blood transfusion programs in the developing countries, while the last article, by Allen and colleagues, describes the role of partnerships between the richer and poorer countries for training and capacity building for developing their hematologic programs.

Hematol Oncol Clin N Am 30 (2016) xiii–xiv
http://dx.doi.org/10.1016/j.hoc.2015.12.003
0889-8588/16/$ – see front matter © 2016 Published by Elsevier Inc.

hemonc.theclinics.com

Since descriptions of the global aspects of hematology are few and far between, we hope that our readers will enjoy this account, particularly those who are considering forming partnerships with the developing countries or North/South partnerships as they are called by the World Health Organization. Already some progress has been made toward these developments and, as reported in the article by Fucharoen and Weatherall, at least a start has been made toward the evolution of South/South partnerships that is between poorer countries who have begun to develop their hematology programs after which they form partnerships with adjacent countries where no progress has been made in this field; the Asian Thalassemia Network is a good example. It is also hoped that these issues will be made available to the major international health agencies and charities, as is clear from several of the articles that financial aid is essential if good hematologic practice can be developed in the poorer countries of the world.

David J. Roberts, DPhil, MRCP, FRCPath
Radcliffe Department of Medicine
National Blood Transfusion Service
University of Oxford
John Radcliffe Hospital
Oxford OX3 9DU, UK

David J. Weatherall, MD, FRCP, FRS
Weatherall Institute of Molecular Medicine
University of Oxford
John Radcliffe Hospital
Oxford OX3 9DS, UK

E-mail addresses:
david.roberts@ndcls.ox.ac.uk (D.J. Roberts)
liz.rose@imm.ox.ac.uk (D.J. Weatherall)

Introduction: The Complexity and Challenge of Preventing, Treating, and Managing Blood Diseases in the Developing Countries

David J. Roberts, DPhil, MRCP, FRCPath[a],*, David J. Weatherall, MD, FRCP, FRS[b]

KEYWORDS

- Hematology • Anemia • Sub-Saharan Africa • Eosinophilia • HIV • Dengue

KEY POINTS

- The diagnosis and management of hematologic disorders in developing countries pose a number of problems not encountered in advanced Western societies.
- The usual clinical features of hematologic disease may be modified to a varying degree by the coexistence of malnutrition, chronic bacterial infection, or parasitic illness.
- Iron deficiency is the major factor in anemia worldwide; numerous other diseases that exacerbate anemia are often operating in the setting of low body iron stores.
- The spectrum of hematologic complications associated with human immunodeficiency virus (HIV) and the high prevalence of infection make HIV testing an essential part of the investigation of cytopenias.
- The pattern of distribution of primary disorders of the blood varies considerably among different populations and some disorders are unique to certain parts of the world.

The diagnosis and management of hematologic disorders in developing countries pose a number of problems that are not encountered in advanced Western societies.[1,2] Although all hematologic conditions can be seen in any population, their clinical features may be modified to a varying degree by the coexistence of malnutrition, chronic bacterial infection, or parasitic illness. Furthermore, many of the common killers, particularly in the tropics, produce their own complicated hematologic

Disclosure Statement: The authors have nothing to disclose.
a Radcliffe Department of Medicine, University of Oxford and National Health Service Blood and Transplant, John Radcliffe Hospital, Level 2, Oxford OX3 9DS, UK; b Weatherall Institute of Molecular Medicine, John Radcliffe Hospital, University of Oxford, Oxford OX3 9DS, UK
* Corresponding author.
E-mail address: david.roberts@ndcls.ox.ac.uk

Hematol Oncol Clin N Am 30 (2016) 233–246
http://dx.doi.org/10.1016/j.hoc.2015.11.001
0889-8588/16/$ – see front matter © 2016 Elsevier Inc. All rights reserved.

manifestations. It is often very difficult to define the clinical features and pathophysiology of a single hematologic disorder in this setting. It, therefore, follows that the study of hematologic disease in these populations presents a particular challenge for hematologists.

The human and material resources available to prevent, diagnose and treat hematologic disease vary widely, not only between countries, but also within countries. In many countries, particularly but not exclusively in newly industrialized countries, there is a long tradition of specialist training and a corresponding breadth and depth of expertise to treat patients with hematologic disease. However, there is a realization that in many parts of the world, there is a gap in knowledge and skills required not simply to treat hematologic problems, but also limited expertise to establish effective polices and training programs for clinical and laboratory hematology. The wider hematologic and scientific community and major donor agencies have responded with a series of initiatives to enhance training and the transfer of skills across the world.

In recent years, it has been possible to start to understand the pathogenesis of some of the hematologic manifestations of systemic disease in children in the Developing World. In this issue of *Hematology/Oncology Clinics of North America*, some of the progress that has been made in understanding and managing the wider aspects of hematology across the world or "global hematology" is reviewed.

PREVALENCE AND MULTIPLE CAUSES OF ANEMIA IN THE DEVELOPING WORLD

Numerous surveys have been conducted to determine the prevalence of anemia in tropical populations. Until recently, it has been very difficult to interpret the results and compare one study with another. It is clear that in many populations the prevalence of anemia in preschool children is extremely high, and in some locations almost 100% of the population is affected. Twenty years ago, the attributable disability-adjusted life-years lost from anemia was estimated to be 35 million healthy life-years.[3]

We now have much more geographically and etiologically defined data on the burden of anemia. Using publicly available data, Kassenbaum and colleagues estimated mild, moderate and severe anemia from 1990 to 2010 for more than 180 countries by sexes and well-defined age groups and attributed the cause of anemia using data from the Global Burden of Diseases, Injuries and Risk Factors 2010 Study[4] and have summarized and updated the findings of this seminal study (in his article on The Global Burden of Anemia, in this issue).

It is certainly difficult to determine the relative importance of different causes of anemia in the tropics. Most surveys have concentrated on only 1 mechanism, such as iron or folate deficiency. However, to get a true picture of the cause of anemia in a particular population, it is necessary to obtain consecutive data over a substantial period (**Table 1**). For example, studies in The Gambia have shown that mean hemoglobin levels in children vary significantly at different times of the year; anemia is much more common in the wet season when malaria transmission is at its highest (**Fig. 1**). This is also the time when diarrhea and malnutrition are most common because heavy rains after many dry months have profound effects on the community, sanitation measures are disrupted and food stores are at a low point in the annual cycle.[5] Although these observations emphasize the multifactorial etiology of anemia, it is clear that iron deficiency, which affects at least 20% of the world's population, is the major factor and that the numerous other diseases that may exacerbate anemia are often operating in the setting of low body iron stores.

The body's response to infection may also reduce iron stores and iron use. Hepcidin is regulated by proinflammatory mediators such as tumor necrosis factor and

Table 1
World Health Organization criteria for hemoglobin concentrations below which anemia is considered to be present in populations at sea level

Age	Hemoglobin Concentration (g/dL)
Children, 6 mo–6 y	11
Children, 6–14 y	12
Adult males	13
Adult females (nonpregnant)	12
Adult females (pregnant)	11

Data from World Health Organization. Nutritional anemias. Report of a WHO group of experts. World Health Organ Tech Rep Ser 1972;503:1–29; with permission.

interleukin-6, which are increased in a wide variety of infections. However, this protective response may contribute to functional iron deficiency and anemia in endemic areas and the interrelationship between iron and infection is explored in more detail (see Pasricha S, Drakesmith H: Iron Deficiency Anemia – Problems in Diagnosis and Prevention at the Population Level, in this issue).

Iron deficiency and anemia are less common in groups that have persisted as hunter–gatherers or the pastoralists who eat blood and meat, such as the Masai in Kenya.[2] In contrast, absorption of nonheme iron, except from breast milk, is comparatively restricted, and so iron deficiency is common in communities whose food is predominantly of vegetable origin.[6] In addition, iron absorption is inhibited by fiber, phytates, phosphates, and polyphenols, which are all found at high levels in the largely vegetarian diets.[6] Loss of iron from chronic hemorrhage secondary to hookworm infection or schistosomiasis further contributes to the high incidence of iron deficiency anemia in the developing world.

Infants of mothers with iron deficiency have low iron stores, their folate status at birth reflects that of their mother, and the folate content of breast milk is diminished by maternal deficiency and maternal malaria.[7–9]

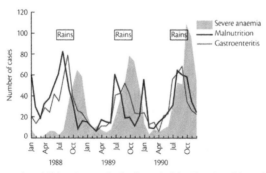

Fig. 1. Admissions to the children's ward of a hospital in The Gambia, where malaria transmission is confined to the rainy season. The incidence of severe malarial anemia corresponds with seasonal epidemics of malaria fever and cerebral malaria. Gastroenteritis and malnutrition also reach a peak incidence in the early part of the rainy season and thus contribute to the multifactorial etiology of the anemia. (*Data from* Brewster DR, Greenwood BM. Seasonal variation of paediatric diseases in The Gambia, West Africa. Ann Trop Paediatr 1993;13:133–46.)

In many populations, anemia may be associated with folate deficiency.[9–11] Again, the reasons are complex and multifactorial. Although intake of folate varies widely among different populations depending on the way in which food is prepared and the temperature at which it is cooked, it is clear that low intake is not necessarily the result of lack of folate in the diet. Loss of appetite associated with recurrent infections such as malaria or tuberculosis is the most important cause of folate deficiency in children[2] and postinfective malabsorption is a particularly common cause of folate deficiency, especially in the Indian subcontinent. Folate deficiency can be exacerbated by the erythroid hyperplasia associated with chronic malarial infection or hemoglobinopathy.[12]

Although nutritional vitamin B_{12} deficiency is uncommon, Indian infants born to mothers with sprue (see Hematologic aspects of malabsorption in the tropics) who are fed breast milk or goat milk containing insufficient vitamin B_{12} may be susceptible to megaloblastic anemia with locomotor complications during the early months of life.[2] This syndrome, which is often fatal, seems to be complicated by a marked predisposition to infection.

Many of the population surveys on the prevalence of anemia in tropical countries have concentrated on 1 particular cause and other illness has not been assessed. Studies in Africa assessing body iron stores, folate levels and the presence of intercurrent infection indicate that chronic recurrent malaria, without other important complicating factors, is the major cause of anemia in these populations.

A major question is whether iron supplementation is the most effective way to prevent anemia in regions where malaria is highly endemic and this is discussed in more depth (see Pasricha S, Drakesmith H: Iron Deficiency Anemia – Problems in Diagnosis and Prevention at the Population Level, and Makani J, Roberts DJ: Hematology in Africa, in this issue).[6] The optimal regime to combine malaria prophylaxis and iron supplementation has not been defined and this dilemma reflects a dichotomy between the optimal protective response to infection and the best physiologic environment for growth, development and recovery. A reduction in iron levels is part of natural host defense against infection, and there is long-standing debate about whether supplementation has adverse consequences, particularly on mortality from infectious diseases.

The outcome of a supplementation program may depend greatly on the pattern of endemic disease in the population and gathering good evidence from well-designed clinical trials to inform policy will undoubtedly be a major focus for future funding and work.

HEMATOLOGIC CHANGES ASSOCIATED WITH SPECIFIC INFECTIONS IN THE TROPICS

Many, if not all, systemic infections are associated with hematologic changes and the common parasitic infections that are widespread across the tropics have a wide variety of hematologic manifestations that may be a presenting feature or form part of a more complex clinical picture.

Malaria

Malaria is the most important parasitic illness of humans and because of its intraerythrocytic life cycle the malarial parasite is particularly prone to cause hematologic manifestations. Anemia caused by ineffective erythropoiesis and increased red blood cell destruction is a common, debilitating and often serious manifestation of many forms of malaria (see Roberts DJ, Field S, Delaney M, et al: Problems and Approaches for Blood Transfusion in the Developing Countries, in this issue).[13]

Visceral Leishmaniasis (Kala-azar)

Leishmaniasis is an infection caused by intracellular protozoan parasites transmitted by various species of sandflies.[14,15] The important hematologic manifestations of leishmanial infection are found in the visceral forms. Severe neutropenia may also occur in young children, and this, together with dyserythropoietic changes in the marrow, marked erythrophagocytosis and bizarre mononuclear infiltrates, may cause confusion with leukemia.

Schistosomiasis

The schistosomes are a group of trematodes that cause major health problems in many parts of the developing world.[16] The most consistent hematologic changes are found in association with *Schistosoma mansoni* infection. The acute phase eosinophilia. As the disease progresses, there may be massive hepatosplenomegaly associated with anemia, neutropenia and thrombocytopenia,[17,18] *Schistosoma haematobium* iron deficiency anemia and/or features of the anemia of chronic disorders.

Trypanosomiasis

Trypanosomal infections are a major cause of ill health throughout the world.[19] American trypanosomiasis is a zoonosis caused by *Trypanosoma cruzi*, which is transmitted to humans in South America by blood-sucking insects. The hematologic changes in Chagas' disease are nonspecific. In the acute phase, mild anemia and lymphocytosis may occur. African trypanosomiasis is caused by *Trypanosoma brucei* and, during the acute phase, normochromic normocytic anemia is present. Occasionally, patients have hemorrhagic manifestations and evidence of disseminated intravascular coagulation.

Hookworm

It has been estimated that more than 900 million people are infected with hookworms, which may cause iron deficiency anemia.[20] A full discussion of the presentation and pathology of anemia associated with infection is given elsewhere (see Roberts DJ: Hematologic Changes Associated with Specific Infections in the Tropics, in this issue).

Complex Hematology of Childhood Human Immunodeficiency Virus Infection in the Developing Countries

Human immunodeficiency virus (HIV) infection provides yet another example of the complex pathogenesis of hematologic problems in the tropics.[21] The virus can infect hematopoietic precursors,[21–23] as well as bone marrow macrophages and stromal fibroblasts, an observation that may explain the marked dyserythropoiesis that is observed commonly in the bone marrow of affected children; however, these changes may also be complicated by opportunistic infection, malnutrition and drug toxicity. Anemia with a low reticulocyte count and a microcytic hypochromic blood picture is common and may reflect both coexistent iron deficiency and the anemia of chronic disorders.[24–26] HIV may cause immune thrombocytopenia early in the course of the disease, but this is not regarded as an adverse prognostic feature. Thrombocytopenia may also be accompanied by microangiopathic hemolytic anemia as part of thrombotic thrombocytopenic purpura, which in the context of HIV infection, responds well to plasma infusion. Later, in addition to the progressive lymphopenia that characterizes acquired immunodeficiency syndrome, both reduced production and increased cellular clearance may contribute to neutropenia and thrombocytopenia.[25,26] Finally, advancing immunodeficiency contributes to a greatly increased risk for lymphoid neoplasms, particularly lymphoma.

The wide spectrum of hematologic complications associated with HIV and the high prevalence of infection make HIV testing an essential part of the investigation of cytopenia in most tropical areas.

TROPICAL EOSINOPHILIA

After anemia, eosinophilia is probably the next most common hematologic abnormality in children in the tropics.[27,28] An increase in eosinophils in bone marrow and peripheral blood, as well as in tissues, is a major feature of infections caused by worms that migrate through extraintestinal organs. Some common causes of eosinophilia in the tropics are summarized in **Box 1**. An absolute increase in the peripheral blood reticulocyte count may occur in any of these conditions listed. However, the term *tropical eosinophilic syndrome* was first used to describe patients with a paroxysmal cough and wheezing, particularly at night, scanty sputum production, weight loss, low-grade fever, lymphadenopathy, and extreme blood eosinophilia (>3000/μL) and is owing to filarial infection.[29,30]

HEMATOLOGIC ASPECTS OF MALABSORPTION IN THE TROPICS

One of the major difficulties in discussing the problem of malabsorption in the tropics is definition.[31] A large proportion of people in tropical climates, both indigenous populations and expatriates who have lived and worked in rural areas, have mild abnormalities of the intestinal mucosa, often associated with impairment of absorption. These structural and functional alterations of the gut have been called *tropical enteropathy*.[32–34] It is likely that they reflect an adaptation to life in the contaminated environment of the tropics with its recurrent enteric infections and peculiarities of diet. Interestingly, similar morphologic lesions have been demonstrated in the colon of otherwise healthy residents of southern India. After expatriates return to temperate climates, these changes in the gut revert to normal.[35]

The more severe malabsorption syndromes, namely sprue and postinfective malabsorption, are associated with chronic diarrhea, wasting and a variety of hematologic

---

Box 1
Causes of eosinophilia in tropical populations

Tissue nematodes
  Wuchereria bancrofti
  Loa loa
  Onchocerca volvulus
  Ankylostoma braziliense
  Strongyloides stercoralis
  Ascaris lumbricoides
  Necator americanus
  Toxocara canis
  Trichinella spiralis

Tissue trematodes
  Schistosoma spp
  Fasciola hepaticum

Tissue cestodes
  Echinococcus granulosus

changes. The term *sprue* was first coined by the English physician Manson while working in China; it is an Anglicization of the Dutch term *indische sprouw*. During the 19th and 20th centuries, tropical sprue was thought to be a disease of expatriates, but it became apparent that similar syndromes commonly occur in indigenous populations. The occurrence of severe malabsorption syndromes is not distributed evenly in the tropical world.[35-37] They are particularly common in the Indian subcontinent, Burma, Malaysia, Vietnam, Borneo, Indonesia, and the Philippines. They are also seen in the West Indies, in parts of Central America (particularly Puerto Rico, Cuba and the Dominican Republic), and in northern parts of South America. There are a few reports from the Middle East and temperate areas. Tropical Africa seems to be spared.

These syndromes are believed to originate from an infection.[38,39] They usually start as an acute attack of diarrhea, which then becomes chronic. Many well-documented epidemics of sprue have been reported both in southern India and in the Philippines among American military personnel. However, despite a vast amount of work, no organism has been isolated that could even approach meeting Koch's postulates. It may be that these disorders can follow infection with a variety of agents, but the reason for the peculiar geographic distribution remains unexplained.

Tropical malabsorption syndromes can occur in individuals of any age. They are characterized by intermittent diarrhea, weight loss and anemia. Varying degrees of mucosal damage are found on biopsy of the small intestine, although an absolutely flat mucosa, as seen in gluten-induced enteropathy, is rare. Hematologic findings in patients with tropical malabsorption syndromes vary considerably. In more advanced disease, megaloblastic anemia is common. It is usually caused by folate deficiency but may also be complicated by vitamin B_{12} deficiency. Frequently, bizarre mixed pictures of iron and folic acid deficiency are found.

Interestingly, although much of the data derive from uncontrolled studies, many of the symptoms and hematologic changes associated with these syndromes can be reversed by a course of oral tetracycline. However, recovery is much more rapid if folate or vitamin B_{12} treatment is given as well.

In a tropical setting, malabsorption can also result from colonization of the small bowel by specific parasites, including *Giardia lamblia*, *Strongyloides stercoralis*, *Cryptosporidium*, and others. Furthermore, abdominal tuberculosis with malabsorption is particularly common, and in Africa HIV infection may be an important cause of malabsorption.[40,41] The local name "slim disease" acknowledges the severe wasting that can occur with HIV infection.[40]

Hematologists without experience in the tropics should be aware that the clinical and hematologic findings of tropical malabsorption syndromes can be extreme. In young children particularly, a good history of diarrheal illness may not always be available, and in many tropical populations recurrent diarrheal illness is the norm anyway. Folate deficiency, as well as producing anemia, may give rise to severe neutropenia and thrombocytopenia with associated infection or bleeding. If intercurrent infection is present, as is often seen in severely affected children, the bone marrow appearance may be deceiving, although there is nearly always some megaloblastic change even if overall the bone marrow is much less hyperplastic than usually observed with folate or B_{12} deficiency in Western settings.

A major diagnostic problem that is often encountered in children returning from the tropics with persistent diarrhea and malabsorption is determining whether they have postinfective malabsorption or celiac disease. If symptoms do not resolve, it may be necessary to initiate a trial of a gluten-free diet and then reintroduce gluten at a later date while monitoring progress with repeated small bowel biopsies.

HEMOSTATIC FAILURE AS A MANIFESTATION OF SYSTEMIC DISEASE IN THE TROPICS

Many tropical infections or other hazards produce serious bleeding disorders. Malaria was considered in a previous section. Here, a few other causes of bleeding disorders that are seen in the tropics are discussed.

Dengue

The dengue viruses are 4 antigenically related but distinct organisms that are transmitted to humans by mosquitos of the species *Aedes aegypti*.[42] The clinical manifestations of this very common infection vary in different parts of the world. In American, African and Indian populations, the disease is characterized by classic dengue fever, but in Southeast Asia a much more serious condition develops in many children, dengue hemorrhagic fever (DHF)/dengue shock syndrome (DSS). The latter develops in infants born to dengue-immune mothers during initial infections or in children older than 1 year during secondary infections. It seems that this curious paradox reflects enhancement of dengue viral infection in mononuclear phagocytes mediated by subneutralizing concentrations of dengue antibody.

The pathophysiologic course of DHF/DSS is quite remarkable.[42,43] Dengue viruses seem to be parasites of mononuclear phagocytes. Furthermore, they use antibody as a specific receptor for gaining entry to these cells. Such antibodies are known as infection-enhancing antibodies. Epidemiologic studies have shown that children 1 year or older always have detectable dengue antibody before acquiring a subsequent infection that results in DHF/DSS. Infants who acquire dengue antibody passively from their mothers are also at risk for development of the syndrome. DHF/DSS is characterized by simultaneous activation of the complement and hemostatic systems, together with a marked increase in vascular permeability.[43–55] It seems that complement activation follows both the classical and alternative pathways. The hemostatic abnormalities include gross thrombocytopenia, prolonged bleeding time, increased prothrombin time, and a reduction in the levels of factors II, V, VII, and IX, together with marked hypofibrinogenemia and an increase in fibrin degradation products. The abnormalities in vascular permeability are characterized by an increased hematocrit, normal or low serum protein levels because of selective loss of albumin, and variable serous effusions.

Precisely what triggers these remarkable events is not clear. However, it seems likely that the mediators are the product of dengue virus–infected mononuclear phagocytes. Studies in Thailand have suggested that low levels of heterotypic neutralizing antibody from a single previous infection prevent the illness in those who acquire dengue 2 infections.[42,45] In contrast, children with circulating dengue-enhancing antibodies but no neutralizing antibodies are at high risk.

Once DHF has been triggered, however, the immune disturbance includes activation of CD4$^+$ and CD8$^+$ T lymphocytes[46] and elevation of tumor necrosis factor and other proinflammatory and procoagulant cytokines.[47] A further factor might be antibodies to plasminogen,[48] thought to arise because of structural homology between plasminogen and the dengue envelope glycoprotein.[49]

The clinical findings of DHF/DSS consist of fever, malaise and anorexia, and about 2 to 5 days later a second phase occurs in which there are widespread hemorrhagic phenomena, including purpura, large spontaneous ecchymoses, and bleeding from previous venipuncture sites. These children then enter a phase of profound shock. The hematologic findings are characterized by a normal or even high hematocrit associated with gross thrombocytopenia and evidence of disseminated intravascular coagulation.[50]

The fact that the most serious pathophysiologic mechanism in this disease is fluid loss rather than hemorrhage has focused attention on the development of treatment regimens similar to those used for the management of severe diarrheal illnesses in children in the tropics. A study in Vietnamese children concluded that initial resuscitation with lactated Ringer solution was appropriate for moderately severe DSS whereas hydroxyethyl starch had fewer adverse reactions than dextran for colloid treatment of severe DSS.[51] Clinical trials of heparin treatment to counteract disseminated intravascular coagulation have not produced impressive results.

Other Viral Hemorrhagic Fevers

Severe hemorrhagic fevers caused by viruses occur throughout the tropical world and are encountered on every continent except Australia and North America.[52] They are the result of RNA viruses of 4 distinct families, each of which is a zoonosis with typical epidemiologic features. They are transmitted by a variety of agents, including ticks and mosquitos. In many instances, the reservoirs and vectors are unknown. These diseases are associated with specific clinical entities in different parts of the world, such as Rift Valley fever, Lassa fever, Argentine hemorrhagic fever, Bolivian hemorrhagic fever, and others.

Many of these conditions are accompanied by hemorrhagic diatheses of varying severity ranging from mild purpura to severe hemostatic failure.[53] As with dengue, shock is a major feature and is often associated with an elevated hematocrit. The bleeding manifestations reflect both increased vascular permeability and consumptive coagulopathy. There have been few extensive coagulation studies performed in patients with these disorders, although disseminated intravascular coagulation has been implicated as the basis for the hemostatic failure.

GEOGRAPHIC VARIABILITY IN THE DISTRIBUTION AND EXPRESSION OF HEMATOLOGIC DISEASE

In addition to the unique hematologic problems caused by disorders that are specific to the tropics or other parts of the developing world, the pattern of distribution of primary disorders of the blood varies considerably among different populations. Furthermore, there are some hematologic syndromes, as yet ill-defined, that are unique to certain parts of the developing world.

Lymphoma and Leukemia

Burkitt's lymphoma is endemic throughout large regions of sub-Saharan Africa and in Papua New Guinea. In Burkitt's classic descriptions of the tumor, he pointed out that its occurrence is related closely to altitude, temperature and rainfall, features that are similar in sub-Saharan Africa and Papua New Guinea. Although this distribution, together with work relating this B-cell tumor to infection with Epstein–Barr virus and evidence for loss of immunologic control of Epstein–Barr virus during acute attacks of malaria,[54,55] relates the prevalence of the tumor to malaria, this is certainly not the whole story. For example, it is not found in Zanzibar, although it is very common in the coastal regions of neighboring Tanzania.

The T-cell leukemia/lymphoma syndrome, first recognized in southern Japan and now known to be owing to infection with human T-cell leukemia/lymphoma virus type 1, has a very restricted distribution in southern Japan and the Caribbean.[56] It is not yet clear which particular lymphocyte populations are involved in the very common histiocytic lymphomas that occur throughout the Middle East and across parts of Central and South America.

The curious syndrome of primary upper intestinal lymphoma (Mediterranean lymphoma) and immunoproliferative disease of the small intestine has to be distinguished from the rare primary intestinal lymphomas that occur sporadically throughout the world, usually in elderly patients.[57,58] In endemic regions, primary upper intestinal lymphoma and immunoproliferative disease of the small intestine occur in much younger age groups, usually of poor socioeconomic background. The pathologic lesions are found predominantly in the upper part of the small intestine and are associated with a clinical picture characterized by malabsorption, which often precedes development of the tumor. In addition, there are considerable variations in age distribution and histologic subtype in different parts of the world. In poorer or less developed countries, Hodgkin's disease occurs at a younger age and is usually the histologic type with a poorer prognosis.[59]

Some interesting differences in rate of occurrence and type of acute leukemia throughout the world are also seen.[54,60] In North America and Europe and in all other westernized populations, acute lymphoblastic leukemia accounts for a high proportion of acute leukemia in children between the ages of 2 and 5. In contrast, acute lymphoblastic leukemia is uncommon in the tropics, particularly in sub-Saharan Africa, where Burkitt's lymphoma is the predominant childhood tumor. On the other hand, in older children the incidence of acute myeloid leukemia and various subtypes of acute lymphoblastic leukemia is similar to that in Western societies.

Hereditary Blood Disorders

The distribution of hemoglobin disorders in the world is described (see Luzzatto L, Nennelli C, Notaro R: Glucose-6-Phosphate Dehydrogenase Deficiency, in this issue). The manifestations of glucose-6-phosphate dehydrogenase (G6PD) deficiency in some developing countries also differ from those seen in the West. The problems of drug-induced hemolysis and favism are discussed in this article. It is important to point out, however, that in parts of Southeast Asia, Greece and Africa, G6PD deficiency seems to be associated with neonatal jaundice.[61–63] This is not a common problem in G6PD deficiency in advanced Western societies. Although this observation was first made more than 30 years ago, the precise mechanism of the neonatal jaundice is not clear. In Singapore, it is enough of a public health problem to have led to routine screening of all newborn babies for G6PD levels.

The high frequency of the hemoglobin disorders and G6PD deficiency reflects relative protection of carriers against malaria. This mechanism is also responsible for the unusually high frequency of ovalocytosis in Melanesia, a condition that is relatively rare in Western populations. Melanesian ovalocytosis is asymptomatic in heterozygotes, although the absence of reported homozygotes suggests that it may have a much more severe phenotype. There is clear evidence that it has reached high frequencies in Melanesia by protection against malaria, particularly cerebral malaria.[64]

Aplastic Anemia

Although more data are needed for confirmation, there is growing evidence that aplastic anemia, particularly in childhood, is much more common in parts of Southeast Asia and South America than in developed Western countries.[65] The ease of availability of potentially toxic agents such as chloramphenicol may be reflected by this finding, but this is probably not the whole story. The possibility exists that it reflects the action of an as yet unidentified infectious agent. This challenging question certainly requires further detailed prospective studies.

Hematologic Disorders Unique to Certain Countries

A number of ill-defined hematologic disorders seem to be common to particular countries. In Thailand, for example, there is a well-recognized disorder called acquired prothrombin complex deficiency, a condition seen mainly in infants who have been breastfed.[66] Despite a great deal of work, the etiology is not yet known, although it is suspected that mothers may have ingested substances antagonistic to prothrombin.

Also in Thailand, a very curious condition called acquired platelet dysfunction with eosinophilia is seen.[67] It is a pediatric disorder characterized by bleeding and ecchymoses. There is associated eosinophilia and abnormal platelet function test results. The etiology is unknown, and current efforts are focused on trying to define a parasitic cause.

In India, an increase has been seen in hemolytic disease of the newborn, which seems to be owing to fetomaternal ABO incompatibility.[68] Evidence showing that this may be related to the administration of tetanus toxoids to pregnant women to prevent the major problem of tetanus neonatorum in that population is increasing; there is a marked increase in the maternal titer of anti-A/anti-B antibodies after the injection of tetanus toxoid.

SUMMARY

The uncertainties and lack of up-to-date clinical and experimental studies and randomized clinical trials that arise in discussion of an outline of global hematology highlight the need for more research and by implication the need for more funding and human resources to understand and tackle these problems. It is hoped that this issue of *Hematology and Oncology Clinics of North America* will not only be informative, but also stimulate thought and provoke action to improve the prevention, diagnosis and treatment of hematologic disorders across the world.

REFERENCES

1. Fleming A, Menendez C. Blood. In: Parry E, Godfrey R, Mabey D, et al, editors. Principles of medicine in Africa. Cambridge (United Kingdom): Cambridge University Press; 1989. p. 924–70.

2. Roberts DJ, Weatherall DJ. Anaemia as a world health problem. In: Warrell D, Cox TM, Firth JD, editors. Oxford textbook of medicine. 5th edition. Oxford (United Kingdom): Oxford University Press; 2015. Available at: http://oxfordmedicine.com/view/10.1093/med/9780199204854.001.1/med-9780199204854-chapter-220503. Accessed July 1, 2015.

3. World Health Organization. World health report 2002. Geneva (Switzerland): World Health Organization; 2002.

4. Kassebaum NJ, Jasrasaria R, Naghavi M, et al. A systematic analysis of global anemia burden from 1990 to 2010. Blood 2014;123(5):615–24.

5. Brewster DR, Greenwood BM. Seasonal variation of paediatric diseases in The Gambia, West Africa. Ann Trop Paediatr 1993;13:133–46.

6. Bothwell TH, Clydesdale FM, Cook JD, et al. The effects of cereals and legumes on iron availability. Washington, DC: International Nutritional Anemia Consultative Group (INACG); 1982.

7. World Health Organization. World health report 2005. Geneva (Switzerland): World Health Organization; 2005. p. 45.

8. Fleming AF. Iron deficiency in the tropics. Clin Haematol 1982;11:365–88.

9. Fleming AF, Ghatoura GBS, Harrison KA, et al. The prevention of anaemia in pregnancy in primigravidae in the guinea savanna of Nigeria. Ann Trop Med Parasitol 1986;80:211–33.

10. Baker SJ. Nutritional anaemias: part 2: tropical Asia. Clin Haematol 1981;10: 843–71.

11. Adam I, Elhassan EM, Haggaz AE, et al. A perspective of the epidemiology of malaria and anaemia and their impact on maternal and perinatal outcomes in Sudan. J Infect Dev Ctries 2011;5(2):83–7.

12. Pitney WR. Anaemia in the tropics. In: Goldberg A, Brain MC, editors. Recent advances in haematology. Edinburgh (Scotland): Churchill Livingstone; 1971. p. 337–56.

13. Lamikanra AA, Brown D, Potocnik A, et al. Malarial anemia: of mice and men. Blood 2007;110(1):18–28.

14. Neva F, Sacks D. Leishmaniasis. In: Warren KS, Mahmoud AAF, editors. Tropical and geographic medicine. New York: McGraw-Hill; 1989. p. 296–308.

15. Herwaldt BL. Leishmaniasis. Lancet 1999;354:1191–9.

16. Mahmoud AAF, Wahab MFA. Schistosomiasis. In: Warren KS, Mahmoud AAF, editors. Tropical and geographic medicine. New York: McGraw-Hill; 1989. p. 458–73.

17. World Health Organization. Progress in assessment of morbidity due to schistosoma haematobium infection: a review of recent literature, WHO/Schisto/87.91. Geneva (Switzerland): World Health Organization; 1987.

18. Miller LH, Warrell DA. Malaria. In: Warren KS, Mahmood AAF, editors. Tropical and geographic medicine. New York: McGraw-Hill; 1989. p. 245–64.

19. Barrett MP, Burchmore RJ, Stich A, et al. The trypanosomiases. Lancet 2003;362: 1469–80.

20. Schad GA, Banwell JG. Hookworms. In: Warren KS, Mahmoud AAF, editors. Tropical and geographic medicine. New York: McGraw-Hill; 1989. p. 379–93.

21. Ellaurie M, Burns ER, Rubinstein A. Hematologic manifestations in pediatric HIV infection: severe anemia as a prognostic factor. Am J Pediatr Hematol Oncol 1990;12:449–53.

22. Folks TM, Kessler SW, Orenstein JM, et al. Infection and replication of HIV-1 in purified progenitor cells of normal human bone marrow. Science 1988;242: 919–22.

23. Zucker-Franklin D, Cao Y. Megakaryocytes of human immunodeficiency virus–infected individuals express viral RNA. Proc Natl Acad Sci U S A 1989;86:5595–9.

24. Tovo PA, De Martino M, Gabiano C, et al. Prognostic factors and survival in children with perinatal HIV-1 infection. The Italian register for HIV infection in children. Lancet 1992;339:1249–53.

25. Perkocha LA, Rodgers GM. Hematologic aspects of human immunodeficiency virus infection: laboratory and clinical considerations. Am J Hematol 1988;29: 94–105.

26. Labrune P, Blanche S, Catherine N, et al. Human immunodeficiency virus–associated thrombocytopenia in infants. Acta Paediatr Scand 1989;78:811–4.

27. Mahmoud AAF. Eosinophilia. In: Warren KS, Mahmoud AAF, editors. Tropical and geographic medicine. New York: McGraw-Hill; 1989. p. 65–70.

28. Ottesen EA. The filariases and tropical eosinophilia. In: Warren KS, Mahmoud AAF, editors. Tropical and geographic medicine. New York: McGraw-Hill; 1989. p. 407–29.

29. Danaraj TJ, Pacheco G, Shanmugaratnam K, et al. The etiology and pathology of eosinophilic lung (tropical eosinophilia). Am J Trop Med Hyg 1966;15:183–9.

30. Joe LK. Occult filariasis: its relationship with tropical pulmonary eosinophilia. Am J Trop Med Hyg 1962;11:646–51.
31. Mathan VI. Gastrointestinal manifestations. In: Warren KS, Mahmoud AAF, editors. Tropical and geographic medicine. New York: McGraw-Hill; 1989. p. 8–15.
32. Baker SJ, Mathan VI. Tropical enteropathy and tropical sprue. Am J Clin Nutr 1972;25:1047–55.
33. Mathan M, Mathan VI. Rectal mucosal morphologic abnormalities in normal subjects in southern India. A tropical colonopathy. Gut 1985;26:710–7.
34. Farthing MJG. Malabsorption in the tropics. In: Weatherall DJ, Ledingham JGG, Warrell DA, editors. Oxford textbook of medicine. Oxford (United Kingdom): Oxford University Press; 1995. p. 14.112–8.
35. Lindenbaum J, Gerson CD, Kent TH. Recovery of small intestinal structure and function after residence in the tropics. I. Studies of peace corps Volunteers. Ann Intern Med 1971;74:218–22.
36. Klipstein FA. Tropical sprue in travelers and expatriates living abroad. Gastroenterology 1981;80:590–600.
37. Klipstein FA, Samloff MI, Schenk EA. Tropical sprue in Haiti. Ann Intern Med 1966; 64:575–94.
38. Klipstein FA, Holdeman LV, Corcino JJ, et al. Enterotoxigenic intestinal bacteria in tropical sprue. Ann Intern Med 1973;79:632–41.
39. Bhat P, Shanthakumari S, Rajan D, et al. Bacterial flora of the gastrointestinal tract in southern Indian control subjects and patients with tropical sprue. Gastroenterology 1972;62:11–21.
40. Serwadda D, Mugerwa RD, Sewankambo NK, et al. Slim disease: a new disease in Uganda and its association with HTLV-III infection. Lancet 1985;2:849–52.
41. Sewankambo N, Mugerwa RD, Goodgame R, et al. Enteropathic AIDS in Uganda: an endoscopic, histological and microbiological study. AIDS 1987;1: 9–13.
42. Halstead SB. Dengue. In: Warren KS, Mahmoud AAF, editors. Tropical and geographic medicine. New York: McGraw-Hill; 1989. p. 675–85.
43. World Health Organization. Dengue hemorrhagic fever: diagnosis, treatment and control. Geneva (Switzerland): World Health Organization; 1986.
44. Bhamarapravati N, Tuchinda P, Boonyapaknavik V. Pathology of Thailand, haemorrhagic fever: a study of 100 autopsy cases. Ann Trop Med Parasitol 1967; 61:500–10.
45. Pathogenetic mechanisms in dengue haemorrhagic fever. Report of an internal collaborative study. Bull World Health Organ 1973;48:117–33.
46. Kurane I, Innis BL, Nimmannitya S, et al. Activation of T lymphocytes in dengue virus infections. High levels of soluble interleukin 2 receptor, soluble CD4, soluble CD8, interleukin 2 and interferon-gamma in sera of children with dengue. J Clin Invest 1991;88:1473–80.
47. Bethell DB, Flobbe K, Cao XT, et al. Pathophysiologic and prognostic role of cytokines in dengue hemorrhagic fever. J Infect Dis 1998;177:778–82.
48. Chungue E, Poli L, Roche C, et al. Correlation between detection of plasminogen cross-reactive antibodies and hemorrhage in dengue virus infection. J Infect Dis 1994;170:1304–7.
49. Markoff LJ, Innis BL, Houghten R, et al. Development of cross-reactive antibodies to plasminogen during the immune response to dengue virus infection. J Infect Dis 1991;164:294–301.

50. Wills BA, Oragui EE, Stephens AC, et al. Coagulation abnormalities in dengue hemorrhagic fever: serial investigations in 167 Vietnamese children with dengue shock syndrome. Clin Infect Dis 2002;35:277–85.
51. Wills BA, Nguyen MD, Ha TL, et al. Comparison of three fluid solutions for resuscitation in dengue shock syndrome. N Engl J Med 2005;353:877–89.
52. McCormick JB, Fisher-Hoch S. Viral hemorrhagic fevers. In: Warren KS, Mahmoud AAF, editors. Tropical and geographic medicine. New York: McGraw-Hill; 1989. p. 700–28.
53. Cosgriff TM. Viruses and hemostasis. Rev Infect Dis 1989;11:S672–88.
54. Hutt MSR, Burkitt DP. The geography of non-infectious disease. Oxford (United Kingdom): Oxford University Press; 1986. p. 98–107.
55. Whittle HC, Brown J, Marsh K, et al. T-cell control of Epstein-Barr virus–infected B cells is lost during P. falciparum malaria. Nature 1984;312:449–50.
56. Blattner WA, Blayney DW, Robert-Guroff M, et al. Epidemiology of human T-cell leukaemia/lymphoma virus. J Infect Dis 1983;147:406–16.
57. Ramot B, Hulu N. Primary intestinal lymphoma and its relation to alpha chain disease. Br J Cancer 1975;11:343–9.
58. Dutz W, Borochovitz D. The two basic forms of primary intestinal lymphoma. In Proceedings of the Symposium on Prevention and Detection of Cancer. New York, Marcel Dekker, 1980.
59. Burn C, Davies JN, Dodge OG, et al. Hodgkin's disease in English and African children. J Natl Cancer Inst 1971;46:37–41.
60. Williams CKO, Folami AO, Laditan AA, et al. Childhood acute leukaemia in a tropical population. Br J Cancer 1982;46:89–94.
61. Bienzle U. Glucose-6-phosphate dehydrogenase deficiency. Part I: tropical Africa. Clin Haematol 1981;10:785–99.
62. Panich V. Glucose-6-phosphate dehydrogenase deficiency. Part 2: tropical Asia. Clin Haematol 1981;10:800–14.
63. Chan MCK. Neonatal jaundice. In: Hendrickse RG, editor. Paediatrics in the tropics. Oxford (United Kingdom): Oxford Medical; 1981. p. 13–26.
64. Allen SJ, O'Donnell A, Alexander NDE, et al. Prevention of cerebral malaria in children in Papua New Guinea by Southeast Asian ovalocytosis band 3. Am J Trop Med Hyg 1999;60:1056–60.
65. Wasi P, Piankijagum A. Geographical variation in blood disease: Southeast Asia. In: Weatherall DJ, Ledingham JGG, Warrell DA, editors. Oxford textbook of medicine. Oxford (United Kingdom): Oxford University Press; 1987. p. 19.266–8.
66. Bhanchet-Isarangkura P. The pathogenesis of acquired prothrombin complex deficiency syndrome (APCD syndrome) in infants. Southeast Asian J Trop Med Public Health 1979;10:350–2.
67. Suvatte V, Mahasandana C, Tanphaichitr V, et al. Acquired platelet dysfunction with eosinophilia: study of platelet function in 62 cases. Southeast Asian J Trop Med Public Health 1979;10:358–67.
68. Mehta BC. Geographical variation in blood disease: India. In: Weatherall DJ, Ledingham JGG, Warrell DA, editors. Oxford textbook of medicine. Oxford (United Kingdom): Oxford University Press; 1987. p. 19.270–3.

The Global Burden of Anemia

Nicholas J. Kassebaum, MD[a,b,*], on behalf of GBD 2013 Anemia Collaborators

KEYWORDS

- Anemia • Iron-deficiency anemia • Burden of disease • Hemoglobinopathies
- Nutrition • Hemoglobin • Global health

KEY POINTS

- Anemia burden is high, affecting 27% of the world's population—1.93 billion people—in 2013. Developing countries account for more than 89% of the burden.
- Preschool children and women of reproductive age are particularly affected by anemia.
- Iron-deficiency anemia is the dominant cause ($\geq$60%) of anemia globally and in most populations, though there are important contributions from multiple other causes.
- Other important causes of anemia include hemoglobinopathies, infections, chronic kidney diseases, gastrointestinal and gynecologic conditions. Patterns vary with respect to age, sex, and geography.
- Individual- and population-level interventions aimed at reducing burden should take into account the context-specific epidemiology of anemia to maximize effectiveness and avoid potential harm.

INTRODUCTION

The primary role of hemoglobin is delivering oxygen to tissues and returning carbon dioxide to the lungs for elimination from the body. Any condition that leads to a shortage of functional hemoglobin or decreased red blood cell (RBC) mass may cause anemia. The pathophysiology of anemia is thus diverse and often multifactorial. Causes can include genetic mutations in hemoglobin genes, acute and chronic blood loss, inadequate nutritional intake, altered RBC morphology leading to shortened RBC life span, infectious processes, or alterations in iron and RBC metabolism secondary to chronic inflammation. A shortage of iron—the core of each hemoglobin molecule— is a common manifestation of many conditions that cause anemia.

Anemia has been associated with increased morbidity and mortality. Symptoms likely result from impaired tissue oxygen delivery and may include weakness, fatigue,

[a] Institute for Health Metrics and Evaluation, University of Washington, Seattle, WA, USA;
[b] Department of Anesthesiology and Pain Medicine, Seattle Children's Hospital, Seattle, WA, USA
* Corresponding author. 2301 5th Avenue, Suite 600, Seattle, WA 98121.
E-mail address: nickjk@uw.edu

Hematol Oncol Clin N Am 30 (2016) 247–308
http://dx.doi.org/10.1016/j.hoc.2015.11.002
0889-8588/16/$ – see front matter © 2016 Elsevier Inc. All rights reserved.

concentration difficulty, or poor work productivity.[1,2] Children may have issues with mental and motor development if they[3-5] or their mothers[6] are anemic. Anemia has been correlated with increased risk of preterm labor, low birth weight,[7,8] child and maternal mortality,[9,10] and may predispose to infection[11] and heart failure.[12] Although many studies have focused on iron-deficiency anemia (IDA), the findings have suggested risk in IDA exceeds that in nonanemic iron deficiency, supporting a primary role for anemia as a risk factor for poor outcomes. Even in high-income settings, anemia has been identified as related to decreased quality of life and physical functioning.[13,14] It has also been shown to be an independent risk factor for fatality in patients undergoing surgical procedures[15] and is associated with increased all-cause mortality in the general population.[16]

Attention to the burden of anemia throughout the world has been increasing. Many early inquiries appropriately focused on populations felt to be at greatest risk—pregnant women and children in low-income countries—because they were believed to be those with the greatest problems with inadequate nutrition, high infectious disease burden, and poor access to routine health care. Subsequent studies have found the prevalence of anemia is nontrivial even in high-income countries,[17,18] in nonpregnant women,[19] and in older adults.[20,21] Additionally, anemia is a common manifestation of conditions such as chronic kidney diseases (CKDs), malignancies, and autoimmune disorders.

This analysis, building on the one previously completed by our group, is intended to serve as a framework for understanding the population-specific epidemiology and pathophysiology of anemia throughout the world. We took advantage of the systematic approach of the Global Burden of Disease (GBD), Injuries and Risk Factors 2013 Study to elucidate levels and trends of anemia-related disability. This includes estimates of prevalence and years lived with disability (YLD) for mild, moderate, severe and total anemia—by underlying cause—in 188 countries, 21 GBD regions, 20 age groups, and both sexes from 1990 to 2013.

METHODS

Anemia burden estimation methods were largely unchanged since GBD 2010. The details of that analysis have been described in detail previously,[22] but will be summarized here with emphasis on the updates since that time.

Estimation of Overall Anemia

Our estimation strategy again began with the calculation of an anemia envelope—a determination of mean hemoglobin as well as sum total of anemia prevalence by severity for each country, age group, and both sexes for each year from 1990 through 2013. The envelope approach avoided double counting while capturing potentially different disease profiles within each population group. We defined a population group as a specific country, sex, age group, and year.

We used population-based surveys of hemoglobin concentration as the primary data input for envelope calculations. These data were not only the most reliable and comparable measures of anemia, coming from national and subnational measurement surveys, but also spanned the most countries and time-periods. Tabulated data from published and unpublished studies, collated by the World Health Organization (WHO) Vitamin and Mineral Nutrition Information System, were used to supplement the dataset. Most used a HemoCue test, adjusted for altitude, and excluded those with terminal or acute medical conditions. Inclusion, exclusion and diagnostic criteria for other studies were similar and can be found in each study. A full list of relevant studies is contained in the Global Health Data Exchange and the Institute for Health Metrics and Evaluation website (available at: www.healthdata.org).

We predicted mean hemoglobin levels for all missing population groups using a mixed-effects linear regression with fixed effects on prevalence of severe underweight (<2 standard deviations below the mean; same as the GBD 2010) and age group and nested random effects on super-region, region, and country/subnational site. For these regressions, we again separated each population into 5 groups: male and female children under 5 years, pregnant females, nonpregnant females, and males over 5 years. The country- and year-specific prevalence of underweight children was obtained from the Institute for Health Metrics and Evaluation causes of death database and had been previously calculated for every year between 1970 and 2013 by using spatial–temporal regression of data from national and subnational measurement surveys.[23]

We adopted different thresholds for defining anemia by age than were used in the GBD 2010 because they do not reflect the hematologic realities of early life. GBD 2010 thresholds had been matched with those used by the WHO in GBD 2000[24], but since then, likely in recognition of the same phenomenon, WHO recommendations have been updated. Our current thresholds match those published by WHO with the exception of those under 1 month of age, where there is no internationally recommended cutoff for diagnosing anemia.[25] The GBD 2010 and the GBD 2013 thresholds are shown in **Table 1**. Our current thresholds match those published by WHO with the exception of those under 1 month of age, where there is no internationally recommended cutoff for diagnosing anemia.[25]

In recognizing the limitations of predicting the prevalence of anemia—especially severe anemia—directly from mean hemoglobin using multiple steps, we instead pooled survey microdata for each population group separately and fitted the pooled data with Weibull distributions. We then performed ordinary least-squares regression of the shape and scale parameters versus all predicted mean hemoglobin values predicted above. The prevalence of mild, moderate, severe, and total anemia was then calculated by determining the area under the Weibull curve for each population group using the hemoglobin thresholds in **Table 1**. After adjusting for estimated prevalence of pregnancy, we finalized the anemia envelope by calculating YLD for each population group. YLD are the product of prevalence times disability weight for each severity of anemia. Disability weights ranged from 0 (no health loss) to 1 (equivalent to death) and were derived from population-representative surveys as described previously.[26,27]

Etiologic Attribution of Anemia Cases

We performed cause-specific attribution on the anemia envelope using the same method as in the GBD 2010. Total "hemoglobin shift" was determined as the difference between the normal and predicted mean hemoglobin levels for each population group. We denoted the normal hemoglobin level as the global 95th percentile of the distribution of mean hemoglobin within each age group, sex, and year. We then determined a total shift for each country in the corresponding age group, sex, and year by finding the difference between the global "normal" and the country-specific predicted mean hemoglobin. Our model of attribution followed that, because the shift is a disease state experienced by 100% of the population, then the sum of cause-specific hemoglobin shifts times the prevalence of each contributing cause should add up to the total. Cause-specific hemoglobin shifts where unchanged from GBD 2010.

We summed shift times prevalence estimates from all causes, compared with the total predicted hemoglobin shift, and proportionally assigned. We distributed the residual envelope among 7 remaining causes. Of note, our IDA estimates include acute

Table 1
Hemoglobin thresholds (g/L) by age, sex, and pregnancy status used in classifying anemia cases as mild, moderate, and severe in GBD 2010 versus 2013

	Severity of Anemia		
Variable	Mild	Moderate	Severe
Severity definitions and corresponding disability weights used to calculate GBD 2010 anemia envelope			
Age <5 y			
Males	110–119	80–109	50–79
Females	110–119	80–109	50–79
Age ≥5 y			
Males	120–129	90–119	60–89
Females, nonpregnant	110–119	80–109	50–79
Females, pregnant	100–109	70–99	40–69
Disability weights			
All cases	0.004 (0.001-0.008)	0.052 (0.034-0.076)	0.149 (0.101-0.209)
Severity definitions and corresponding disability weights used to calculate GBD 2013 anemia envelope			
Age <1 mo			
Males	130–149	90–129	<90
Females	130–149	90–129	<90
Age 1 mo–5 y			
Males	100–109	70–99	<70
Females	100–109	70–99	<70
Age 5–14 y			
Males	110–114	80–109	<80
Females	110–114	80–109	<80
Age ≥5 y			
Males	110–129	80–109	<80
Females, nonpregnant	110–119	80–109	<80
Females, pregnant	100–109	70–99	<70
Disability weights			
All cases	0.005 (0.002–0.011)	0.058 (0.038–0.086)	0.164 (0.112–0.228)

Global Burden of Disease (GBD) 2010 definitions for each severity were based on GBD 2000. Subsequent revisions to World Health Organization hemoglobin threshold recommendations led to changes in the GBD 2013 definitions as shown in the lower panel. Cutoffs for mild, moderate, and severe anemia vary by age, sex, and pregnancy status. Disability weights were determined via a worldwide health survey. Additional surveys were administered for GBD 2013, which resulted in slight changes to disability weight values.

and chronic hemorrhagic states for which supplementation may be helpful, but poor nutritional intake is not the only underlying problem. A few causes in this category, namely, hookworm, schistosomiasis, upper gastrointestinal bleeding, and gynecologic conditions, were considered separately from IDA because there was enough data from the GBD 2013 to do so. Distribution of anemia burden to IDA only after assignment to "known" causes avoided double counting of these cases. Most other causes of anemia not specifically considered were included in the "other" categories.

Two changes in the GBD 2013 analysis affected the etiology-specific anemia estimates. First, and most important, we identified an inconsistency in this cause-specific attribution method where the total number of cases of anemia owing to a condition was not bounded to be less than the total number of cases of the condition itself. We have introduced a method in this analysis to ensure that bounds are included. Second, inherent in our method of determining "normal" hemoglobin is the fact that 5% of population groups will have zero, or negative, total shift. In these cases, or when the sum of all causes' shift–times–prevalence estimates exceeded the total shift, we assigned the denominator to be equal to the sum of the numerators. Subsequent review of findings from National Health and Nutrition Examination Survey III suggested that the implicit assumption of zero residual—and therefore zero IDA—in the GBD 2010 approach was implausible.[28,29] Based on the published rates of IDA seen in these analyses, we therefore introduced a minimum of 10% of all anemia to be assigned to residual causes in the GBD 2013.

To disaggregate marginal estimates of anemia severity and etiology into a complete set of prevalence estimates for etiology/severity pairs, we developed a new method for the GBD 2013 that used techniques from Bayesian contingency table modeling.[30,31] The model combined marginal estimates on the row sums (total etiology prevalence for each cause) and column sums (total anemia prevalence by severity [mild, moderate, or severe]) with priors on the mean hemoglobin shift for each etiology and priors on the rank order of variation of severity (ie, anemia owing to malaria is expected to vary most between cases of all etiologies, whereas anemias owing to sickle cell disorders are expected to be some of the least variable in severity). We used nonlinear optimization to find the maximum a posteriori point estimate for 50 samples from estimated posterior distributions on the marginal values (etiology and severity estimates) independently for each population group, and then scaled and shifted these estimates to ensure that updated marginal row sums were all nonzero and the updated column sums matched the original draws exactly.

Uncertainty and Aggregation

The final result of our analysis was estimates of mild, moderate, and severe anemia by cause for each of 20 age groups, 188 countries, 21 GBD regions, and both sexes in 1990, 1995, 2000, 2005, 2010, and 2013. Uncertainty was propagated using Monte Carlo simulation techniques by taking 1000 draws of each quantity calculated for each population group. Aggregations by geography, age, cause, and sex were made at the draw level assuming uncorrelated uncertainty. The uncertainty interval around each quantity, at each level of aggregation, is presented as the 2.5th and 97.5th centile of the draws, which can be interpreted as a 95% uncertainty interval (UI).

RESULTS

Our dataset for estimating the anemia envelope covered 996 separate surveys from 161 countries and contained more than 4 times as many data points as it did in the GBD 2010 (9899 vs 2425), notably including data from Turkey and India as well as subnational data from the United Kingdom, China, and Mexico.

The global age-standardized prevalence of anemia was 27.0% in 2013, down from 33.3% in 1990, a decrease of approximately 21% (**Fig. 1**). Largely owing to population growth, the total number of cases worldwide actually increased somewhat over this

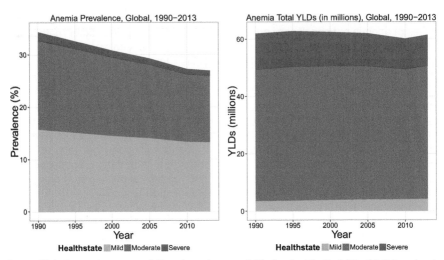

Fig. 1. Global prevalence rate (%) and total years of life lived with disability (YLDs) owing to anemia for both sexes combined from 1990 to 2013. (*Left*) Global prevalence rate of anemia, by severity, for all ages combined. (*Right*) Total YLDs globally; also by severity. A majority of anemia cases are mild and moderate, but a majority of the disability is owing to moderate and severe anemia.

time period. There were a total of 1.93 billion people with anemia in 2013 (compared with 1.83 billion in 1990), including 950 million cases of mild anemia, 906 million cases of moderate anemia, and 75.6 million cases of severe anemia. The total global number of YLDs also changed very little, decreasing from 62,023,831 (95% UI, 41,591,487–89,266,761) to 61,525,570 (95% UI, 41,020,763–88,730,696) for both sexes combined.

Geographic differences in anemia burden are readily apparent (**Fig. 2**). The age-standardized prevalence rates of anemia in 2013 were greatest in central and western sub-Saharan Africa at 45.1% and 43.2%, respectively, although the greatest number of cases was in South Asia. Four countries with highest prevalence were Afghanistan, Chad, Mali, and Yemen, all of which had anemia age-standardized prevalence rates in excess of 50% in 2013, although this is an improvement from 1990 when more than 20 countries had anemia prevalence rates of greater than 50%. Anemia was nontrivial in all countries. Chile, Venezuela, Canada, and Ukraine were the lowest globally, although in each case the age-standardized anemia prevalence was still greater than 14%. Country-specific anemia prevalence and YLDs for 1990 and 2013 is shown in **Table 2**.

Analysis of YLD rates shows that anemia burden is even more concentrated in many of the highest prevalence countries, especially in western and central sub-Saharan Africa (**Fig. 3**, top panel), because cases in those locations tend to be more severe, likely reflecting the wide variety of anemia-causing conditions that are highly prevalent there. Analyzing changes in age-standardized YLD rates from 1990 to 2013, a metric to disentangle changes in disease severity from those in total anemia prevalence further demonstrates geographic heterogeneity (see **Fig. 3**, bottom panel). Global change in absolute YLD rates was -24.0%. The biggest gains were seen in the GBD regions of South Asia, East Asia, Southeast Asia, and Eastern sub-Saharan Africa where absolute YLD rates changed by -50.5%, -44.8%, -31.7% and -21.1%, respectively. High income countries had a collective YLD rate change of only -3.0%, although

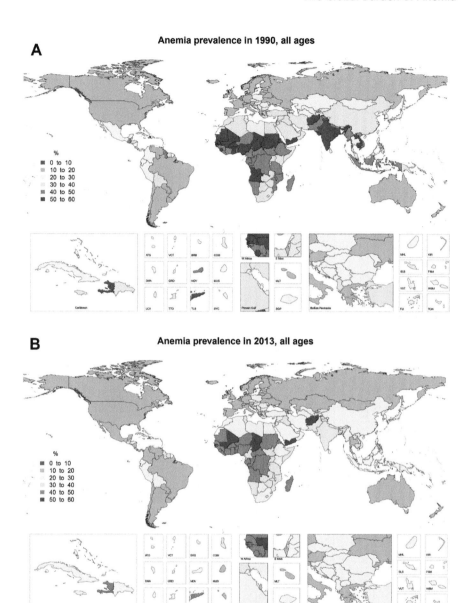

Fig. 2. All ages anemia prevalence rate (%) in 1990 (*A*) and 2013 (*B*). The maps demonstrate the anemia prevalence comparing 1990 with 2013 for all ages combined. This is the final result of the Global Burden of Disease (GBD) 2013 analysis. As can be seen, there has been substantial progress in many countries since 1990, especially in East, Southeast and South Asia, North Africa and the Middle East, and Eastern sub-Saharan Africa. Anemia prevalence is nontrivial in all locations because no country has a prevalence rate of less than 10%. ATG, Antigua and Barbuda; BRB, Barbados; COM, Comoros; DMA, Dominica; FJI, Fiji; FSM, Federated States of Micronesia; GRD, Grenada; KIR, Kiribati; LCA, Saint Lucia; MDV, Maldives; MHL, Marshall Islands; MLT, Malta; MUS, Mauritius; SGP, Singapore; SLB, Solomon Islands; SYC, Seychelles; TLS, Timor-Leste; TON, Tonga; TTO, Trinidad and Tobago; VCT, Saint Vincent and the Grenadines; VUT, Vanuatu; WSM, Samoa.

Table 2
Global, regional, and national levels of anemia burden in 2013

Location	Year	Sex	Prevalent Cases of Mild Anemia	Prevalent Cases of Moderate Anemia	Prevalent Cases of Severe Anemia	Age-Standardized Prevalence (per 100,000)	Total YLDs	Age-Standardized YLDs (per 100,000)
Global	1990	Both sexes	839,101,225.4 (838,208,707.5–839,955,789.6)	901,120,023.0 (899,990,318.7–902,046,164.5)	88,720,927.6 (88,552,510.9–88,859,872.5)	33,299.5 (33,263.5–33,331.5)	62,023,831.1 (41,591,487.1–89,266,761.4)	1,091.9 (732.3–1,569.5)
	2013	Both sexes	950,135,190.5 (949,030,314.0–951,108,861.0)	905,501,750.5 (904,278,930.0–906,519,016.7)	75,565,628.1 (75,357,541.3–75,721,856.5)	26,991.8 (26,960.4–27,018.7)	61,525,569.8 (41,020,762.8–88,730,696.2)	859.3 (573.2–1,238.6)
Developing	1990	Both sexes	717,671,655.0 (716,867,100.8–718,498,928.4)	803,792,125.1 (802,749,357.9–804,607,118.1)	82,149,100.0 (81,975,156.7–82,287,958.6)	37,954.4 (37,911.8–37,989.9)	55,406,696.0 (37,199,421.0–79,697,035.6)	1,248.7 (839.0–1,792.5)
	2013	Both sexes	816,531,244.4 (815,466,757.9–817,478,531.6)	809,200,194.2 (808,094,426.7–810,128,652.7)	69,480,441.4 (69,275,554.2–69,633,255.2)	28,704.2 (28,668.2–28,734.0)	54,943,619.1 (36,684,321.5–79,166,056.1)	915.7 (611.5–1,318.6)
Developed	1990	Both sexes	121,429,570.4 (121,222,264.7–121,614,940.7)	97,327,897.8 (97,066,039.9–97,597,282.9)	6,571,827.5 (6,553,301.2–6,588,472.7)	19,748.7 (19,713.1–19,784.2)	6,617,135.1 (4,406,509.6–9,587,496.3)	599.9 (398.9–868.8)
	2013	Both sexes	133,603,946.0 (133,431,595.0–133,779,611.7)	96,301,556.3 (96,037,352.6–96,515,838.6)	6,085,186.7 (6,067,444.4–6,101,388.3)	19,269.5 (19,240.8–19,295.1)	6,581,950.7 (4,387,351.3–9,536,709.7)	580.8 (386.0–843.0)
Southeast Asia, East Asia, and Oceania	1990	Both sexes	272,843,162.9 (272,517,508.7–273,114,891.9)	259,280,129.5 (258,953,407.3–259,543,749.3)	21,568,299.3 (21,540,572.5–21,598,183.2)	32,915.7 (32,880.9–32,943.1)	17,333,763.7 (11,541,978.2–25,090,126.5)	1,002.1 (668.0–1,449.8)
	2013	Both sexes	248,399,344.4 (248,087,264.3–248,675,600.5)	203,469,039.8 (203,237,374.8–203,682,641.4)	14,075,627.6 (14,055,440.6–14,097,074.5)	23,542.3 (23,517.6–23,563.2)	13,503,538.9 (8,943,371.5–19,685,329.7)	708.2 (469.9–1,028.8)
East Asia	1990	Both sexes	185,710,649.9 (185,467,649.2–185,906,403.8)	166,410,635.6 (166,187,371.7–166,593,443.7)	12,806,104.4 (12,787,096.2–12,826,907.3)	30,393.7 (30,361.4–30,419.3)	11,048,546.0 (7,337,047.3–16,046,122.5)	908.5 (604.1–1,317.2)
	2013	Both sexes	160,676,128.6 (160,442,997.7–160,882,358.4)	124,256,712.2 (124,094,331.3–124,412,866.0)	8,089,471.4 (8,076,864.8–8,101,249.7)	22,066.1 (22,040.5–22,088.4)	8,240,350.8 (5,446,745.7–12,043,703.1)	662.0 (438.9–962.9)

Region	Year	Sex						
China	1990	Both sexes	180,178,918.6 (179,944,201.7–180,368,073.8)	161,341,194.3 (161,124,102.3–161,518,767.0)	12,415,638.4 (12,397,214.2–12,436,710.6)	30,501.6 (30,469.3–30,527.1)	10,711,188.4 (7,112,678.7–15,556,170.5)	911.3 (605.9–1,321.3)
	2013	Both sexes	154,517,804.0 (154,288,559.5–154,716,500.1)	119,303,240.2 (119,142,419.2–119,454,208.3)	7,742,259.4 (7,729,815.8–7,753,758.6)	21,954.7 (21,929.0–21,976.5)	7,909,598.3 (5,226,886.8–11,563,249.7)	658.2 (436.4–957.6)
North Korea	1990	Both sexes	3,391,424.3 (3,384,778.8–3,398,259.8)	3,084,557.1 (3,077,947.5–3,089,529.7)	245,759.9 (244,771.8–247,432.4)	33,541.5 (33,487.5–33,587.3)	205,501.4 (136,769.5–298,361.6)	1,024.5 (682.6–1,483.8)
	2013	Both sexes	3,820,259.5 (3,813,691.0–3,825,353.2)	3,222,264.6 (3,216,318.0–3,227,823.4)	239,662.3 (238,710.8–240,670.3)	30,056.5 (30,005.5–30,099.1)	214,485.8 (142,313.4–310,981.2)	909.3 (604.2–1,317.6)
Taiwan	1990	Both sexes	2,140,307.0 (2,135,513.9–2,143,997.3)	1,984,884.2 (1,979,936.2–1,989,970.2)	144,706.1 (144,359.0–144,965.7)	21,134.8 (21,095.4–21,171.6)	131,856.2 (88,025.9–191,590.3)	634.5 (423.4–921.8)
	2013	Both sexes	2,338,065.1 (2,331,317.8–2,343,939.8)	1,731,207.4 (1,721,647.9–1,739,302.5)	107,549.6 (107,056.7–107,958.1)	20,109.6 (20,047.9–20,160.5)	116,266.7 (77,736.1–169,281.4)	610.5 (407.5–883.4)
Southeast Asia	1990	Both sexes	86,149,050.0 (86,047,549.0–86,252,013.6)	91,700,835.0 (91,567,083.4–91,805,536.5)	8,656,438.7 (8,639,493.1–8,672,081.8)	40,055.8 (40,011.3–40,097.9)	6,206,884.6 (4,150,478.1–8,952,476.3)	1,258.4 (844.5–1,811.5)
	2013	Both sexes	86,391,594.5 (86,282,467.9–86,488,515.8)	77,709,847.0 (77,610,065.5–77,800,783.6)	5,864,052.2 (5,849,391.2–5,878,256.5)	26,806.3 (26,774.7–26,836.7)	5,163,748.2 (3,432,159.2–7,501,408.1)	804.1 (535.1–1,166.2)
Cambodia	1990	Both sexes	2,061,813.3 (2,058,386.9–2,069,946.7)	2,958,193.4 (2,950,675.1–2,961,684.1)	393,544.4 (392,411.5–394,659.2)	59,404.3 (59,290.9–59,512.1)	207,816.8 (140,641.1–295,986.6)	2,116.6 (1,449.0–3,008.7)
	2013	Both sexes	2,815,221.3 (2,810,036.8–2,820,586.6)	2,943,217.8 (2,936,418.0–2,948,611.4)	267,096.9 (265,738.5–268,213.9)	39,106.9 (39,044.5–39,162.7)	197,913.5 (132,501.3–285,981.3)	1,243.9 (834.5–1,793.9)

(continued on next page)

Table 2
(continued)

Location	Year	Sex	Prevalent Cases of Mild Anemia	Prevalent Cases of Moderate Anemia	Prevalent Cases of Severe Anemia	Age-Standardized Prevalence (per 100,000)	Total YLDs	Age-Standardized YLDs (per 100,000)
Indonesia	1990	Both sexes	34,871,513.8 (34,819,231.2–34,945,635.5)	36,636,877.7 (36,542,150.4–36,688,203.0)	3,417,771.1 (3,404,677.9–3,429,301.8)	41,592.6 (41,526.5–41,653.8)	2,486,375.5 (1,657,028.9–3,591,988.0)	1,304.2 (871.7–1,877.7)
	2013	Both sexes	34,609,446.1 (34,539,775.1–34,664,356.1)	31,522,620.1 (31,467,501.5–31,578,171.8)	2,402,193.1 (2,390,571.6–2,411,038.6)	27,369.6 (27,320.0–27,414.6)	2,101,004.5 (1,396,800.0–3,051,889.8)	818.1 (544.0–1,186.0)
Laos	1990	Both sexes	915,673.6 (914,560.0–917,613.1)	1,111,371.6 (1,109,287.9–1,112,722.1)	120,198.5 (119,616.2–120,573.8)	50,284.9 (50,207.8–50,352.9)	76,864.9 (51,515.7–110,503.6)	1,678.9 (1,129.3–2,408.3)
	2013	Both sexes	1,183,417.0 (1,181,368.4–1,185,151.2)	1,178,914.9 (1,176,790.4–1,180,745.9)	100,864.8 (99,998.6–101,416.5)	35,846.1 (35,784.7–35,895.4)	79,188.3 (52,735.8–114,371.3)	1,093.7 (729.4–1,579.1)
Malaysia	1990	Both sexes	2,877,959.4 (2,872,965.5–2,883,472.2)	2,885,387.5 (2,879,711.6–2,889,153.2)	238,036.4 (237,307.4–238,785.7)	31,888.7 (31,835.9–31,936.7)	192,696.2 (128,562.5–278,681.7)	956.9 (637.8–1,384.3)
	2013	Both sexes	3,062,031.2 (3,038,827.8–3,077,982.4)	2,718,241.6 (2,693,914.6–2,737,495.7)	187,727.5 (186,126.9–188,866.1)	20,366.7 (20,224.9–20,475.0)	178,786.7 (118,223.5–260,389.2)	603.8 (399.6–878.7)
Maldives	1990	Both sexes	45,957.4 (45,881.8–46,030.2)	54,740.5 (54,656.9–54,803.7)	5,695.2 (5,664.3–5,718.8)	48,534.4 (48,462.3–48,596.3)	3,775.8 (2,528.8–5,439.2)	1,581.8 (1,062.6–2,273.2)
	2013	Both sexes	52,331.4 (52,252.8–52,383.1)	46,985.5 (46,905.2–47,059.8)	3,595.4 (3,565.3–3,613.7)	29,909.7 (29,866.4–29,942.4)	3,130.6 (2,080.2–4,548.6)	892.8 (594.2–1,297.4)
Myanmar	1990	Both sexes	8,355,107.3 (8,335,273.3–8,370,629.8)	9,039,293.4 (8,985,513.5–9,056,607.6)	860,098.9 (853,475.2–863,673.9)	42,806.8 (42,673.3–42,880.9)	611,447.5 (409,900.0–878,704.9)	1,346.9 (905.4–1,935.5)
	2013	Both sexes	7,535,176.1 (7,523,390.5–7,544,097.6)	6,554,959.2 (6,543,636.7–6,567,104.5)	480,968.8 (476,203.9–482,937.0)	27,836.3 (27,794.4–27,873.8)	434,239.1 (288,182.8–631,172.2)	831.3 (552.7–1,205.8)

Philippines	1990	Both sexes	10,715,626.0 (10,699,274.6–10,729,089.4)	11,224,111.2 (11,207,776.5–11,237,570.5)	973,241.3 (969,850.1–976,348.6)	35,466.7 (35,415.8–35,513.1)	749,518.1 (500,563.5–1,081,332.8)	1,064.6 (711.9–1,537.1)
	2013	Both sexes	13,759,337.1 (13,732,473.9–13,780,931.2)	13,279,133.5 (13,256,612.4–13,301,210.4)	1,038,786.8 (1,036,072.1–1,041,569.8)	27,476.0 (27,423.7–27,519.5)	881,368.1 (586,376.2–1,281,441.3)	814.1 (541.9–1,182.4)
Sri Lanka	1990	Both sexes	3,053,759.8 (3,048,478.6–3,060,024.9)	3,060,485.1 (3,053,114.5–3,065,656.6)	267,265.5 (265,911.3–268,364.4)	36,555.1 (36,494.0–36,613.8)	205,967.2 (137,620.4–298,286.3)	1,132.5 (756.2–1,638.4)
	2013	Both sexes	2,777,895.1 (2,772,264.4–2,782,739.2)	2,483,388.4 (2,478,502.1–2,488,171.3)	179,876.1 (179,241.7–180,444.2)	25,864.0 (25,817.7–25,908.5)	164,704.6 (109,212.4–238,933.1)	788.3 (523.1–1,142.7)
Thailand	1990	Both sexes	8,018,299.0 (8,003,328.1–8,029,778.0)	7,458,609.3 (7,446,706.0–7,471,114.6)	576,550.1 (572,454.8–579,424.9)	28,102.6 (28,059.2–28,143.3)	497,685.7 (331,359.1–721,705.8)	840.8 (559.6–1,219.5)
	2013	Both sexes	6,730,494.8 (6,712,526.6–6,744,684.0)	5,281,975.2 (5,265,395.9–5,298,618.9)	340,135.8 (334,011.4–342,552.4)	19,921.7 (19,872.6–19,964.4)	352,441.2 (234,572.0–513,271.4)	599.7 (399.1–870.8)
Timor-Leste	1990	Both sexes	170,781.8 (170,556.4–170,979.1)	195,392.9 (195,169.4–195,649.3)	22,658.1 (22,565.9–22,730.5)	50,915.9 (50,866.5–50,965.3)	13,765.6 (9,226.2–19,754.0)	1,733.0 (1,168.1–2,475.7)
	2013	Both sexes	217,413.6 (217,154.3–217,588.9)	234,105.8 (233,881.4–234,321.8)	22,702.8 (22,615.9–22,767.6)	39,923.8 (39,882.1–39,958.4)	15,976.4 (10,666.4–23,055.5)	1,208.2 (806.6–1,742.7)
Vietnam	1990	Both sexes	14,945,546.7 (14,925,923.6–14,977,731.9)	16,959,274.5 (16,925,270.4–16,981,212.9)	1,770,581.2 (1,765,646.7–1,776,719.0)	48,626.2 (48,561.2–48,692.1)	1,153,066.1 (776,726.8–1,655,719.7)	1,578.6 (1,067.7–2,266.7)
	2013	Both sexes	13,528,685.3 (13,502,560.7–13,550,805.0)	11,361,620.6 (11,339,379.2–11,384,058.6)	832,335.4 (825,600.3–836,906.0)	28,788.8 (28,740.1–28,833.3)	748,044.6 (495,542.2–1,088,428.7)	854.4 (567.3–1,240.8)

(continued on next page)

Table 2
(continued)

Location	Year	Sex	Prevalent Cases of Mild Anemia	Prevalent Cases of Moderate Anemia	Prevalent Cases of Severe Anemia	Age-Standardized Prevalence (per 100,000)	Total YLDs	Age-Standardized YLDs (per 100,000)
Oceania	1990	Both sexes	983,462.9 (981,819.4–984,995.4)	1,168,658.8 (1,166,889.4–1,170,074.1)	105,756.3 (105,470.4–106,035.5)	32,241.0 (32,190.4–32,281.3)	78,333.0 (52,212.2–113,119.0)	1,044.7 (697.0–1,506.3)
	2013	Both sexes	1,331,621.3 (1,329,589.0–1,333,329.7)	1,502,480.7 (1,500,562.7–1,504,109.4)	122,104.0 (121,684.0–122,461.1)	26,462.4 (26,424.1–26,494.6)	99,439.9 (66,307.2–143,977.7)	846.8 (564.0–1,224.8)
Fiji	1990	Both sexes	80,902.3 (80,675.1–81,064.1)	92,492.1 (92,315.2–92,640.0)	7,109.2 (7,066.1–7,144.1)	22,472.1 (22,424.3–22,515.3)	6,079.9 (4,047.5–8,820.3)	713.8 (475.0–1,033.4)
	2013	Both sexes	86,409.7 (86,177.2–86,604.0)	89,959.1 (89,644.6–90,191.6)	6,410.2 (6,362.4–6,445.1)	20,454.5 (20,396.9–20,501.5)	5,914.4 (3,924.7–8,570.5)	651.6 (432.5–943.3)
Kiribati	1990	Both sexes	8,675.9 (8,656.6–8,693.8)	9,988.7 (9,970.2–10,003.6)	785.0 (780.8–790.8)	25,013.2 (24,962.8–25,058.2)	653.7 (434.1–943.5)	794.1 (527.6–1,144.3)
	2013	Both sexes	10,834.1 (10,803.0–10,858.0)	11,745.9 (11,721.2–11,770.2)	873.7 (870.5–876.8)	22,175.3 (22,117.5–22,221.8)	769.6 (513.9–1,116.1)	705.7 (472.0–1,022.8)
Marshall Islands	1990	Both sexes	5,260.5 (5,249.2–5,269.7)	6,031.0 (6,018.5–6,040.2)	457.3 (454.1–459.5)	22,173.3 (22,126.1–22,214.1)	394.9 (262.9–573.8)	704.8 (469.1–1,019.8)
	2013	Both sexes	7,299.2 (7,281.8–7,312.7)	8,147.3 (8,133.5–8,160.8)	610.3 (607.7–612.9)	21,622.1 (21,574.5–21,662.6)	534.6 (356.7–774.1)	687.8 (459.4–994.5)
Federated States of Micronesia	1990	Both sexes	12,295.8 (12,269.7–12,321.0)	14,794.9 (14,765.1–14,817.3)	1,227.2 (1,219.2–1,237.4)	26,367.2 (26,313.1–26,415.3)	981.2 (654.4–1,419.3)	842.9 (561.9–1,220.6)
	2013	Both sexes	11,394.3 (11,366.4–11,418.6)	12,845.0 (12,820.3–12,869.1)	995.0 (987.3–999.3)	22,975.2 (22,922.9–23,020.2)	848.1 (566.1–1,231.5)	733.3 (489.1–1,063.0)
Papua New Guinea	1990	Both sexes	674,178.0 (672,989.0–675,367.7)	813,596.2 (812,252.6–814,659.3)	76,370.2 (76,117.7–76,600.4)	35,852.4 (35,788.9–35,903.1)	54,780.0 (36,543.1–79,023.8)	1,167.0 (779.9–1,680.8)
	2013	Both sexes	969,186.2 (967,435.5–970,545.2)	1,113,088.8 (1,111,548.0–1,114,336.2)	92,455.0 (92,069.5–92,773.6)	28,055.7 (28,008.8–28,094.0)	73,768.2 (49,237.6–106,861.0)	897.2 (598.1–1,297.6)

Samoa	1990	Both sexes	16,357.0 (16,273.0– 16,407.1)	18,728.7 (18,624.8– 18,799.5)	1,379.8 (1,366.2– 1,390.8)	19,236.9 (19,145.9– 19,306.9)	1,230.4 (814.3– 1,788.9)	614.3 (405.8–892.8)
	2013	Both sexes	17,782.1 (17,717.3– 17,826.1)	20,161.9 (20,041.4– 20,242.1)	1,471.6 (1,454.7– 1,483.4)	18,548.6 (18,469.5– 18,610.0)	1,327.2 (886.8– 1,932.3)	593.0 (396.9–862.7)
Solomon Islands	1990	Both sexes	43,317.0 (43,195.6– 43,385.7)	52,180.8 (52,096.3– 52,241.6)	4,407.4 (4,380.3– 4,427.8)	28,354.9 (28,299.8– 28,394.3)	3,461.7 (2,306.2– 5,008.6)	903.1 (601.5– 1,305.2)
	2013	Both sexes	67,213.4 (67,093.0– 67,302.1)	77,745.4 (77,645.3– 77,838.7)	6,146.1 (6,119.4– 6,166.6)	24,354.1 (24,314.4– 24,387.2)	5,123.7 (3,418.4– 7,419.1)	774.1 (515.0– 1,117.5)
Tonga	1990	Both sexes	11,053.4 (11,013.4– 11,082.6)	13,173.7 (13,123.9– 13,207.2)	1,057.4 (1,050.2– 1,065.4)	24,291.6 (24,212.6– 24,347.3)	872.5 (581.0– 1,265.9)	799.6 (533.6– 1,159.2)
	2013	Both sexes	11,567.6 (11,535.5– 11,592.4)	13,666.8 (13,614.1– 13,701.2)	1,078.6 (1,070.5– 1,085.1)	23,264.3 (23,195.4– 23,321.5)	905.3 (605.0– 1,310.7)	765.0 (511.3– 1,108.8)
Vanuatu	1990	Both sexes	18,815.4 (18,779.9– 18,844.8)	22,377.7 (22,341.9– 22,413.1)	1,836.8 (1,819.0– 1,845.5)	25,991.1 (25,945.3– 26,032.1)	1,483.3 (988.0– 2,146.7)	827.1 (549.4– 1,196.8)
	2013	Both sexes	28,793.4 (28,739.7– 28,828.8)	32,534.6 (32,479.8– 32,582.2)	2,536.6 (2,506.9– 2,548.2)	23,705.0 (23,664.9– 23,738.0)	2,144.2 (1,428.4– 3,106.5)	753.3 (501.4– 1,091.3)
Central Europe, Eastern Europe, and Central Asia	1990	Both sexes	41,741,255.5 (41,611,512.1– 41,844,040.4)	38,532,521.1 (38,329,850.2– 38,714,797.3)	2,697,951.8 (2,684,969.1– 2,708,351.9)	20,360.2 (20,285.1– 20,425.2)	2,694,007.0 (1,800,541.5– 3,887,837.8)	662.9 (443.1–956.9)
	2013	Both sexes	40,421,690.1 (40,319,418.7– 40,503,455.0)	32,955,222.6 (32,822,062.4– 33,085,403.9)	2,095,222.3 (2,085,642.5– 2,102,686.1)	19,822.1 (19,770.6– 19,866.1)	2,319,146.1 (1,549,886.5– 3,353,069.3)	640.2 (426.7–927.3)
Central Asia	1990	Both sexes	7,474,993.9 (7,453,138.1– 7,493,734.1)	8,268,778.3 (8,188,616.2– 8,295,200.1)	627,090.4 (623,667.8– 629,367.3)	22,248.1 (22,150.3– 22,318.1)	562,890.0 (377,222.3– 810,728.5)	745.7 (501.2– 1,071.7)
	2013	Both sexes	8,325,012.9 (8,301,378.1– 8,346,296.6)	8,431,508.5 (8,397,190.7– 8,457,310.9)	595,608.5 (591,415.6– 598,045.6)	20,525.7 (20,462.2– 20,582.2)	579,072.9 (386,645.7– 840,116.0)	689.1 (461.3–998.1)
Armenia	1990	Both sexes	347,426.9 (345,392.2– 349,094.7)	369,277.9 (365,387.9– 371,979.9)	26,320.5 (25,903.4– 26,637.3)	20,549.6 (20,371.6– 20,677.6)	25,408.3 (16,944.3– 36,872.8)	694.5 (463.7– 1,006.2)
	2013	Both sexes	270,998.2 (268,943.5– 272,849.1)	256,589.5 (253,629.3– 258,847.2)	17,176.7 (16,860.0– 17,361.0)	19,424.5 (19,255.8– 19,556.8)	18,095.7 (12,046.3– 26,294.3)	658.7 (437.6–958.1)

(continued on next page)

Table 2
(continued)

Location	Year	Sex	Prevalent Cases of Mild Anemia	Prevalent Cases of Moderate Anemia	Prevalent Cases of Severe Anemia	Age-Standardized Prevalence (per 100,000)	Total YLDs	Age-Standardized YLDs (per 100,000)
Azerbaijan	1990	Both sexes	861,947.0 (858,410.0–865,387.0)	1,013,535.8 (1,009,119.4–1,017,221.2)	84,578.0 (84,084.1–85,042.0)	26,971.5 (26,849.5–27,076.1)	69,131.5 (46,398.5–99,779.3)	935.5 (630.3–1,344.7)
	2013	Both sexes	1,050,215.2 (1,044,892.3–1,054,112.5)	1,105,202.7 (1,098,894.1–1,109,941.1)	84,081.2 (83,495.2–84,517.7)	24,524.8 (24,400.1–24,619.2)	75,848.9 (51,042.8–109,482.3)	847.1 (569.5–1,220.7)
Georgia	1990	Both sexes	496,629.7 (494,475.5–498,474.1)	483,101.0 (475,908.5–486,610.6)	32,350.7 (31,904.8–32,628.9)	18,936.7 (18,793.8–19,029.7)	33,211.5 (22,078.7–47,876.4)	624.8 (415.5–901.2)
	2013	Both sexes	386,390.5 (384,523.8–388,028.0)	336,401.7 (333,848.8–339,134.3)	20,943.1 (20,727.7–21,137.7)	18,541.1 (18,456.7–18,622.7)	23,730.3 (15,948.7–34,025.9)	615.5 (410.8–883.5)
Kazakhstan	1990	Both sexes	1,605,736.2 (1,592,634.9–1,617,342.7)	1,685,036.4 (1,602,849.1–1,703,435.3)	119,920.3 (117,202.9–121,577.2)	20,214.8 (19,774.9–20,410.6)	115,781.6 (77,652.3–166,431.7)	677.8 (454.7–972.7)
	2013	Both sexes	1,534,185.4 (1,522,933.0–1,542,553.0)	1,498,369.7 (1,483,449.6–1,510,421.7)	100,297.0 (98,161.5–101,495.0)	19,222.8 (19,080.5–19,344.2)	103,893.3 (69,469.9–150,805.1)	645.3 (431.6–935.7)
Kyrgyzstan	1990	Both sexes	478,206.3 (476,380.5–479,898.9)	528,735.0 (526,246.2–530,799.4)	39,558.0 (39,273.6–39,719.8)	21,867.3 (21,751.8–21,967.9)	35,817.2 (23,894.2–51,647.3)	725.3 (484.9–1,044.0)
	2013	Both sexes	543,258.0 (540,356.0–545,505.8)	554,612.1 (549,955.5–557,640.6)	38,401.9 (37,925.3–38,724.3)	19,740.9 (19,605.7–19,856.0)	37,854.4 (25,251.2–54,794.8)	660.9 (443.8–954.0)

Mongolia	1990	Both sexes	213,551.9 (211,561.6–214,393.4)	230,587.0 (228,689.7–231,757.6)	16,772.2 (16,574.4–16,897.1)	17,835.7 (17,687.4–17,937.9)	15,763.0 (10,489.2–22,707.2)	587.2 (391.0–844.0)
	2013	Both sexes	221,005.0 (219,560.9–222,024.8)	206,809.7 (204,524.9–208,723.5)	13,560.4 (13,368.8–13,694.9)	15,349.8 (15,218.3–15,454.2)	14,535.3 (9,769.2–21,091.1)	516.5 (347.3–747.5)
Tajikistan	1990	Both sexes	653,565.2 (651,567.5–655,323.2)	750,331.9 (747,960.9–752,340.1)	59,094.6 (58,682.4–59,328.3)	24,577.6 (24,477.2–24,672.6)	50,725.9 (33,738.2–73,397.6)	813.9 (544.5–1,177.5)
	2013	Both sexes	986,362.5 (983,465.2–988,712.3)	1,062,704.6 (1,059,708.3–1,065,541.2)	80,744.2 (80,205.8–81,046.4)	24,097.1 (24,013.0–24,174.2)	71,682.8 (47,928.8–103,813.9)	792.4 (530.2–1,143.4)
Turkmenistan	1990	Both sexes	407,908.2 (406,148.6–409,345.6)	461,590.5 (459,560.8–463,290.4)	35,184.5 (35,020.1–35,299.3)	22,251.7 (22,120.1–22,343.6)	31,246.0 (20,856.1–45,461.4)	740.3 (497.2–1,072.3)
	2013	Both sexes	519,986.6 (517,192.9–522,094.4)	534,401.8 (531,148.7–537,308.5)	38,002.9 (37,756.6–38,192.5)	20,465.0 (20,323.3–20,582.5)	36,646.8 (24,381.6–53,134.3)	687.0 (457.0–990.8)
Uzbekistan	1990	Both sexes	2,410,022.5 (2,402,124.9–2,416,020.3)	2,746,582.8 (2,737,475.1–2,753,732.2)	213,311.5 (212,315.0–214,083.6)	23,592.3 (23,493.4–23,674.2)	185,805.0 (124,188.0–267,591.3)	782.2 (524.9–1,124.4)
	2013	Both sexes	2,812,611.5 (2,801,377.2–2,821,942.6)	2,876,416.8 (2,864,343.4–2,888,427.2)	202,401.0 (200,837.9–203,661.8)	20,004.7 (19,920.5–20,078.0)	196,785.6 (131,780.4–285,419.7)	667.0 (447.5–965.0)
Central Europe	1990	Both sexes	15,529,394.0 (15,504,389.4–15,553,786.5)	12,627,915.7 (12,587,852.4–12,660,594.4)	912,996.1 (911,602.2–914,364.2)	23,939.0 (23,888.9–23,983.3)	876,516.1 (587,478.2–1,267,822.4)	728.7 (488.3–1,054.3)
	2013	Both sexes	14,886,038.5 (14,857,649.9–14,913,721.1)	10,284,649.6 (10,241,897.1–10,324,824.9)	659,383.4 (657,709.2–660,960.0)	23,191.9 (23,143.9–23,238.1)	725,712.0 (483,875.9–1,053,241.2)	706.2 (471.0–1,022.8)

(continued on next page)

Table 2
(continued)

Location	Year	Sex	Prevalent Cases of Mild Anemia	Prevalent Cases of Moderate Anemia	Prevalent Cases of Severe Anemia	Age-Standardized Prevalence (per 100,000)	Total YLDs	Age-Standardized YLDs (per 100,000)
Albania	1990	Both sexes	588,393.5 (587,209.7–589,472.3)	529,186.0 (527,832.7–530,270.9)	44,774.7 (44,600.4–44,883.3)	33,553.7 (33,470.8–33,630.3)	36,397.6 (24,312.1–52,740.9)	1,007.9 (674.8–1,455.8)
	2013	Both sexes	509,559.4 (508,526.4–510,540.1)	382,934.7 (381,313.4–384,405.8)	28,853.8 (28,757.8–28,915.3)	29,476.7 (29,401.6–29,549.1)	26,633.7 (17,692.8–38,590.1)	879.8 (583.8–1,275.2)
Bosnia and Herzegovina	1990	Both sexes	638,341.8 (636,175.8–640,153.9)	523,389.3 (520,728.4–525,713.8)	38,767.0 (38,680.9–38,852.8)	27,209.8 (27,098.4–27,302.0)	36,099.6 (24,081.6–52,151.9)	829.0 (553.9–1,196.2)
	2013	Both sexes	474,059.5 (472,457.1–475,548.1)	339,490.6 (336,486.9–342,185.0)	22,492.8 (22,343.8–22,605.0)	23,192.1 (23,103.5–23,274.7)	23,991.3 (15,924.4–34,681.7)	707.8 (470.3–1,022.1)
Bulgaria	1990	Both sexes	1,083,260.7 (1,078,976.5–1,088,172.8)	827,841.6 (821,670.6–834,079.4)	57,552.1 (57,368.6–57,738.4)	23,122.0 (23,029.2–23,227.1)	58,294.0 (38,791.7–83,687.1)	706.8 (470.1–1,017.1)
	2013	Both sexes	900,780.6 (896,406.9–904,038.0)	601,845.6 (596,650.5–607,181.5)	37,528.6 (37,314.1–37,682.9)	22,840.3 (22,758.9–22,922.4)	42,762.4 (28,307.6–61,672.6)	696.0 (462.4–1,007.5)
Croatia	1990	Both sexes	565,490.1 (563,623.4–567,058.0)	433,893.1 (430,985.8–436,383.4)	29,710.2 (29,585.3–29,803.3)	22,326.5 (22,238.9–22,397.0)	30,401.9 (20,371.6–44,044.5)	682.4 (457.2–989.2)
	2013	Both sexes	513,610.1 (511,985.1–514,948.2)	354,150.3 (350,814.0–357,165.7)	22,550.1 (22,380.9–22,692.4)	22,126.4 (22,039.3–22,200.2)	25,340.2 (16,893.5–36,459.0)	677.5 (450.2–979.0)
Czech Republic	1990	Both sexes	1,228,016.6 (1,222,267.5–1,233,375.3)	969,015.1 (961,633.5–976,747.6)	68,305.3 (67,990.1–68,550.8)	22,557.9 (22,453.1–22,672.0)	67,765.2 (45,318.6–97,664.1)	688.9 (460.7–992.3)
	2013	Both sexes	1,312,551.4 (1,308,608.5–1,315,549.0)	894,225.7 (887,461.5–900,439.0)	56,458.3 (56,187.6–56,660.5)	22,925.3 (22,850.9–22,989.2)	62,988.3 (42,045.6–90,695.4)	695.7 (463.5–1,004.6)

Country	Year	Sex						
Hungary	1990	Both sexes	1,283,935.4 (1,278,769.1–1,288,631.7)	995,587.3 (989,122.2–1,001,759.0)	69,199.3 (68,928.1–69,438.9)	23,337.2 (23,247.5–23,422.9)	69,682.9 (46,979.6–100,440.3)	712.6 (479.9–1,028.9)
	2013	Both sexes	1,235,360.2 (1,229,934.0–1,240,367.6)	851,121.6 (844,033.9–858,737.6)	54,047.4 (53,743.5–54,270.6)	22,904.3 (22,815.8–22,994.0)	60,478.9 (40,694.1–87,136.6)	701.1 (469.5–1,011.9)
Macedonia	1990	Both sexes	248,314.7 (247,477.3–249,191.2)	207,893.0 (206,859.4–208,819.4)	15,212.3 (15,164.7–15,248.7)	23,541.4 (23,450.0–23,632.8)	14,396.6 (9,549.5–20,839.4)	717.2 (476.0–1,036.6)
	2013	Both sexes	256,280.4 (255,367.8–257,206.9)	182,815.3 (181,211.0–184,268.7)	12,120.6 (12,065.9–12,172.1)	22,846.4 (22,745.4–22,943.2)	12,905.2 (8,617.2–18,647.6)	696.7 (466.0–1,006.1)
Montenegro	1990	Both sexes	73,489.7 (73,263.7–73,677.1)	61,478.6 (61,168.4–61,793.7)	4,490.8 (4,475.4–4,504.2)	23,155.1 (23,063.9–23,236.5)	4,246.9 (2,847.2–6,159.5)	702.9 (471.2–1,019.3)
	2013	Both sexes	76,818.1 (76,546.8–77,047.2)	57,035.4 (56,625.0–57,409.9)	3,874.2 (3,857.4–3,886.8)	23,198.8 (23,106.3–23,278.7)	3,997.7 (2,688.6–5,807.9)	706.1 (474.8–1,024.9)
Poland	1990	Both sexes	4,645,104.9 (4,628,971.3–4,657,870.4)	3,893,375.7 (3,865,254.6–3,916,318.0)	282,889.8 (282,147.3–283,668.1)	23,245.5 (23,147.7–23,327.7)	268,899.1 (180,231.0–388,588.6)	706.5 (473.4–1,021.2)
	2013	Both sexes	4,733,795.6 (4,710,409.9–4,750,267.9)	3,212,294.3 (3,177,640.1–3,242,682.4)	200,791.5 (199,624.8–201,918.3)	22,813.1 (22,709.3–22,899.7)	225,925.6 (150,273.9–327,505.2)	693.5 (462.6–1,003.7)
Romania	1990	Both sexes	3,105,162.1 (3,098,138.8–3,112,503.4)	2,491,303.2 (2,480,029.2–2,504,234.6)	180,229.9 (179,689.1–180,612.7)	25,263.3 (25,188.0–25,346.8)	172,406.7 (114,739.6–249,174.7)	765.5 (509.6–1,107.3)
	2013	Both sexes	2,778,670.8 (2,769,687.2–2,784,797.3)	1,940,869.6 (1,920,737.0–1,954,330.8)	125,830.8 (125,130.0–126,388.6)	23,747.9 (23,645.5–23,819.6)	136,783.3 (91,283.2–198,752.0)	722.6 (482.0–1,051.5)
Serbia	1990	Both sexes	1,177,208.7 (1,172,903.3–1,180,170.8)	959,484.4 (954,097.4–964,501.2)	68,909.2 (68,611.1–69,150.5)	22,987.6 (22,891.2–23,063.1)	67,058.3 (44,938.8–97,318.5)	703.5 (471.0–1,021.2)
	2013	Both sexes	1,168,068.0 (1,162,690.3–1,172,494.2)	834,179.2 (825,854.0–841,217.4)	55,150.2 (54,849.0–55,441.3)	22,930.4 (22,812.5–23,023.2)	59,229.3 (39,674.9–85,083.6)	701.4 (467.2–1,010.2)

(continued on next page)

Table 2
(continued)

Location	Year	Sex	Prevalent Cases of Mild Anemia	Prevalent Cases of Moderate Anemia	Prevalent Cases of Severe Anemia	Age-Standardized Prevalence (per 100,000)	Total YLDs	Age-Standardized YLDs (per 100,000)
Slovakia	1990	Both sexes	646,964.9 (645,104.8–648,691.6)	542,436.1 (539,619.6–545,162.4)	39,431.5 (39,247.7–39,581.0)	23,428.5 (23,339.6–23,508.3)	37,468.8 (25,072.9–54,282.8)	712.3 (476.7–1,032.1)
	2013	Both sexes	671,627.7 (669,505.0–673,432.4)	461,391.0 (458,564.5–464,277.5)	28,760.8 (28,625.6–28,867.5)	22,973.9 (22,902.7–23,040.3)	32,355.3 (21,563.0–46,866.5)	700.1 (466.5–1,014.3)
Slovenia	1990	Both sexes	245,711.0 (244,905.0–246,362.8)	193,032.1 (191,692.9–194,345.6)	13,524.0 (13,463.6–13,563.2)	23,410.7 (23,312.1–23,500.1)	13,398.6 (8,998.8–19,287.1)	711.7 (477.3–1,025.5)
	2013	Both sexes	254,856.9 (253,615.8–256,053.4)	172,296.4 (170,527.5–174,019.5)	10,924.2 (10,835.0–10,981.5)	22,659.1 (22,558.4–22,750.9)	12,320.7 (8,230.7–17,855.2)	691.7 (464.2–1,002.7)
Eastern Europe	1990	Both sexes	18,736,867.6 (18,630,095.4–18,817,836.3)	17,635,827.1 (17,466,193.2–17,790,198.3)	1,157,865.3 (1,146,129.2–1,167,171.1)	17,702.0 (17,595.0–17,800.0)	1,254,600.9 (839,601.8–1,809,219.1)	597.1 (399.5–861.1)
	2013	Both sexes	17,210,638.7 (17,143,872.1–17,264,952.3)	14,239,064.5 (14,137,994.3–14,335,558.6)	840,230.3 (833,256.0–846,102.2)	17,428.0 (17,359.1–17,484.5)	1,014,361.2 (677,963.4–1,468,178.0)	578.1 (384.2–839.9)
Belarus	1990	Both sexes	883,188.3 (877,403.7–888,805.7)	839,260.0 (828,777.3–847,655.4)	55,347.8 (54,276.4–56,046.3)	18,167.3 (18,006.6–18,295.2)	58,658.6 (39,365.9–84,715.1)	604.9 (405.5–873.2)
	2013	Both sexes	800,675.3 (796,218.1–804,332.7)	664,977.9 (657,414.9–672,078.2)	39,030.0 (38,490.3–39,421.0)	17,862.4 (17,740.9–17,958.1)	47,064.4 (31,353.4–67,966.2)	591.0 (393.2–857.5)
Estonia	1990	Both sexes	138,838.7 (137,996.1–139,641.2)	130,566.3 (129,182.9–131,787.5)	8,560.2 (8,429.3–8,645.5)	18,523.6 (18,389.9–18,647.1)	9,134.5 (6,131.7–13,156.9)	616.7 (413.2–890.0)
	2013	Both sexes	114,411.8 (113,581.3–115,068.9)	96,415.9 (94,931.0–97,771.9)	5,856.8 (5,784.1–5,906.3)	17,900.9 (17,772.3–18,010.6)	6,875.8 (4,586.6–9,828.4)	593.2 (394.6–853.5)

Country	Year	Sex						
Latvia	1990	Both sexes	230,809.3 (229,499.1–232,138.2)	213,622.2 (211,819.9–215,290.3)	13,620.3 (13,428.2–13,756.5)	18,212.7 (18,117.9–18,308.3)	14,995.5 (9,991.8–21,585.3)	608.3 (405.2–876.9)
	2013	Both sexes	172,789.8 (171,574.2–173,879.1)	144,694.7 (143,093.4–146,171.7)	8,524.9 (8,417.4–8,611.1)	17,966.7 (17,858.0–18,054.0)	10,334.5 (6,965.5–14,843.1)	597.2 (399.9–864.3)
Lithuania	1990	Both sexes	319,333.5 (316,996.1–321,258.3)	299,776.2 (296,976.6–302,703.1)	19,724.0 (19,452.9–19,932.7)	18,047.1 (17,923.1–18,168.5)	21,039.4 (14,046.9–30,341.4)	602.1 (402.6–869.6)
	2013	Both sexes	250,454.6 (249,116.5–251,651.7)	208,771.2 (206,057.1–211,048.5)	12,368.7 (12,204.7–12,485.8)	17,829.6 (17,722.4–17,924.2)	14,894.4 (10,076.1–21,469.1)	592.5 (396.9–854.8)
Moldova	1990	Both sexes	443,851.9 (441,490.2–445,937.4)	474,533.1 (471,884.2–476,709.3)	34,244.0 (33,837.4–34,528.1)	21,698.0 (21,588.6–21,795.2)	32,147.1 (21,522.2–46,577.6)	728.2 (488.1–1,054.8)
	2013	Both sexes	353,830.6 (352,155.6–355,400.0)	335,457.6 (333,703.3–337,031.6)	22,516.7 (22,331.3–22,656.3)	21,970.2 (21,883.0–22,052.2)	22,727.0 (15,176.1–32,872.9)	733.0 (488.6–1,059.4)
Russia	1990	Both sexes	13,049,161.2 (12,956,927.2–13,118,580.5)	12,419,744.6 (12,270,317.2–12,544,911.3)	821,870.8 (811,901.3–829,524.4)	18,532.1 (18,393.8–18,651.7)	884,463.0 (593,506.1–1,280,192.6)	628.5 (420.9–909.0)
	2013	Both sexes	12,375,903.9 (12,311,962.9–12,424,639.6)	10,417,162.2 (10,310,244.7–10,514,772.1)	622,150.9 (615,370.9–627,850.9)	18,154.1 (18,068.8–18,231.0)	738,888.8 (495,032.0–1,072,774.1)	602.8 (401.8–878.0)
Ukraine	1990	Both sexes	3,671,684.5 (3,639,293.2–3,693,070.2)	3,258,324.6 (3,202,532.5–3,302,497.0)	204,498.3 (199,068.3–207,967.9)	14,878.9 (14,699.9–15,004.2)	234,162.8 (156,789.3–336,699.6)	494.7 (330.8–712.5)
	2013	Both sexes	3,142,572.8 (3,122,475.3–3,160,930.5)	2,371,585.2 (2,335,775.5–2,407,391.8)	129,782.3 (127,348.3–131,317.1)	14,681.5 (14,539.0–14,772.1)	173,576.4 (116,390.9–249,749.6)	483.4 (324.7–700.0)

(continued on next page)

Table 2
(continued)

Location	Year	Sex	Prevalent Cases of Mild Anemia	Prevalent Cases of Moderate Anemia	Prevalent Cases of Severe Anemia	Age-Standardized Prevalence (per 100,000)	Total YLDs	Age-Standardized YLDs (per 100,000)
High-income	1990	Both sexes	91,083,813.6 (90,934,394.6– 91,220,399.2)	71,010,515.5 (70,802,445.3– 71,188,011.9)	4,779,754.2 (4,764,654.3– 4,792,742.3)	19,455.7 (19,420.7– 19,485.4)	4,750,004.7 (3,158,561.6– 6,903,728.9)	577.2 (383.6–837.5)
	2013	Both sexes	106,261,799.2 (106,115,450.4– 106,405,045.0)	76,176,751.0 (75,923,182.7– 76,373,988.3)	4,877,227.5 (4,861,252.6– 4,891,994.6)	18,928.0 (18,895.1– 18,954.3)	5,138,029.7 (3,424,410.0– 7,449,343.7)	560.3 (372.4–813.5)
High-income Asia Pacific	1990	Both sexes	21,842,239.3 (21,810,745.1– 21,875,604.9)	18,315,673.7 (18,284,192.5– 18,339,200.6)	1,291,750.7 (1,287,209.1– 1,296,859.2)	25,637.2 (25,603.5– 25,667.9)	1,210,186.9 (801,663.6– 1,761,995.2)	773.7 (512.3– 1,123.8)
	2013	Both sexes	23,505,546.2 (23,468,556.2– 23,544,072.2)	17,270,792.0 (17,240,503.0– 17,296,910.4)	1,109,057.1 (1,105,955.6– 1,111,934.8)	24,798.8 (24,768.5– 24,826.0)	1,132,997.1 (752,872.2– 1,660,163.9)	744.2 (494.1– 1,085.3)
Brunei	1990	Both sexes	32,427.8 (32,349.7– 32,500.3)	31,239.6 (31,174.2– 31,296.6)	2,322.5 (2,311.9– 2,331.5)	23,859.9 (23,806.4– 23,901.8)	2,065.4 (1,367.3– 3,009.6)	704.8 (467.4– 1,026.9)
	2013	Both sexes	50,486.6 (50,374.0– 50,584.3)	44,108.9 (44,026.3– 44,186.4)	3,160.4 (3,148.4– 3,174.5)	23,867.1 (23,824.1– 23,906.7)	2,921.3 (1,934.9– 4,261.1)	708.3 (469.9– 1,032.0)
Japan	1990	Both sexes	15,304,862.2 (15,276,324.3– 15,336,802.4)	12,525,738.3 (12,496,325.8– 12,547,346.8)	855,481.0 (851,116.9– 859,315.9)	24,653.1 (24,606.3– 24,693.7)	826,793.1 (548,013.1– 1,205,088.7)	746.4 (494.4– 1,085.1)
	2013	Both sexes	16,200,919.3 (16,163,135.7– 16,236,192.1)	11,904,218.9 (11,877,595.7– 11,927,601.1)	753,867.5 (751,312.1– 756,264.3)	24,114.6 (24,070.4– 24,152.3)	780,477.6 (518,821.9– 1,142,286.1)	728.7 (483.5– 1,063.7)
South Korea	1990	Both sexes	6,141,168.2 (6,130,792.0– 6,152,572.4)	5,453,549.0 (5,442,215.7– 5,461,755.5)	412,330.1 (410,599.3– 414,693.9)	28,408.5 (28,365.3– 28,449.3)	361,117.0 (238,899.2– 524,647.4)	846.8 (561.1– 1,228.9)
	2013	Both sexes	6,771,595.1 (6,760,228.3– 6,783,253.3)	4,956,905.4 (4,945,833.4– 4,967,774.3)	328,096.6 (326,392.4– 329,476.0)	26,438.4 (26,399.2– 26,476.4)	325,517.8 (216,182.4– 477,185.2)	782.8 (521.2– 1,139.3)

	Year								
Singapore	1990	Both sexes	363,781.1 (362,879.4–364,543.2)	305,146.7 (304,417.9–305,767.5)	21,617.1 (21,497.0–21,689.7)	26,061.9 (26,004.8–26,109.6)	20,211.4 (13,385.1–29,554.8)	777.7 (516.5–1,132.5)
	2013	Both sexes	482,545.2 (481,588.0–483,226.8)	365,558.8 (364,832.3–366,131.6)	23,932.5 (23,836.3–23,993.6)	24,186.0 (24,138.5–24,218.1)	24,080.3 (15,948.2–35,302.7)	720.4 (478.9–1,049.9)
Australasia	1990	Both sexes	2,041,156.3 (2,032,590.0–2,047,135.1)	1,619,514.3 (1,611,464.4–1,626,396.2)	110,824.2 (110,080.8–111,416.1)	19,018.6 (18,947.3–19,081.0)	108,353.0 (72,006.0–156,822.3)	562.4 (374.0–814.8)
	2013	Both sexes	2,832,044.5 (2,818,340.1–2,842,268.7)	2,067,253.7 (2,049,505.9–2,079,664.8)	133,335.1 (132,333.7–134,143.2)	18,791.6 (18,689.1–18,862.3)	139,093.9 (93,186.7–201,867.4)	555.7 (372.0–806.5)
Australia	1990	Both sexes	1,709,728.7 (1,701,081.9–1,715,183.8)	1,361,353.2 (1,353,902.1–1,367,307.7)	93,269.2 (92,605.1–93,827.9)	19,132.9 (19,049.9–19,196.0)	91,068.5 (60,531.5–132,169.8)	567.0 (377.1–822.0)
	2013	Both sexes	2,390,187.1 (2,376,327.3–2,400,388.1)	1,749,618.9 (1,731,914.3–1,761,874.7)	112,916.2 (111,912.1–113,670.2)	18,897.1 (18,778.0–18,982.8)	117,663.2 (78,979.7–170,545.0)	559.9 (374.7–811.4)
New Zealand	1990	Both sexes	331,427.6 (328,418.9–332,927.4)	258,161.0 (254,807.0–259,888.1)	17,555.0 (17,248.5–17,760.7)	18,436.1 (18,227.3–18,529.6)	17,284.5 (11,555.4–25,144.5)	539.2 (360.8–785.5)
	2013	Both sexes	441,857.3 (437,875.2–444,005.8)	317,634.8 (314,348.9–320,256.8)	20,418.9 (20,124.6–20,654.5)	18,229.2 (18,011.6–18,332.8)	21,430.7 (14,307.8–31,139.8)	533.6 (355.3–777.1)
Western Europe	1990	Both sexes	38,670,348.8 (38,534,656.8–38,765,224.8)	28,256,886.0 (28,077,514.5–28,403,568.4)	1,838,611.6 (1,828,621.2–1,846,945.3)	19,230.4 (19,156.3–19,288.7)	1,899,009.9 (1,263,821.3–2,753,933.5)	564.6 (375.7–819.3)
	2013	Both sexes	43,617,259.7 (43,488,872.7–43,709,623.2)	29,626,464.5 (29,411,043.1–29,781,578.9)	1,854,599.7 (1,843,600.1–1,865,783.6)	18,986.0 (18,914.1–19,036.4)	2,009,946.2 (1,339,892.1–2,910,261.9)	556.9 (370.0–808.2)
Andorra	1990	Both sexes	5,007.7 (4,974.1–5,036.0)	3,651.8 (3,590.7–3,691.4)	237.4 (232.3–240.9)	19,027.0 (18,804.5–19,159.3)	247.7 (164.5–360.7)	562.0 (373.0–817.2)
	2013	Both sexes	8,068.3 (8,014.8–8,113.3)	5,495.6 (5,406.8–5,565.3)	342.8 (335.1–350.1)	18,962.5 (18,751.6–19,095.3)	374.2 (249.2–542.5)	558.1 (372.2–811.9)

(continued on next page)

Table 2
(continued)

Location	Year	Sex	Prevalent Cases of Mild Anemia	Prevalent Cases of Moderate Anemia	Prevalent Cases of Severe Anemia	Age-Standardized Prevalence (per 100,000)	Total YLDs	Age-Standardized YLDs (per 100,000)
Austria	1990	Both sexes	775,909.0 (770,767.5–780,345.8)	559,568.3 (540,695.3–567,031.8)	35,917.7 (35,138.9–36,379.3)	19,199.4 (18,830.0–19,351.4)	37,903.5 (25,470.5–54,760.7)	566.9 (378.0–824.9)
	2013	Both sexes	873,442.4 (868,018.2–878,070.6)	578,469.7 (565,045.8–586,512.3)	35,049.5 (34,264.3–36,198.7)	19,100.0 (18,848.1–19,228.1)	39,985.7 (26,376.3–57,759.6)	566.1 (374.3–824.0)
Belgium	1990	Both sexes	1,008,873.6 (1,003,857.9–1,012,883.8)	733,041.1 (723,752.4–739,868.9)	47,448.2 (46,906.6–48,002.6)	19,251.7 (19,136.3–19,329.7)	49,612.5 (33,129.3–71,782.5)	568.5 (378.7–821.6)
	2013	Both sexes	1,145,620.0 (1,137,735.4–1,151,454.6)	787,691.3 (775,478.5–799,297.4)	49,669.5 (48,941.2–50,501.6)	19,098.9 (18,942.6–19,197.5)	53,979.2 (36,260.9–77,831.5)	563.7 (377.4–817.5)
Cyprus	1990	Both sexes	68,928.4 (68,703.2–69,131.1)	58,164.4 (57,927.6–58,433.2)	4,101.6 (4,054.5–4,129.4)	19,603.4 (19,541.8–19,666.0)	3,898.5 (2,592.3–5,653.0)	581.3 (386.6–843.1)
	2013	Both sexes	88,346.6 (88,007.6–88,737.3)	62,004.1 (61,584.1–62,475.2)	3,924.9 (3,880.9–3,947.9)	19,339.7 (19,277.8–19,417.2)	4,210.3 (2,800.3–6,124.8)	575.6 (384.9–833.9)
Denmark	1990	Both sexes	521,946.5 (518,967.3–524,425.8)	368,826.8 (363,100.3–372,639.3)	23,169.1 (22,777.5–23,499.5)	19,147.1 (18,967.5–19,272.5)	25,018.5 (16,666.7–36,204.9)	564.6 (376.7–818.6)
	2013	Both sexes	573,906.0 (569,461.6–577,530.5)	401,396.0 (392,597.2–408,377.0)	25,659.8 (25,007.7–26,320.4)	19,027.7 (18,800.1–19,183.5)	27,405.9 (18,277.5–39,863.6)	559.6 (372.8–816.4)
Finland	1990	Both sexes	422,768.0 (420,392.3–424,337.1)	309,724.6 (307,556.8–311,939.3)	20,515.9 (20,312.3–20,609.9)	16,356.8 (16,280.2–16,412.6)	21,197.4 (14,075.3–30,674.7)	485.1 (322.2–702.0)
	2013	Both sexes	469,420.7 (466,754.5–471,752.2)	308,719.6 (305,627.7–311,903.0)	19,244.3 (19,021.5–19,414.0)	16,245.6 (16,176.6–16,310.1)	21,917.9 (14,628.9–31,293.3)	485.9 (323.9–701.4)

France	1990	Both sexes	5,446,713.0 (5,420,328.6–5,469,123.3)	4,038,903.6 (4,006,476.4–4,068,177.7)	268,622.4 (264,940.8–271,053.6)	18,116.6 (18,034.3–18,194.3)	275,595.2 (183,749.7–400,622.0)	535.2 (356.7–777.3)
	2013	Both sexes	6,149,028.9 (6,115,641.8–6,187,176.3)	4,334,285.0 (4,296,791.4–4,374,897.8)	282,671.5 (279,239.2–285,404.0)	17,846.1 (17,779.0–17,912.2)	300,653.8 (200,463.4–434,059.7)	528.7 (351.7–767.0)
Germany	1990	Both sexes	8,190,915.9 (8,105,535.0–8,237,747.9)	5,718,198.5 (5,563,671.9–5,817,113.4)	355,307.0 (349,187.6–360,101.5)	19,633.3 (19,360.2–19,793.2)	384,267.5 (257,242.6–552,774.5)	576.7 (384.2–835.5)
	2013	Both sexes	8,609,962.4 (8,535,625.3–8,652,725.9)	5,548,520.2 (5,360,259.7–5,661,568.1)	332,077.8 (325,858.2–339,194.8)	19,345.2 (19,053.5–19,505.2)	377,943.8 (253,049.3–547,207.1)	568.0 (379.2–827.4)
Greece	1990	Both sexes	1,085,146.0 (1,080,732.6–1,089,069.8)	815,480.8 (810,578.9–820,037.6)	55,724.1 (55,106.5–56,089.7)	20,274.9 (20,199.7–20,335.8)	55,258.8 (36,845.9–80,619.7)	598.2 (399.0–870.7)
	2013	Both sexes	1,178,249.9 (1,172,549.9–1,183,669.7)	784,347.1 (776,486.2–792,957.2)	49,196.5 (48,561.0–49,685.3)	19,602.1 (19,529.0–19,678.7)	54,047.2 (36,108.3–78,183.6)	580.0 (386.3–843.7)
Iceland	1990	Both sexes	25,999.6 (25,805.2–26,118.3)	21,317.7 (21,156.9–21,439.0)	1,476.9 (1,456.9–1,493.7)	19,325.0 (19,202.8–19,403.7)	1,425.7 (949.4–2,071.6)	568.0 (378.3–825.1)
	2013	Both sexes	32,452.6 (32,135.1–32,611.4)	24,071.9 (23,774.4–24,294.1)	1,584.7 (1,559.4–1,604.4)	19,154.8 (18,950.6–19,256.7)	1,622.9 (1,080.6–2,362.7)	562.9 (374.4–820.7)
Ireland	1990	Both sexes	357,860.0 (354,680.8–359,847.3)	308,757.0 (301,860.9–312,183.5)	22,274.1 (22,015.5–22,479.7)	19,264.0 (19,022.2–19,410.6)	20,728.6 (13,807.9–29,940.6)	567.0 (376.9–819.9)
	2013	Both sexes	464,892.7 (459,807.2–468,104.9)	352,788.6 (344,709.0–359,080.5)	23,469.8 (23,103.2–23,848.6)	19,077.0 (18,800.5–19,253.3)	23,862.8 (15,817.4–34,377.5)	562.3 (373.4–812.2)
Israel	1990	Both sexes	460,982.9 (456,628.2–463,697.1)	414,550.1 (408,284.2–418,179.6)	30,200.8 (29,664.5–30,501.9)	19,259.9 (19,066.9–19,397.6)	27,897.2 (18,509.4–40,388.2)	571.7 (379.5–827.6)
	2013	Both sexes	792,319.6 (785,565.3–796,196.6)	667,230.0 (658,637.4–672,575.1)	46,780.3 (46,126.2–47,272.6)	19,159.7 (18,984.5–19,272.7)	44,962.3 (29,942.8–65,326.3)	567.5 (377.5–823.9)

(continued on next page)

Table 2
(continued)

Location	Year	Sex	Prevalent Cases of Mild Anemia	Prevalent Cases of Moderate Anemia	Prevalent Cases of Severe Anemia	Age-Standardized Prevalence (per 100,000)	Total YLDs	Age-Standardized YLDs (per 100,000)
Italy	1990	Both sexes	5,688,383.2 (5,667,986.7–5,707,594.2)	4,064,799.1 (4,040,572.7–4,085,986.6)	265,029.3 (262,546.9–266,546.5)	19,165.2 (19,113.9–19,212.1)	269,714.1 (178,835.4–393,641.9)	559.3 (371.2–812.5)
	2013	Both sexes	6,371,104.4 (6,347,846.5–6,397,764.3)	4,189,151.9 (4,155,310.9–4,225,954.9)	260,731.5 (257,914.9–263,680.2)	19,054.5 (18,993.9–19,109.6)	278,730.2 (186,479.8–404,043.5)	554.7 (369.3–805.9)
Luxembourg	1990	Both sexes	38,242.1 (37,991.0–38,435.2)	27,197.6 (26,628.1–27,574.4)	1,698.3 (1,655.8–1,732.7)	19,143.8 (18,891.7–19,302.4)	1,836.4 (1,229.7–2,677.6)	564.5 (377.9–823.8)
	2013	Both sexes	54,261.5 (53,922.2–54,535.7)	37,893.4 (36,874.5–38,503.1)	2,407.2 (2,353.9–2,457.7)	18,962.1 (18,730.0–19,110.0)	2,578.7 (1,726.2–3,728.6)	557.9 (373.0–802.9)
Malta	1990	Both sexes	38,246.2 (37,968.1–38,430.2)	31,355.1 (30,837.3–31,649.8)	2,166.9 (2,126.9–2,196.0)	19,426.3 (19,205.8–19,558.9)	2,102.1 (1,403.5–3,051.9)	572.9 (382.8–831.2)
	2013	Both sexes	43,139.9 (42,890.4–43,333.1)	28,582.3 (27,817.2–28,971.0)	1,793.1 (1,754.1–1,822.5)	19,078.4 (18,777.9–19,184.0)	1,942.9 (1,294.1–2,833.3)	560.1 (373.6–815.5)
Netherlands	1990	Both sexes	1,529,951.3 (1,521,889.8–1,536,317.2)	1,114,297.4 (1,100,700.2–1,122,318.7)	70,714.4 (69,683.2–71,692.2)	19,518.3 (19,392.1–19,597.8)	74,916.5 (49,412.5–107,892.4)	575.0 (380.6–830.6)
	2013	Both sexes	1,740,514.0 (1,730,311.7–1,748,714.5)	1,227,307.4 (1,211,039.7–1,240,101.4)	78,225.7 (76,871.9–79,768.8)	19,251.7 (19,118.3–19,343.7)	83,919.1 (56,241.5–122,530.8)	568.7 (378.0–832.3)
Norway	1990	Both sexes	430,119.9 (428,263.9–431,833.2)	313,464.5 (311,418.3–315,034.2)	20,262.4 (20,023.6–20,554.7)	19,087.2 (19,010.2–19,142.8)	20,570.6 (13,567.0–30,052.3)	551.2 (364.7–802.3)
	2013	Both sexes	513,713.4 (511,282.1–516,180.2)	365,384.1 (362,108.3–367,797.4)	23,377.8 (23,056.9–23,798.5)	18,941.7 (18,835.9–19,010.3)	24,095.4 (16,060.9–35,126.8)	547.3 (362.8–796.1)

Portugal	1990 Both sexes	993,414.9 (985,720.3–999,092.3)	773,643.3 (764,334.1–780,290.2)	52,929.3 (52,227.5–53,474.6)	19,095.0 (18,903.5–19,209.2)	52,224.2 (35,027.2–75,874.2)	564.8 (378.1–821.5)
	2013 Both sexes	1,075,657.0 (1,070,002.0–1,080,675.1)	730,302.0 (720,014.7–738,613.6)	45,662.9 (45,054.8–46,351.2)	18,904.1 (18,757.9–18,983.1)	50,042.6 (33,426.2–72,049.6)	558.7 (372.4–808.4)
Spain	1990 Both sexes	4,035,921.3 (3,994,779.3–4,065,167.8)	3,089,177.9 (3,026,435.5–3,116,424.7)	206,267.8 (203,728.2–209,216.2)	19,777.1 (19,584.9–19,906.6)	203,696.3 (135,973.2–296,867.8)	572.0 (381.7–833.6)
	2013 Both sexes	4,966,007.7 (4,931,761.3–4,990,857.1)	3,320,990.4 (3,257,995.9–3,351,095.4)	200,650.4 (197,343.4–208,225.7)	19,425.6 (19,274.7–19,540.9)	218,518.4 (144,996.5–318,757.7)	560.2 (372.3–814.3)
Sweden	1990 Both sexes	879,252.5 (873,219.3–884,003.7)	625,992.5 (616,077.1–632,559.3)	39,487.5 (38,764.8–40,067.1)	19,162.2 (18,942.8–19,294.5)	42,451.3 (28,326.8–61,747.4)	564.8 (376.1–822.0)
	2013 Both sexes	988,924.5 (983,340.9–993,398.8)	678,255.4 (665,305.0–686,979.8)	42,389.4 (41,458.6–43,177.4)	19,081.4 (18,863.4–19,205.0)	46,149.7 (30,705.2–66,263.6)	560.0 (373.7–810.1)
Switzerland	1990 Both sexes	679,201.8 (675,785.5–682,501.4)	479,171.1 (471,959.9–484,887.5)	30,467.8 (30,067.4–30,868.7)	19,149.4 (19,032.5–19,251.4)	32,262.0 (21,634.2–46,738.2)	561.9 (376.2–812.8)
	2013 Both sexes	827,036.8 (822,001.8–830,784.4)	549,874.0 (537,935.2–557,748.9)	33,831.9 (33,212.0–34,514.9)	19,109.0 (18,960.8–19,211.0)	37,131.8 (24,834.7–54,090.7)	559.1 (372.1–811.6)
United Kingdom	1990 Both sexes	5,942,605.6 (5,915,434.1–5,959,707.5)	4,355,887.9 (4,303,299.7–4,385,568.1)	282,541.9 (278,553.1–285,102.2)	19,515.8 (19,337.4–19,609.6)	294,054.7 (195,066.4–428,499.5)	575.1 (382.0–838.5)
	2013 Both sexes	6,600,939.0 (6,578,110.1–6,617,571.9)	4,609,474.9 (4,555,018.1–4,641,020.4)	293,692.8 (289,576.5–296,510.6)	19,251.9 (19,081.2–19,339.8)	313,551.6 (208,816.8–454,452.5)	566.5 (376.1–824.9)

(continued on next page)

Table 2
(continued)

Location	Year	Sex	Prevalent Cases of Mild Anemia	Prevalent Cases of Moderate Anemia	Prevalent Cases of Severe Anemia	Age-Standardized Prevalence (per 100,000)	Total YLDs	Age-Standardized YLDs (per 100,000)
Southern Latin America	1990	Both sexes	3,920,504.8 (3,904,421.2-3,935,320.3)	3,946,360.5 (3,923,309.2-3,966,100.9)	278,788.1 (276,532.9-280,445.2)	16,089.3 (16,018.1-16,157.7)	263,986.7 (176,116.7-383,023.5)	510.6 (340.2-739.7)
	2013	Both sexes	4,754,530.4 (4,737,245.9-4,770,057.0)	4,398,908.8 (4,373,375.3-4,422,755.3)	291,654.6 (289,429.5-293,267.3)	15,522.4 (15,458.3-15,580.6)	296,152.2 (196,583.0-428,935.6)	494.0 (328.1-715.4)
Argentina	1990	Both sexes	2,699,170.9 (2,684,876.4-2,710,756.4)	2,748,168.1 (2,727,744.9-2,765,133.1)	196,378.2 (194,272.5-197,824.2)	16,649.7 (16,553.5-16,732.2)	183,919.6 (122,971.8-267,204.5)	529.0 (353.2-767.4)
	2013	Both sexes	3,280,959.1 (3,267,156.0-3,293,740.0)	3,084,841.7 (3,061,250.5-3,105,566.2)	206,652.3 (204,629.2-208,110.5)	16,085.8 (15,999.6-16,162.2)	207,183.5 (137,532.3-299,800.4)	511.9 (339.8-740.6)
Chile	1990	Both sexes	956,554.8 (951,334.4-960,712.3)	944,790.0 (938,748.6-950,246.5)	64,919.1 (64,138.1-65,635.2)	14,391.4 (14,313.8-14,462.7)	63,092.7 (41,874.6-91,367.2)	456.1 (303.0-660.7)
	2013	Both sexes	1,191,308.3 (1,185,285.2-1,196,299.5)	1,058,260.6 (1,048,365.5-1,066,615.0)	68,084.4 (67,296.7-68,715.4)	13,981.7 (13,907.0-14,047.7)	71,628.2 (47,818.2-104,465.9)	444.2 (296.4-646.7)
Uruguay	1990	Both sexes	264,625.1 (263,378.2-265,661.3)	253,265.7 (251,488.0-254,796.5)	17,481.9 (17,308.3-17,588.4)	17,204.7 (17,116.0-17,278.3)	16,965.2 (11,293.3-24,547.3)	544.8 (362.7-788.8)
	2013	Both sexes	282,034.4 (280,766.1-283,103.9)	255,616.4 (253,109.0-257,433.5)	16,906.0 (16,657.8-17,067.1)	16,677.9 (16,575.0-16,749.3)	17,327.5 (11,619.5-25,139.9)	531.2 (356.3-771.7)
High-income North America	1990	Both sexes	24,609,564.4 (24,557,839.0-24,657,768.1)	18,872,081.1 (18,805,539.8-18,940,055.5)	1,259,779.5 (1,249,109.1-1,264,666.8)	16,801.3 (16,764.6-16,836.7)	1,268,468.3 (844,332.0-1,848,491.6)	495.2 (329.7-719.1)
	2013	Both sexes	31,552,418.5 (31,483,373.5-31,616,433.0)	22,813,332.0 (22,697,817.8-22,911,282.9)	1,488,580.9 (1,479,729.7-1,496,456.5)	16,773.0 (16,737.7-16,808.1)	1,559,840.4 (1,041,759.2-2,254,251.7)	496.4 (330.4-718.0)

	Year	Sex						
Canada	1990	Both sexes	1,951,937.4 (1,942,568.6–1,961,961.1)	1,627,596.7 (1,616,898.9–1,636,031.5)	104,434.6 (103,172.1–105,725.7)	14,385.2 (14,319.1–14,443.2)	110,473.6 (73,705.6–159,331.8)	446.4 (298.3–644.7)
	2013	Both sexes	2,463,157.6 (2,450,917.6–2,473,180.2)	1,808,409.9 (1,796,167.1–1,822,467.3)	108,130.1 (107,345.7–108,814.2)	14,274.5 (14,222.0–14,321.6)	124,874.4 (83,610.7–181,028.6)	441.8 (295.1–640.7)
United States	1990	Both sexes	22,652,315.3 (22,601,377.3–22,700,375.0)	17,240,356.5 (17,175,081.8–17,306,760.1)	1,155,066.6 (1,144,354.8–1,159,516.3)	17,074.1 (17,036.6–17,112.4)	1,157,717.9 (770,572.9–1,687,740.9)	500.7 (333.3–728.1)
	2013	Both sexes	29,083,601.7 (29,014,429.9–29,151,337.8)	21,000,827.3 (20,884,770.3–21,101,540.1)	1,380,183.8 (1,371,228.1–1,388,056.7)	17,057.7 (17,019.1–17,098.1)	1,434,687.1 (957,548.1–2,074,547.3)	502.3 (334.2–726.2)
Latin America and Caribbean	1990	Both sexes	42,911,725.0 (42,703,991.5–43,042,155.2)	46,100,041.4 (45,769,852.2–46,280,907.4)	3,675,445.1 (3,639,954.5–3,695,871.0)	21,840.3 (21,743.0–21,903.6)	3,127,640.1 (2,091,548.1–4,519,421.5)	700.7 (469.6–1,011.8)
	2013	Both sexes	52,639,465.4 (52,420,318.8–52,828,336.1)	51,116,184.9 (50,794,607.3–51,368,105.5)	3,746,592.9 (3,707,985.2–3,770,655.9)	19,278.8 (19,189.5–19,358.0)	3,505,007.6 (2,339,161.1–5,053,678.2)	623.2 (416.5–897.3)
Caribbean	1990	Both sexes	5,938,743.8 (5,930,111.1–5,947,202.1)	6,199,108.0 (6,190,004.7–6,207,389.1)	571,154.8 (567,486.2–574,110.3)	34,728.5 (34,683.1–34,771.9)	428,480.0 (286,814.3–616,316.8)	1,134.1 (760.5–1,629.4)
	2013	Both sexes	6,898,142.0 (6,887,287.2–6,908,126.7)	6,554,901.6 (6,545,172.3–6,563,892.4)	554,742.0 (550,744.0–557,840.1)	31,618.5 (31,574.8–31,660.3)	452,787.4 (302,762.9–652,169.7)	1,020.3 (682.4–1,468.9)
Antigua and Barbuda	1990	Both sexes	8,801.1 (8,773.7–8,822.2)	8,338.0 (8,310.6–8,358.4)	647.0 (634.6–653.1)	28,751.3 (28,667.4–28,817.5)	568.0 (378.8–820.2)	899.2 (600.4–1,297.6)
	2013	Both sexes	12,588.0 (12,551.5–12,614.9)	11,302.3 (11,270.2–11,327.6)	843.6 (833.8–851.6)	27,762.2 (27,691.4–27,821.0)	772.1 (513.7–1,113.5)	869.0 (579.0–1,252.5)
The Bahamas	1990	Both sexes	35,390.2 (35,308.5–35,464.7)	34,565.7 (34,476.7–34,657.0)	2,731.9 (2,608.6–2,770.7)	27,549.9 (27,472.8–27,612.3)	2,379.1 (1,589.0–3,434.7)	869.5 (581.3–1,252.3)
	2013	Both sexes	51,234.4 (50,995.4–51,435.5)	42,756.9 (42,582.3–42,899.9)	3,116.4 (3,026.5–3,174.9)	26,828.7 (26,733.9–26,911.8)	2,973.2 (1,995.4–4,283.0)	845.9 (568.5–1,214.9)

(continued on next page)

Table 2
(continued)

Location	Year	Sex	Prevalent Cases of Mild Anemia	Prevalent Cases of Moderate Anemia	Prevalent Cases of Severe Anemia	Age-Standardized Prevalence (per 100,000)	Total YLDs	Age-Standardized YLDs (per 100,000)
Barbados	1990	Both sexes	37,580.2 (37,451.5–37,668.9)	33,392.8 (33,295.2–33,474.6)	2,506.7 (2,451.0–2,530.2)	28,817.2 (28,727.7–28,881.5)	2,283.3 (1,524.4–3,312.5)	904.8 (604.4–1,310.8)
	2013	Both sexes	39,705.2 (39,538.4–39,845.5)	32,021.6 (31,925.8–32,102.1)	2,270.4 (2,245.9–2,293.3)	27,271.9 (27,193.4–27,340.6)	2,219.8 (1,490.0–3,208.0)	854.3 (573.0–1,233.7)
Belize	1990	Both sexes	29,056.0 (28,996.5–29,125.1)	31,804.7 (31,739.0–31,862.9)	2,680.6 (2,660.8–2,695.6)	31,100.2 (31,026.7–31,176.0)	2,151.4 (1,439.5–3,114.4)	968.2 (649.1–1,397.4)
	2013	Both sexes	47,786.0 (47,653.5–47,886.3)	47,725.0 (47,621.1–47,821.7)	3,827.1 (3,797.3–3,856.2)	29,129.4 (29,061.2–29,186.8)	3,239.6 (2,153.1–4,700.7)	907.0 (604.7–1,315.7)
Cuba	1990	Both sexes	1,580,506.4 (1,575,874.5–1,584,728.2)	1,351,667.6 (1,347,508.6–1,354,773.0)	100,670.8 (99,423.2–101,449.1)	29,345.4 (29,269.3–29,408.4)	92,270.9 (61,655.5–133,327.8)	913.0 (610.7–1,315.9)
	2013	Both sexes	1,591,646.0 (1,586,201.7–1,596,586.6)	1,238,237.9 (1,234,911.8–1,241,315.8)	86,747.8 (85,819.9–87,369.0)	27,371.8 (27,311.8–27,429.5)	85,599.3 (57,172.6–123,984.5)	851.2 (567.7–1,231.0)
Dominica	1990	Both sexes	9,213.1 (9,191.3–9,233.4)	8,901.6 (8,880.1–8,925.3)	685.7 (665.0–693.7)	26,720.4 (26,653.9–26,781.2)	608.2 (408.1–878.4)	835.0 (561.8–1,202.3)
	2013	Both sexes	9,287.5 (9,263.9–9,306.9)	8,293.4 (8,273.0–8,315.3)	621.1 (607.7–631.2)	26,105.3 (26,046.9–26,165.7)	570.8 (381.1–825.4)	815.7 (544.7–1,179.8)
Dominican Republic	1990	Both sexes	1,135,834.3 (1,133,054.5–1,138,216.7)	1,182,297.9 (1,179,555.2–1,184,694.6)	99,622.0 (97,418.9–100,469.9)	31,773.3 (31,682.0–31,838.4)	80,804.2 (53,893.4–116,681.6)	995.3 (663.7–1,435.6)
	2013	Both sexes	1,472,016.0 (1,467,696.7–1,475,046.9)	1,390,019.9 (1,386,328.4–1,392,820.9)	109,277.8 (107,492.9–110,608.7)	28,061.2 (27,976.6–28,119.4)	95,551.6 (64,103.5–137,473.9)	880.0 (591.0–1,262.1)
Grenada	1990	Both sexes	16,629.0 (16,602.6–16,655.9)	16,634.1 (16,598.7–16,667.6)	1,406.9 (1,377.5–1,420.5)	34,481.8 (34,408.1–34,548.9)	1,135.8 (761.1–1,636.4)	1,067.2 (718.6–1,534.7)
	2013	Both sexes	17,196.3 (17,154.4–17,232.9)	14,880.1 (14,842.9–14,918.6)	1,175.2 (1,151.1–1,195.4)	31,531.8 (31,459.3–31,599.7)	1,028.9 (688.2–1,482.5)	972.8 (651.5–1,400.6)

	Year	Sex						
Guyana	1990	Both sexes	137,840.4 (137,542.2–138,227.9)	148,006.1 (147,622.1–148,295.4)	14,215.3 (14,113.1–14,270.1)	41,703.4 (41,610.8–41,791.2)	10,187.8 (6,819.1–14,672.7)	1,362.9 (913.5–1,961.1)
	2013	Both sexes	128,156.3 (127,850.0–128,406.0)	138,191.2 (137,941.4–138,417.1)	12,339.5 (12,261.7–12,405.1)	34,391.2 (34,316.1–34,458.4)	9,442.0 (6,299.4–13,622.9)	1,099.2 (737.3–1,582.6)
Haiti	1990	Both sexes	1,483,355.4 (1,480,690.6–1,487,982.4)	1,918,393.1 (1,913,567.1–1,921,500.4)	218,620.2 (216,488.3–219,994.0)	50,174.9 (50,064.8–50,277.8)	135,177.5 (90,780.5–193,913.6)	1,762.5 (1,187.3–2,518.2)
	2013	Both sexes	1,963,466.5 (1,959,492.1–1,966,763.1)	2,236,910.4 (2,232,899.7–2,240,651.2)	224,121.1 (222,203.1–225,824.6)	42,607.4 (42,528.4–42,681.1)	155,139.7 (104,084.9–223,088.7)	1,436.1 (966.0–2,062.3)
Jamaica	1990	Both sexes	361,467.5 (360,653.5–362,250.5)	366,215.1 (365,312.3–366,990.7)	30,141.7 (29,290.8–30,505.5)	30,366.4 (30,288.7–30,431.2)	25,077.8 (16,777.7–36,210.9)	958.8 (642.9–1,380.8)
	2013	Both sexes	398,737.6 (397,364.0–399,653.4)	366,060.6 (364,951.7–367,002.4)	28,342.2 (27,418.2–28,753.4)	28,300.9 (28,205.3–28,366.9)	25,112.3 (16,754.8–36,200.0)	888.1 (592.5–1,279.6)
Saint Lucia	1990	Both sexes	21,558.2 (21,515.7–21,603.7)	22,036.8 (21,983.5–22,078.8)	1,804.7 (1,769.8–1,819.5)	30,881.8 (30,812.4–30,943.9)	1,490.0 (993.8–2,142.5)	960.1 (643.0–1,379.1)
	2013	Both sexes	26,364.8 (26,273.2–26,432.1)	23,132.7 (23,067.9–23,187.5)	1,742.9 (1,717.2–1,759.5)	28,531.8 (28,446.7–28,596.9)	1,588.0 (1,058.4–2,292.7)	892.1 (595.0–1,286.7)
Saint Vincent and the Grenadines	1990	Both sexes	16,736.9 (16,698.7–16,768.7)	17,616.3 (17,572.3–17,646.1)	1,492.5 (1,472.0–1,503.4)	31,920.2 (31,838.5–31,982.1)	1,198.4 (801.0–1,729.9)	999.4 (669.1–1,442.5)
	2013	Both sexes	15,520.7 (15,472.0–15,557.7)	13,795.6 (13,758.3–13,828.1)	1,044.7 (1,034.2–1,053.7)	28,064.7 (27,991.6–28,127.0)	946.7 (631.1–1,370.0)	876.0 (584.5–1,266.8)
Suriname	1990	Both sexes	70,033.9 (69,862.4–70,227.2)	69,801.3 (69,623.5–69,936.3)	6,011.8 (5,939.1–6,046.8)	35,288.3 (35,201.8–35,364.0)	4,758.4 (3,186.4–6,873.3)	1,105.6 (742.3–1,592.9)
	2013	Both sexes	83,795.1 (83,569.6–83,965.8)	77,382.4 (77,198.2–77,533.1)	6,168.5 (6,117.3–6,217.4)	31,146.7 (31,071.9–31,206.5)	5,294.1 (3,536.2–7,630.2)	974.2 (650.8–1,403.0)

(continued on next page)

Table 2 (*continued*)

Location	Year	Sex	Prevalent Cases of Mild Anemia	Prevalent Cases of Moderate Anemia	Prevalent Cases of Severe Anemia	Age-Standardized Prevalence (per 100,000)	Total YLDs	Age-Standardized YLDs (per 100,000)
Trinidad and Tobago	1990	Both sexes	179,140.0 (178,597.8–179,614.5)	178,902.2 (178,428.9–179,314.0)	14,435.2 (14,223.7–14,598.4)	29,410.1 (29,331.8–29,486.6)	12,211.0 (8,188.4–17,703.5)	920.4 (615.5–1,329.3)
	2013	Both sexes	185,962.1 (185,228.9–186,561.1)	154,638.9 (154,108.6–155,100.6)	11,087.7 (10,935.5–11,200.4)	27,312.0 (27,228.5–27,386.2)	10,641.7 (7,111.9–15,403.8)	854.0 (571.1–1,235.0)
Andean Latin America	1990	Both sexes	4,618,222.1 (4,607,096.6–4,628,420.8)	5,687,409.6 (5,676,193.7–5,696,377.5)	483,780.9 (482,404.4–484,914.2)	25,020.3 (24,959.5–25,071.8)	384,622.3 (256,395.4–553,457.0)	847.4 (568.3–1,219.2)
	2013	Both sexes	5,883,485.1 (5,863,266.6–5,900,842.4)	6,670,009.0 (6,636,303.0–6,690,540.5)	518,491.0 (513,063.3–521,656.3)	22,168.8 (22,087.1–22,230.7)	454,300.9 (302,822.4–656,719.7)	757.9 (505.9–1,093.9)
Bolivia	1990	Both sexes	893,010.0 (890,878.5–895,767.0)	1,265,211.3 (1,262,004.2–1,267,325.6)	128,881.0 (128,510.5–129,268.3)	29,522.8 (29,443.1–29,597.0)	87,713.8 (58,900.8–125,541.3)	1,064.6 (716.4–1,526.3)
	2013	Both sexes	1,236,047.1 (1,230,900.1–1,239,722.2)	1,630,994.0 (1,623,937.4–1,635,127.0)	149,087.7 (148,065.3–149,725.3)	26,106.4 (26,012.4–26,176.7)	111,723.3 (74,543.4–160,625.8)	932.4 (622.5–1,340.4)
Ecuador	1990	Both sexes	1,294,060.6 (1,290,173.2–1,298,532.5)	1,580,850.8 (1,576,637.8–1,584,138.3)	134,546.0 (133,746.3–135,111.1)	26,989.0 (26,899.5–27,066.0)	106,914.8 (71,328.5–154,214.1)	913.1 (609.1–1,317.3)
	2013	Both sexes	1,702,894.1 (1,697,887.4–1,707,958.1)	1,904,618.4 (1,899,350.4–1,909,751.4)	146,145.4 (145,489.6–146,683.9)	23,074.5 (23,005.6–23,138.9)	129,585.0 (86,485.1–187,389.0)	784.4 (524.7–1,132.3)
Peru	1990	Both sexes	2,431,151.5 (2,423,304.0–2,439,480.9)	2,841,347.5 (2,832,693.0–2,848,153.7)	220,353.8 (219,301.2–221,087.1)	22,670.1 (22,590.8–22,747.2)	189,993.7 (126,656.5–273,267.2)	746.1 (500.3–1,072.7)
	2013	Both sexes	2,944,544.0 (2,930,083.2–2,957,754.1)	3,134,396.7 (3,109,726.6–3,151,403.8)	223,257.9 (218,806.2–225,868.8)	20,283.3 (20,162.6–20,380.5)	212,992.6 (142,665.4–308,810.8)	678.3 (454.8–980.5)

Location	Year	Sex						
Central Latin America	1990	Both sexes	19,133,876.5 (19,069,418.7–19,182,093.8)	20,220,046.8 (20,136,035.3–20,274,140.9)	1,621,518.8 (1,614,033.9–1,626,666.6)	22,805.8 (22,737.6–22,856.8)	1,367,223.9 (913,631.7–1,977,547.4)	715.0 (477.9–1,031.3)
	2013	Both sexes	24,431,029.6 (24,247,487.4–24,535,719.4)	23,343,421.8 (23,140,957.7–23,495,804.1)	1,726,159.0 (1,712,910.9–1,737,200.1)	19,739.6 (19,590.9–19,838.4)	1,595,451.2 (1,064,379.0–2,312,758.1)	624.4 (417.5–903.4)
Colombia	1990	Both sexes	3,713,050.6 (3,669,731.6–3,741,896.6)	3,782,072.5 (3,720,335.7–3,812,499.2)	290,576.7 (285,438.2–293,554.3)	22,134.7 (21,883.7–22,283.2)	254,852.0 (170,135.8–368,139.7)	686.2 (460.3–989.9)
	2013	Both sexes	4,778,030.0 (4,598,647.7–4,847,795.8)	4,379,709.8 (4,187,493.9–4,485,973.8)	310,934.1 (298,436.4–319,573.3)	19,510.4 (18,776.3–19,875.3)	298,207.9 (198,855.3–434,377.0)	609.1 (406.9–885.4)
Costa Rica	1990	Both sexes	289,562.6 (286,781.9–290,628.7)	291,915.8 (288,185.5–293,957.7)	21,676.1 (21,469.3–21,772.4)	18,341.9 (18,170.5–18,435.9)	19,731.0 (13,202.5–28,584.3)	573.2 (384.5–829.0)
	2013	Both sexes	435,200.5 (432,308.4–436,809.1)	381,094.3 (375,753.4–384,758.0)	26,213.4 (25,973.7–26,358.9)	17,805.4 (17,627.8–17,919.6)	26,348.4 (17,555.4–38,151.2)	563.9 (376.0–814.5)
El Salvador	1990	Both sexes	744,093.0 (742,061.7–746,519.2)	923,800.4 (920,936.8–925,585.0)	88,097.9 (87,790.2–88,362.9)	32,198.1 (32,114.8–32,272.9)	62,960.0 (42,258.8–90,530.1)	1,095.9 (737.4–1,571.9)
	2013	Both sexes	824,626.1 (822,331.4–826,708.5)	942,974.3 (940,651.1–945,314.4)	82,966.4 (82,660.4–83,221.9)	29,214.3 (29,139.3–29,287.2)	64,118.0 (42,957.1–91,816.0)	995.8 (667.1–1,424.1)
Guatemala	1990	Both sexes	1,670,040.5 (1,666,664.1–1,673,715.0)	1,864,783.2 (1,859,821.7–1,867,471.4)	179,424.6 (178,977.4–180,207.5)	41,291.4 (41,198.2–41,376.4)	126,580.3 (84,961.4–182,417.7)	1,289.5 (870.5–1,850.6)
	2013	Both sexes	2,544,892.7 (2,536,366.5–2,550,015.3)	2,675,207.9 (2,666,190.6–2,680,102.3)	234,426.6 (233,419.9–235,172.5)	34,575.5 (34,445.0–34,652.5)	181,313.1 (121,047.6–261,514.9)	1,072.1 (720.8–1,542.0)

(continued on next page)

Table 2
(continued)

Location	Year	Sex	Prevalent Cases of Mild Anemia	Prevalent Cases of Moderate Anemia	Prevalent Cases of Severe Anemia	Age-Standardized Prevalence (per 100,000)	Total YLDs	Age-Standardized YLDs (per 100,000)
Honduras	1990	Both sexes	763,829.4 (762,151.3–765,248.9)	801,053.6 (799,228.1–802,407.8)	67,388.9 (67,098.7–67,621.5)	31,091.9 (30,996.9–31,166.6)	54,008.8 (36,089.2–78,085.7)	932.0 (625.3–1,344.7)
	2013	Both sexes	1,020,980.6 (1,014,010.0–1,026,064.7)	957,859.6 (945,858.3–967,266.4)	73,528.5 (72,564.4–74,263.2)	24,168.6 (23,968.3–24,336.6)	64,928.6 (43,407.3–93,886.4)	724.8 (485.7–1,046.9)
Mexico	1990	Both sexes	9,570,893.6 (9,545,210.0–9,588,307.7)	10,135,055.4 (10,094,687.4–10,155,406.5)	791,596.6 (786,606.7–794,169.6)	22,258.7 (22,197.9–22,295.9)	685,402.4 (457,589.6–991,448.8)	700.1 (467.1–1,010.9)
	2013	Both sexes	11,604,867.2 (11,568,412.6–11,630,086.4)	11,113,280.8 (11,057,117.9–11,144,276.0)	792,755.8 (786,663.5–796,011.8)	18,922.2 (18,847.7–18,969.1)	760,373.6 (507,699.1–1,100,584.6)	602.1 (402.2–870.1)
Nicaragua	1990	Both sexes	475,633.9 (474,116.7–476,891.5)	519,756.3 (517,455.5–522,036.4)	41,347.7 (41,179.4–41,517.8)	22,063.9 (21,973.2–22,141.7)	34,472.1 (23,236.4–49,796.1)	648.3 (437.5–924.0)
	2013	Both sexes	598,185.1 (593,359.9–603,623.9)	567,861.8 (560,866.1–574,178.0)	41,603.8 (41,121.4–42,084.4)	18,980.9 (18,799.8–19,153.2)	38,585.7 (25,874.8–55,617.1)	582.9 (391.3–838.0)
Panama	1990	Both sexes	262,495.4 (261,007.3–263,725.5)	265,242.5 (263,283.6–266,765.2)	20,157.1 (20,025.7–20,259.9)	20,762.9 (20,649.7–20,846.5)	17,890.1 (11,976.2–25,856.7)	643.9 (431.0–929.3)
	2013	Both sexes	382,761.5 (375,081.7–387,234.1)	351,468.5 (342,913.3–358,387.0)	25,226.3 (24,596.1–25,721.5)	19,385.6 (18,987.0–19,670.8)	24,051.8 (16,055.3–34,857.4)	605.7 (405.2–877.2)

	Year	Sex						
Venezuela	1990	Both sexes	1,644,277.5 (1,614,671.5–1,672,558.5)	1,636,367.2 (1,610,063.0–1,670,614.0)	121,253.3 (119,183.5–123,407.5)	15,270.5 (15,052.8–15,507.1)	111,327.3 (74,797.4–162,256.7)	470.7 (316.4–681.6)
	2013	Both sexes	2,241,485.9 (2,181,355.8–2,281,628.6)	1,973,964.9 (1,910,588.6–2,046,597.6)	138,504.2 (134,515.4–143,371.7)	14,007.8 (13,629.9–14,355.7)	137,524.1 (91,347.9–198,872.0)	436.5 (290.2–630.9)
Tropical Latin America	1990	Both sexes	13,220,882.7 (13,034,568.9–13,327,194.0)	13,993,477.0 (13,729,045.1–14,152,340.2)	998,990.6 (967,631.3–1,017,564.2)	16,892.7 (16,674.9–17,026.9)	947,313.9 (631,364.7–1,374,494.0)	544.2 (363.1–786.7)
	2013	Both sexes	15,426,808.6 (15,284,747.2–15,544,259.0)	14,547,852.4 (14,310,424.4–14,696,682.8)	947,200.9 (918,882.9–962,969.0)	15,257.5 (15,069.2–15,384.1)	1,002,468.1 (669,697.8–1,442,087.1)	496.0 (331.7–712.9)
Brazil	1990	Both sexes	12,861,292.1 (12,676,605.2–12,966,254.7)	13,595,547.9 (13,334,661.0–13,751,878.4)	970,135.2 (939,161.2–988,576.1)	16,919.3 (16,699.0–17,055.9)	920,493.6 (613,646.9–1,335,499.1)	544.9 (363.6–787.8)
	2013	Both sexes	14,889,578.1 (14,749,941.4–15,006,240.3)	13,998,035.1 (13,770,275.7–14,145,406.7)	908,913.4 (882,332.8–924,268.5)	15,247.8 (15,056.5–15,378.3)	965,059.3 (644,703.1–1,387,392.3)	495.7 (331.5–712.0)
Paraguay	1990	Both sexes	359,590.6 (355,008.8–361,716.9)	397,929.1 (389,362.4–401,289.5)	28,855.4 (27,955.8–29,278.6)	15,898.4 (15,684.0–16,012.4)	26,820.3 (17,851.2–38,992.3)	517.7 (346.3–750.6)
	2013	Both sexes	537,230.5 (532,612.3–539,397.3)	549,817.4 (535,857.9–555,115.4)	38,287.5 (36,647.9–38,975.4)	15,480.1 (15,265.6–15,582.5)	37,408.7 (24,972.8–54,216.7)	503.1 (335.3–728.7)
North Africa and Middle East	1990	Both sexes	50,945,834.8 (50,878,767.9–51,004,121.9)	56,166,967.3 (56,096,038.7–56,222,508.9)	4,957,998.8 (4,947,921.7–4,968,630.8)	32,756.6 (32,713.4–32,793.5)	3,766,788.6 (2,515,159.2–5,440,566.0)	1,010.0 (676.0–1,456.4)
	2013	Both sexes	71,231,000.5 (71,135,176.5–71,317,287.2)	68,788,986.2 (68,701,152.6–68,866,185.9)	5,584,631.8 (5,571,567.9–5,596,303.0)	28,353.0 (28,322.0–28,381.3)	4,594,913.2 (3,055,766.9–6,646,118.0)	872.4 (581.2–1,261.2)

(continued on next page)

Table 2
(continued)

Location	Year Sex	Prevalent Cases of Mild Anemia	Prevalent Cases of Moderate Anemia	Prevalent Cases of Severe Anemia	Age-Standardized Prevalence (per 100,000)	Total YLDs	Age-Standardized YLDs (per 100,000)
Algeria	1990 Both sexes	3,816,842.8 (3,809,789.3–3,825,361.7)	4,228,533.4 (4,219,188.9–4,234,590.4)	353,815.8 (352,357.2–355,172.8)	29,658.1 (29,591.1–29,712.6)	281,566.1 (188,122.9–407,567.7)	898.5 (600.3–1,299.2)
	2013 Both sexes	5,157,278.3 (5,147,597.5–5,166,450.3)	4,642,047.0 (4,631,397.0–4,651,334.0)	335,432.4 (333,484.4–337,343.2)	25,948.2 (25,900.9–25,992.7)	306,735.1 (203,504.6–446,707.6)	783.0 (520.5–1,137.5)
Bahrain	1990 Both sexes	73,812.1 (73,669.4–73,963.2)	76,561.0 (76,349.9–76,788.1)	6,997.6 (6,773.5–7,102.6)	31,836.5 (31,770.7–31,895.8)	5,253.3 (3,530.8–7,578.1)	1,027.1 (691.3–1,477.2)
	2013 Both sexes	175,858.3 (175,462.0–176,234.2)	160,552.3 (160,125.3–160,948.5)	14,117.1 (13,631.0–14,348.4)	28,885.6 (28,835.9–28,930.7)	11,086.5 (7,441.6–15,913.1)	929.1 (623.8–1,329.9)
Egypt	1990 Both sexes	8,860,823.8 (8,842,398.4–8,886,812.2)	9,673,875.5 (9,642,457.6–9,690,364.8)	831,694.9 (827,829.6–838,030.9)	32,906.7 (32,820.9–32,979.2)	645,815.7 (431,452.3–932,099.0)	1,025.7 (686.6–1,480.2)
	2013 Both sexes	11,609,428.9 (11,583,595.9–11,630,385.1)	11,597,126.8 (11,572,394.4–11,617,717.7)	918,878.0 (915,095.4–922,201.7)	28,989.9 (28,930.0–29,041.9)	769,570.4 (512,865.3–1,113,636.3)	897.8 (598.7–1,297.3)
Iran	1990 Both sexes	8,659,325.8 (8,646,338.5–8,670,242.9)	9,367,288.7 (9,353,770.9–9,378,780.8)	790,430.2 (786,307.0–793,768.6)	30,740.3 (30,685.1–30,789.7)	624,664.9 (417,628.6–904,496.0)	905.9 (603.7–1,313.6)
	2013 Both sexes	9,192,375.4 (9,170,815.6–9,208,771.9)	7,544,080.1 (7,524,942.4–7,561,072.1)	516,376.2 (513,794.0–518,089.4)	23,035.1 (22,992.5–23,072.3)	497,980.2 (330,648.3–723,404.7)	676.5 (450.1–980.3)

Iraq	1990	Both sexes	2,712,130.1 (2,707,236.1–2,717,480.9)	3,037,040.2 (3,031,086.7–3,041,299.4)	261,174.4 (258,984.0–262,807.7)	31,843.7 (31,777.3–31,900.9)	202,819.5 (135,395.8–293,607.4)	967.8 (647.6–1,399.0)
	2013	Both sexes	4,973,410.0 (4,964,795.7–4,980,040.2)	5,276,367.1 (5,268,059.6–5,283,280.6)	436,710.5 (433,071.8–439,138.6)	29,941.3 (29,886.5–29,985.0)	352,033.1 (235,144.7–510,786.3)	909.6 (608.7–1,317.8)
Jordan	1990	Both sexes	454,606.2 (453,860.8–455,412.8)	518,840.9 (517,968.7–519,452.2)	44,187.3 (43,994.3–44,404.9)	28,000.3 (27,941.3–28,047.7)	34,539.2 (23,013.8–49,976.5)	850.4 (567.0–1,231.0)
	2013	Both sexes	934,576.8 (932,810.8–936,109.5)	936,352.4 (934,481.3–937,827.5)	72,427.6 (71,925.1–72,758.3)	26,099.9 (26,051.5–26,138.9)	61,909.4 (40,980.5–89,822.5)	794.8 (527.0–1,150.4)
Kuwait	1990	Both sexes	278,197.9 (277,668.7–278,785.8)	267,312.2 (266,748.5–267,779.2)	21,321.0 (21,240.1–21,398.4)	26,833.8 (26,785.3–26,880.7)	17,855.9 (11,857.5–25,872.1)	779.8 (518.9–1,132.5)
	2013	Both sexes	409,003.0 (408,425.2–409,589.7)	324,182.9 (323,519.0–324,811.5)	23,216.1 (23,105.1–23,309.8)	23,622.8 (23,587.3–23,657.6)	21,666.7 (14,340.3–31,643.1)	680.9 (451.9–989.8)
Lebanon	1990	Both sexes	353,648.4 (352,809.9–354,419.7)	360,149.5 (359,288.7–360,855.5)	27,886.8 (27,743.1–28,031.9)	26,040.0 (25,974.6–26,092.4)	23,650.6 (15,825.0–34,188.9)	788.1 (527.7–1,137.7)
	2013	Both sexes	606,318.9 (605,038.7–607,463.1)	524,199.6 (522,929.3–525,373.0)	37,612.1 (37,420.0–37,793.1)	25,417.0 (25,372.3–25,458.2)	34,687.9 (23,101.2–50,198.2)	773.7 (515.6–1,118.4)
Libya	1990	Both sexes	559,178.2 (558,018.6–560,515.4)	606,427.7 (605,093.9–607,379.1)	49,594.9 (48,989.0–49,925.5)	26,125.5 (26,064.6–26,177.1)	40,338.5 (26,932.7–58,502.2)	781.8 (520.2–1,132.4)
	2013	Both sexes	807,051.1 (805,442.9–808,447.7)	763,063.8 (761,569.2–764,381.9)	57,471.0 (56,866.2–57,800.3)	26,000.1 (25,950.1–26,043.3)	50,613.0 (33,732.8–73,415.8)	785.8 (524.8–1,139.1)

(continued on next page)

Table 2
(continued)

Location	Year	Sex	Prevalent Cases of Mild Anemia	Prevalent Cases of Moderate Anemia	Prevalent Cases of Severe Anemia	Age-Standardized Prevalence (per 100,000)	Total YLDs	Age-Standardized YLDs (per 100,000)
Morocco	1990	Both sexes	3,798,889.6 (3,790,833.7– 3,807,124.4)	4,096,148.3 (4,087,921.2– 4,102,358.6)	345,905.8 (343,611.8– 347,731.7)	31,742.1 (31,676.8– 31,798.3)	273,141.4 (182,392.5– 394,121.0)	968.0 (647.1– 1,395.3)
	2013	Both sexes	4,665,117.1 (4,656,941.0– 4,672,845.5)	4,284,233.5 (4,277,021.1– 4,291,419.7)	321,133.8 (318,158.0– 322,770.7)	28,177.9 (28,132.6– 28,222.4)	283,183.9 (188,053.9– 411,402.6)	853.1 (567.2– 1,237.6)
Palestine	1990	Both sexes	291,064.6 (290,570.0– 291,590.2)	329,286.2 (328,722.4– 329,696.2)	26,899.7 (26,778.7– 27,074.4)	27,582.6 (27,522.3– 27,635.8)	21,809.8 (14,525.6– 31,617.4)	832.3 (553.9– 1,204.4)
	2013	Both sexes	559,740.6 (558,786.3– 560,589.5)	595,904.5 (594,941.2– 596,794.9)	47,279.2 (47,123.1– 47,428.4)	25,762.4 (25,713.0– 25,807.8)	39,503.5 (26,352.4– 57,203.1)	777.3 (517.5– 1,124.3)
Oman	1990	Both sexes	317,479.8 (317,014.6– 317,953.6)	341,988.2 (341,453.5– 342,482.0)	30,631.2 (30,305.9– 30,815.4)	35,588.4 (35,528.7– 35,642.2)	23,060.3 (15,350.0– 33,282.1)	1,069.0 (716.3– 1,538.8)
	2013	Both sexes	483,640.0 (482,929.1– 484,308.1)	376,985.5 (376,214.7– 377,654.5)	28,268.0 (27,734.5– 28,609.9)	26,719.4 (26,680.6– 26,753.0)	25,477.0 (16,975.6– 36,900.3)	786.6 (526.0– 1,134.3)
Qatar	1990	Both sexes	54,928.3 (54,860.4– 54,989.6)	45,656.5 (45,582.8– 45,721.8)	3,416.1 (3,396.0– 3,433.1)	22,389.4 (22,359.6– 22,414.8)	3,054.3 (2,025.0– 4,442.3)	640.6 (425.9–928.2)
	2013	Both sexes	210,064.2 (209,797.3– 210,257.6)	125,481.4 (125,204.4– 125,769.0)	8,269.0 (8,236.2– 8,296.1)	20,411.6 (20,386.9– 20,433.8)	8,520.4 (5,616.6– 12,564.8)	583.8 (387.9–850.7)
Saudi Arabia	1990	Both sexes	2,554,370.7 (2,550,534.5– 2,558,788.4)	2,645,914.4 (2,639,524.8– 2,653,644.5)	227,770.6 (221,941.6– 230,551.1)	31,760.6 (31,697.5– 31,818.2)	179,059.5 (119,610.3– 258,075.0)	949.3 (636.5– 1,367.9)
	2013	Both sexes	3,688,488.2 (3,682,139.2– 3,694,102.6)	3,329,647.6 (3,322,347.1– 3,335,751.5)	262,499.9 (252,834.9– 266,737.9)	25,478.4 (25,422.8– 25,524.1)	225,631.9 (150,688.6– 326,408.8)	762.3 (509.6– 1,100.4)

Syria	1990	Both sexes	1,936,073.5 (1,932,879.7–1,939,295.8)	2,202,104.0 (2,198,536.6–2,204,844.8)	190,827.4 (189,704.2–192,006.6)	32,254.4 (32,194.8–32,306.9)	146,522.9 (97,796.7–211,711.3)	968.1 (647.5–1,397.1)
	2013	Both sexes	2,995,762.7 (2,991,178.7–3,000,167.2)	3,032,303.4 (3,027,727.7–3,036,825.1)	241,584.1 (239,986.6–242,525.3)	27,585.6 (27,548.9–27,622.8)	200,884.1 (133,736.8–290,686.1)	827.6 (551.5–1,199.4)
Tunisia	1990	Both sexes	1,132,214.6 (1,129,883.1–1,134,557.0)	1,181,461.7 (1,179,072.6–1,183,428.5)	95,380.7 (94,563.2–96,072.2)	28,084.1 (28,024.1–28,134.9)	78,709.6 (52,405.8–113,894.2)	851.3 (566.8–1,232.2)
	2013	Both sexes	1,384,440.8 (1,381,363.4–1,387,051.4)	1,197,197.5 (1,193,863.7–1,200,001.0)	84,369.9 (83,839.7–84,809.2)	24,951.5 (24,899.6–24,997.3)	79,327.0 (52,639.0–115,457.7)	756.6 (502.8–1,098.9)
Turkey	1990	Both sexes	7,995,034.3 (7,978,788.7–8,012,062.3)	8,240,303.5 (8,221,706.4–8,251,609.2)	669,134.6 (666,432.2–671,593.2)	30,089.5 (30,030.3–30,143.5)	547,121.9 (366,404.5–793,083.8)	914.3 (612.4–1,325.2)
	2013	Both sexes	9,395,772.0 (9,379,645.4–9,410,221.3)	8,540,659.9 (8,527,691.7–8,552,710.0)	620,104.3 (617,792.6–622,108.7)	25,076.9 (25,039.7–25,111.5)	563,057.1 (374,568.9–818,363.6)	758.6 (504.9–1,101.5)
United Arab Emirates	1990	Both sexes	271,902.9 (271,571.2–272,215.0)	231,790.3 (231,390.0–232,110.7)	18,774.8 (18,634.5–18,878.7)	29,526.4 (29,484.6–29,565.6)	15,602.6 (10,365.5–22,615.7)	853.9 (569.9–1,234.3)
	2013	Both sexes	1,155,442.2 (1,153,636.6–1,157,023.9)	758,283.5 (756,449.3–759,869.5)	51,520.4 (50,992.9–51,839.1)	25,441.0 (25,405.0–25,472.8)	51,053.6 (33,906.6–74,936.4)	737.8 (493.6–1,069.1)
Yemen	1990	Both sexes	2,441,119.4 (2,437,185.1–2,449,189.3)	3,198,996.9 (3,187,981.4–3,203,281.5)	346,640.9 (345,142.0–349,184.8)	49,602.3 (49,484.1–49,701.7)	220,562.6 (147,553.9–316,604.4)	1,664.8 (1,118.6–2,384.4)
	2013	Both sexes	5,305,270.0 (5,298,665.9–5,312,045.5)	6,366,823.4 (6,357,722.0–6,375,407.8)	699,324.3 (697,604.3–701,071.7)	50,813.6 (50,745.8–50,879.1)	442,192.9 (296,559.6–636,199.2)	1,714.1 (1,153.1–2,457.2)

(continued on next page)

Table 2
(continued)

Location	Year	Sex	Prevalent Cases of Mild Anemia	Prevalent Cases of Moderate Anemia	Prevalent Cases of Severe Anemia	Age-Standardized Prevalence (per 100,000)	Total YLDs	Age-Standardized YLDs (per 100,000)
South Asia	1990	Both sexes	250,534,908.3 (250,163,550.5–251,141,169.4)	311,017,380.4 (310,342,024.7–311,427,364.2)	37,085,993.0 (36,949,764.8–37,188,025.7)	53,600.1 (53,501.4–53,686.7)	21,931,897.7 (14,751,353.7–31,334,203.7)	1,874.4 (1,266.1–2,669.2)
	2013	Both sexes	283,437,229.8 (282,888,457.1–283,888,687.3)	283,419,709.9 (282,907,232.9–283,916,295.1)	24,828,081.6 (24,676,215.7–24,941,750.4)	35,755.9 (35,693.7–35,815.2)	19,207,951.5 (12,843,105.6–27,610,019.2)	1,130.9 (756.8–1,623.5)
Afghanistan	1990	Both sexes	2,685,507.9 (2,682,916.6–2,691,890.9)	3,721,215.5 (3,714,592.1–3,724,661.6)	463,669.7 (462,654.7–464,669.0)	57,402.7 (57,325.5–57,489.7)	262,726.9 (176,943.8–374,725.1)	2,051.4 (1,392.0–2,912.2)
	2013	Both sexes	6,452,643.1 (6,446,490.8–6,459,348.9)	8,288,074.0 (8,280,277.6–8,295,777.4)	926,905.5 (924,586.4–928,889.6)	51,072.5 (51,016.7–51,130.4)	575,290.0 (386,497.3–825,710.8)	1,717.1 (1,161.7–2,458.2)
Bangladesh	1990	Both sexes	24,912,860.0 (24,864,012.6–24,994,350.3)	34,909,928.0 (34,810,075.6–34,959,451.6)	4,782,565.0 (4,771,293.0–4,792,239.2)	60,678.3 (60,546.0–60,801.4)	2,524,039.7 (1,705,123.1–3,585,871.9)	2,254.0 (1,528.6–3,192.6)
	2013	Both sexes	29,369,953.7 (29,302,141.7–29,429,322.8)	29,449,553.0 (29,385,453.0–29,521,574.4)	2,664,553.5 (2,651,849.8–2,677,622.8)	39,348.3 (39,259.7–39,435.1)	1,994,019.8 (1,333,001.9–2,874,179.6)	1,239.5 (828.4–1,780.0)
Bhutan	1990	Both sexes	81,930.4 (81,764.9–82,124.8)	92,036.7 (91,805.9–92,181.2)	7,882.3 (7,841.5–7,910.6)	31,466.3 (31,380.6–31,534.7)	6,170.7 (4,130.7–8,924.5)	977.7 (655.2–1,410.9)
	2013	Both sexes	76,122.9 (74,663.0–76,550.3)	74,245.1 (72,676.4–74,769.0)	5,349.9 (5,256.1–5,395.0)	20,515.8 (20,137.5–20,638.8)	4,954.5 (3,297.2–7,198.7)	641.5 (427.3–931.4)
India	1990	Both sexes	197,484,225.5 (197,146,527.7–198,074,869.6)	242,764,403.3 (242,131,839.6–243,121,155.8)	28,911,010.3 (28,772,479.2–29,006,790.4)	54,189.2 (54,074.1–54,291.3)	17,124,429.9 (11,520,720.0–24,457,190.0)	1,896.5 (1,281.3–2,699.5)
	2013	Both sexes	215,706,218.1 (215,258,354.4–216,083,184.4)	212,827,806.1 (212,383,414.6–213,251,012.7)	18,525,569.5 (18,380,241.1–18,629,697.7)	35,744.5 (35,675.1–35,810.1)	14,440,372.7 (9,649,495.6–20,755,590.4)	1,131.8 (757.8–1,624.4)

	Year	Sex					
Nepal	1990	Both sexes	3,787,669.8 (3,782,162.1–3,794,798.0)	4,379,260.7 (4,372,301.7–4,384,760.6)	445,527.7 (444,623.6–446,309.0)	46,536.2 (46,458.2–46,612.8)	300,037.7 (201,110.3–431,413.7)	1,505.3 (1,010.1–2,160.4)
	2013	Both sexes	4,671,257.9 (4,661,886.7–4,678,192.6)	4,737,408.4 (4,731,125.4–4,743,304.9)	402,863.3 (401,713.6–403,910.8)	34,427.0 (34,371.1–34,473.2)	317,721.5 (212,078.0–459,017.5)	1,047.3 (696.8–1,514.0)
Pakistan	1990	Both sexes	21,582,714.6 (21,545,993.0–21,625,072.7)	25,150,536.0 (25,107,712.3–25,184,918.0)	2,475,338.0 (2,465,719.8–2,482,502.3)	42,706.6 (42,617.0–42,787.4)	1,714,492.7 (1,148,332.5–2,469,076.3)	1,373.7 (923.7–1,970.7)
	2013	Both sexes	27,161,034.1 (27,100,434.9–27,212,548.3)	28,042,623.4 (27,990,980.2–28,092,652.2)	2,302,840.0 (2,288,204.2–2,312,991.1)	30,694.5 (30,635.0–30,747.3)	1,875,593.0 (1,254,378.5–2,709,539.8)	954.7 (637.9–1,378.2)
Sub-Saharan Africa	1990	Both sexes	89,040,525.3 (88,898,291.6–89,127,145.2)	119,012,467.9 (118,880,037.9–119,160,979.7)	13,955,485.4 (13,868,657.0–13,999,980.3)	42,080.4 (42,028.8–42,125.7)	8,419,729.3 (5,669,257.1–11,988,879.5)	1,456.6 (985.6–2,071.6)
	2013	Both sexes	147,744,661.0 (147,576,626.5–147,888,295.0)	189,575,856.0 (189,363,382.9–189,748,395.3)	20,358,244.3 (20,238,275.9–20,423,531.8)	36,315.8 (36,273.9–36,348.6)	13,256,982.9 (8,892,691.9–18,928,345.7)	1,237.2 (833.0–1,766.4)
Central Sub-Saharan Africa	1990	Both sexes	10,779,192.9 (10,748,089.1–10,795,138.7)	13,888,708.2 (13,854,073.6–13,929,190.4)	1,550,849.9 (1,528,488.7–1,561,417.6)	48,541.2 (48,442.7–48,633.9)	967,429.9 (651,239.2–1,374,680.6)	1,663.8 (1,126.3–2,358.4)
	2013	Both sexes	19,907,991.8 (19,876,522.1–19,937,898.8)	24,830,871.1 (24,789,360.7–24,865,088.1)	2,641,819.4 (2,609,248.5–2,655,512.9)	45,090.3 (45,011.9–45,161.4)	1,724,435.3 (1,156,488.3–2,455,378.2)	1,515.8 (1,021.3–2,154.0)
Angola	1990	Both sexes	2,342,842.3 (2,330,370.9–2,350,222.5)	3,136,500.3 (3,125,469.1–3,153,169.1)	383,108.9 (378,166.7–385,877.1)	56,977.6 (56,810.6–57,156.4)	222,187.8 (149,751.4–314,625.3)	2,070.7 (1,406.0–2,920.4)
	2013	Both sexes	3,892,961.6 (3,884,611.4–3,899,775.2)	4,517,405.5 (4,507,280.1–4,526,289.7)	428,233.7 (421,791.6–431,556.6)	39,931.4 (39,846.2–40,005.8)	309,071.9 (206,772.2–443,365.7)	1,297.2 (871.4–1,853.5)

(continued on next page)

Table 2
(continued)

Location	Year	Sex	Prevalent Cases of Mild Anemia	Prevalent Cases of Moderate Anemia	Prevalent Cases of Severe Anemia	Age-Standardized Prevalence (per 100,000)	Total YLDs	Age-Standardized YLDs (per 100,000)
Central African Republic	1990	Both sexes	602,129.5 (599,623.1–602,954.1)	746,986.3 (745,892.0–748,156.6)	79,602.2 (78,708.8–80,085.1)	47,828.7 (47,737.0–47,899.0)	51,488.8 (34,739.2–73,557.0)	1,613.6 (1,093.5–2,295.7)
	2013	Both sexes	964,924.3 (962,792.0–966,363.7)	1,170,965.7 (1,168,819.6–1,172,851.8)	125,967.4 (124,353.2–126,661.1)	48,220.8 (48,117.1–48,299.4)	81,348.0 (54,644.9–116,268.0)	1,643.5 (1,107.2–2,344.1)
Congo	1990	Both sexes	434,352.1 (429,520.5–436,165.4)	583,434.5 (581,747.3–585,088.9)	63,962.7 (62,816.8–64,473.1)	43,227.3 (43,035.1–43,375.2)	40,555.8 (27,249.7–57,824.4)	1,519.4 (1,026.0–2,156.1)
	2013	Both sexes	778,435.7 (776,519.5–779,675.7)	1,019,582.2 (1,017,691.0–1,021,393.5)	106,941.3 (105,235.4–107,579.4)	40,410.1 (40,310.6–40,489.5)	70,627.1 (47,394.5–101,200.8)	1,414.1 (953.1–2,018.7)
Democratic Republic of the Congo	1990	Both sexes	7,125,940.7 (7,100,248.9–7,139,926.8)	9,081,767.3 (9,050,252.6–9,113,766.8)	985,947.5 (964,302.2–994,667.2)	46,634.4 (46,501.5–46,756.1)	629,394.3 (424,371.7–894,357.5)	1,564.2 (1,060.7–2,223.6)
	2013	Both sexes	13,827,331.3 (13,800,898.2–13,853,705.5)	17,594,030.9 (17,558,512.9–17,621,538.5)	1,925,321.5 (1,893,735.0–1,936,557.8)	46,951.5 (46,845.9–47,041.2)	1,226,619.5 (822,875.6–1,744,437.9)	1,586.1 (1,069.1–2,249.3)
Equatorial Guinea	1990	Both sexes	80,293.9 (80,108.1–80,474.7)	90,148.9 (89,936.1–90,461.7)	9,226.0 (9,003.9–9,329.1)	46,668.5 (46,546.3–46,770.7)	6,232.9 (4,192.1–8,928.4)	1,561.3 (1,054.3–2,229.0)
	2013	Both sexes	117,921.3 (117,552.7–118,178.9)	127,580.3 (127,058.9–127,955.5)	10,848.1 (10,472.6–10,963.2)	31,657.9 (31,529.4–31,741.5)	8,680.5 (5,808.1–12,486.6)	1,016.9 (685.4–1,457.3)
Gabon	1990	Both sexes	193,634.4 (193,006.3–194,147.4)	249,870.8 (249,197.6–251,014.3)	29,002.8 (28,586.5–29,198.5)	49,452.0 (49,311.4–49,575.6)	17,570.2 (11,851.7–24,963.5)	1,770.3 (1,199.5–2,506.2)
	2013	Both sexes	326,417.6 (325,752.4–326,961.9)	401,306.6 (400,585.1–402,031.0)	44,507.4 (43,866.0–44,772.3)	45,865.5 (45,776.1–45,945.4)	28,088.4 (18,964.6–40,075.5)	1,608.6 (1,090.3–2,285.2)

Eastern Sub-Saharan Africa	1990	Both sexes	30,641,447.7 (30,599,833.0–30,672,075.5)	40,295,837.0 (40,250,545.0–40,336,252.6)	4,208,706.4 (4,198,468.6–4,217,785.6)	35,621.3 (35,577.4–35,656.9)	2,780,443.3 (1,865,408.1–3,982,776.3)	1,192.5 (803.1–1,704.3)
	2013	Both sexes	50,127,608.4 (50,073,010.2–50,175,435.3)	63,556,993.7 (63,473,733.3–63,620,243.8)	5,942,691.4 (5,925,087.3–5,956,032.9)	29,062.2 (29,029.3–29,091.8)	4,325,199.2 (2,892,741.8–6,215,770.5)	965.6 (647.6–1,384.0)
Burundi	1990	Both sexes	737,078.4 (734,102.4–739,550.3)	893,310.5 (888,373.2–897,910.7)	76,514.2 (75,227.1–77,394.4)	23,747.8 (23,672.9–23,816.6)	60,007.1 (40,218.4–86,320.1)	748.5 (500.2–1,079.2)
	2013	Both sexes	1,415,707.6 (1,412,429.4–1,418,869.1)	1,656,301.9 (1,649,015.4–1,661,843.0)	145,249.0 (143,426.6–146,359.2)	25,922.9 (25,845.1–25,992.2)	112,388.8 (75,251.7–162,719.5)	819.3 (548.7–1,181.8)
Comoros	1990	Both sexes	58,955.2 (58,852.4–59,046.1)	74,905.4 (74,790.9–75,006.3)	6,818.0 (6,795.0–6,832.6)	29,519.8 (29,452.9–29,568.9)	5,074.3 (3,388.8–7,299.5)	971.6 (649.7–1,393.4)
	2013	Both sexes	102,740.4 (102,502.1–102,930.8)	126,315.6 (126,098.3–126,523.5)	11,198.5 (11,153.4–11,234.1)	28,483.9 (28,406.0–28,546.7)	8,552.7 (5,735.6–12,316.5)	939.8 (632.3–1,354.5)
Djibouti	1990	Both sexes	80,983.2 (80,723.8–81,210.7)	101,588.0 (101,285.1–101,798.0)	9,236.8 (9,198.9–9,276.1)	29,230.0 (29,131.6–29,303.2)	6,897.9 (4,615.8–9,930.3)	966.6 (647.9–1,389.5)
	2013	Both sexes	131,012.3 (130,628.2–131,319.7)	146,941.1 (146,561.4–147,272.5)	13,111.7 (13,003.5–13,164.6)	31,638.6 (31,542.7–31,719.8)	10,015.1 (6,699.2–14,419.3)	1,045.2 (701.4–1,500.8)
Eritrea	1990	Both sexes	648,904.4 (647,679.6–651,459.0)	892,740.1 (888,707.0–894,101.5)	107,379.5 (107,082.4–107,708.8)	47,750.5 (47,624.1–47,861.8)	63,221.8 (42,510.1–90,233.1)	1,663.5 (1,121.8–2,366.1)
	2013	Both sexes	1,103,450.8 (1,100,205.5–1,105,767.9)	1,403,285.8 (1,400,646.2–1,405,806.0)	145,689.4 (145,162.8–146,060.8)	39,056.6 (38,952.3–39,143.1)	96,979.0 (64,966.6–139,135.0)	1,312.2 (881.7–1,877.6)
Ethiopia	1990	Both sexes	8,198,618.9 (8,182,482.5–8,212,110.1)	9,965,301.5 (9,947,862.5–9,981,394.7)	1,029,148.8 (1,025,599.8–1,032,237.8)	35,394.7 (35,310.2–35,465.7)	689,633.3 (462,352.0–988,736.7)	1,123.9 (755.9–1,611.1)
	2013	Both sexes	12,346,102.2 (12,319,878.2–12,367,307.2)	14,391,354.8 (14,344,120.7–14,429,957.3)	1,279,836.6 (1,274,224.1–1,284,206.9)	25,605.5 (25,528.1–25,664.4)	976,830.8 (654,020.4–1,400,903.4)	808.7 (543.6–1,160.8)

(continued on next page)

Table 2
(continued)

Location	Year	Sex	Prevalent Cases of Mild Anemia	Prevalent Cases of Moderate Anemia	Prevalent Cases of Severe Anemia	Age-Standardized Prevalence (per 100,000)	Total YLDs	Age-Standardized YLDs (per 100,000)
Kenya	1990	Both sexes	3,467,083.1 (3,456,023.7–3,473,930.6)	4,551,630.0 (4,541,109.6–4,560,967.9)	426,300.5 (419,237.3–429,835.0)	30,662.6 (30,571.2–30,735.2)	309,491.0 (207,176.7–444,967.8)	1,013.1 (679.2–1,449.6)
	2013	Both sexes	5,581,201.1 (5,568,201.7–5,590,173.9)	6,823,546.2 (6,810,630.9–6,836,250.8)	573,007.7 (562,925.3–577,774.2)	24,981.1 (24,915.6–25,031.3)	460,039.2 (308,057.4–664,567.5)	825.3 (554.1–1,189.2)
Madagascar	1990	Both sexes	2,186,819.1 (2,182,248.0–2,189,586.1)	2,683,162.4 (2,680,072.6–2,687,594.5)	281,939.5 (279,682.8–283,219.6)	41,149.7 (41,083.6–41,217.9)	185,248.2 (124,457.8–264,359.3)	1,328.4 (891.6–1,895.7)
	2013	Both sexes	4,251,781.9 (4,245,259.4–4,256,822.1)	5,060,968.1 (5,053,547.8–5,067,823.9)	519,550.4 (513,168.1–521,986.6)	40,312.2 (40,245.1–40,373.0)	349,664.5 (234,329.2–501,652.0)	1,308.3 (878.0–1,873.0)
Malawi	1990	Both sexes	1,556,360.6 (1,550,686.7–1,559,201.9)	2,227,167.6 (2,223,510.7–2,232,448.0)	258,813.4 (257,416.6–259,710.6)	37,321.2 (37,227.3–37,395.7)	156,410.4 (105,476.1–223,019.6)	1,295.4 (875.6–1,845.7)
	2013	Both sexes	2,244,952.4 (2,240,839.6–2,248,006.3)	3,128,396.2 (3,122,845.9–3,132,304.1)	317,316.0 (315,086.8–318,451.1)	29,291.9 (29,220.1–29,344.8)	215,443.2 (144,151.3–309,387.3)	1,011.9 (680.1–1,449.3)
Mauritius	1990	Both sexes	143,263.5 (143,014.8–143,499.7)	131,920.0 (131,664.2–132,172.4)	9,933.1 (9,868.7–9,990.8)	26,658.8 (26,614.4–26,701.5)	8,771.9 (5,805.2–12,699.3)	798.4 (529.0–1,154.2)
	2013	Both sexes	122,218.8 (121,843.3–122,559.3)	99,815.6 (99,321.2–100,149.2)	6,570.7 (6,528.5–6,604.4)	19,742.2 (19,675.1–19,788.1)	6,638.1 (4,402.4–9,661.7)	595.4 (394.9–867.1)
Mozambique	1990	Both sexes	2,367,555.4 (2,358,588.2–2,375,267.2)	3,724,324.8 (3,715,669.2–3,734,240.0)	470,784.9 (469,539.7–473,236.9)	45,506.1 (45,373.2–45,635.0)	264,514.9 (178,485.9–375,084.8)	1,722.6 (1,166.8–2,425.6)
	2013	Both sexes	3,919,071.8 (3,908,204.8–3,926,410.8)	5,824,599.1 (5,812,806.2–5,834,376.9)	621,206.4 (618,518.6–623,285.0)	36,678.9 (36,568.3–36,772.8)	400,296.6 (268,618.6–571,773.4)	1,335.3 (901.4–1,893.5)

	Year	Both sexes					
Rwanda	1990	Both sexes	1,064,778.7 (1,061,405.6–1,066,954.0)	1,314,625.0 (1,308,033.5–1,317,672.1)	115,865.3 (115,113.6–116,344.5)	29,217.6 (29,127.8–29,286.0)	88,470.2 (58,923.8–127,375.5)	926.8 (620.6–1,335.4)
	2013	Both sexes	1,438,223.3 (1,433,746.8–1,442,369.6)	1,660,638.2 (1,653,502.0–1,666,580.6)	132,879.6 (132,106.5–133,478.4)	23,357.7 (23,255.6–23,449.1)	111,070.3 (74,343.8–160,274.2)	744.2 (497.5–1,071.5)
Seychelles	1990	Both sexes	6,862.1 (6,843.3–6,870.7)	6,964.4 (6,949.9–6,978.0)	510.1 (506.1–512.6)	18,856.5 (18,823.1–18,885.8)	459.3 (305.2–668.2)	568.2 (376.7–824.6)
	2013	Both sexes	8,115.5 (8,097.5–8,128.3)	6,845.0 (6,826.6–6,860.2)	441.5 (437.9–443.6)	17,199.4 (17,163.8–17,226.0)	451.7 (298.9–656.4)	520.8 (345.3–755.1)
Somalia	1990	Both sexes	962,311.4 (959,531.8–964,477.9)	1,210,677.6 (1,207,742.3–1,213,519.6)	111,585.4 (111,090.0–111,894.0)	30,597.9 (30,514.7–30,674.7)	81,969.4 (54,806.4–117,948.1)	1,007.3 (675.7–1,447.3)
	2013	Both sexes	1,710,982.7 (1,707,722.1–1,713,463.3)	2,232,257.9 (2,228,865.0–2,235,219.7)	221,413.1 (220,593.5–222,013.5)	34,867.0 (34,788.8–34,931.3)	152,806.1 (102,342.8–219,159.6)	1,155.5 (777.7–1,658.9)
Tanzania	1990	Both sexes	4,281,259.6 (4,263,001.7–4,294,759.1)	6,016,615.3 (5,993,548.9–6,026,862.1)	654,587.3 (651,290.4–657,146.4)	39,293.6 (39,156.6–39,404.5)	417,066.0 (280,073.6–596,295.4)	1,380.6 (928.6–1,967.8)
	2013	Both sexes	7,064,406.9 (7,046,944.4–7,077,001.6)	9,550,905.6 (9,532,977.9–9,567,514.5)	911,190.6 (902,162.4–917,890.2)	31,336.7 (31,251.3–31,403.0)	650,796.7 (434,744.3–934,844.1)	1,085.2 (727.2–1,557.2)
Uganda	1990	Both sexes	2,674,331.3 (2,669,159.7–2,678,320.8)	3,684,123.2 (3,678,990.6–3,688,268.7)	371,886.5 (370,124.9–373,116.6)	32,727.5 (32,658.3–32,785.4)	250,643.5 (168,287.2–359,650.6)	1,096.0 (737.4–1,569.6)
	2013	Both sexes	5,022,958.1 (5,013,564.5–5,030,552.9)	6,857,498.7 (6,846,117.2–6,867,443.8)	631,526.6 (628,596.5–633,492.1)	27,171.7 (27,107.1–27,225.5)	463,214.4 (309,845.2–665,649.6)	915.3 (614.0–1,312.5)
Zambia	1990	Both sexes	1,139,897.6 (1,137,134.3–1,141,902.6)	1,448,661.0 (1,445,696.4–1,452,522.6)	132,446.1 (129,112.5–133,598.4)	29,838.7 (29,758.0–29,910.1)	98,189.4 (65,792.1–140,945.0)	979.3 (654.5–1,402.7)
	2013	Both sexes	1,945,537.2 (1,942,028.3–1,948,030.1)	2,468,995.7 (2,464,604.3–2,473,831.5)	215,028.7 (209,607.9–216,686.0)	26,310.8 (26,252.3–26,360.0)	166,319.6 (111,335.1–239,990.5)	864.4 (579.0–1,241.6)

(continued on next page)

Table 2 (continued)

Location	Year	Sex	Prevalent Cases of Mild Anemia	Prevalent Cases of Moderate Anemia	Prevalent Cases of Severe Anemia	Age-Standardized Prevalence (per 100,000)	Total YLDs	Age-Standardized YLDs (per 100,000)
Southern Sub-Saharan Africa	1990	Both sexes	8,084,397.0 (8,066,636.0–8,102,575.2)	8,875,349.5 (8,854,795.7–8,889,088.0)	750,356.3 (748,530.1–753,620.2)	31,269.4 (31,186.3–31,336.0)	599,500.4 (401,004.9–861,736.8)	993.4 (668.4–1,425.3)
	2013	Both sexes	10,130,466.8 (10,106,789.3–10,150,394.3)	10,262,962.4 (10,242,246.8–10,283,157.9)	805,802.3 (803,807.1–807,437.8)	27,402.2 (27,343.2–27,455.8)	692,461.9 (462,410.4–997,765.0)	870.5 (582.3–1,252.0)
Botswana	1990	Both sexes	226,680.0 (226,133.0–227,277.1)	264,809.9 (264,083.0–265,269.7)	23,562.4 (23,436.6–23,659.6)	34,274.1 (34,168.6–34,356.1)	17,947.9 (11,981.3–25,841.3)	1,096.3 (733.2–1,577.8)
	2013	Both sexes	265,222.1 (263,649.2–266,112.6)	272,007.6 (269,245.3–273,039.5)	21,256.1 (21,013.0–21,365.4)	26,493.2 (26,307.7–26,585.4)	18,279.5 (12,241.9–26,485.6)	833.8 (559.7–1,203.5)
Lesotho	1990	Both sexes	246,146.8 (245,534.1–246,815.4)	277,692.5 (277,062.3–278,191.8)	23,562.1 (23,414.1–23,752.2)	31,398.4 (31,301.6–31,488.3)	18,753.4 (12,540.9–26,961.9)	991.8 (665.4–1,427.9)
	2013	Both sexes	276,709.2 (275,821.4–277,484.4)	288,115.6 (287,324.3–288,755.9)	22,823.3 (22,721.2–22,884.3)	26,936.8 (26,844.8–27,015.7)	19,389.7 (12,967.5–27,972.0)	845.5 (568.3–1,217.8)
Namibia	1990	Both sexes	256,951.8 (256,329.2–257,635.4)	300,285.7 (299,166.6–300,817.8)	28,105.9 (28,002.1–28,199.7)	39,023.2 (38,893.2–39,118.9)	20,468.3 (13,705.2–29,565.2)	1,261.5 (846.1–1,812.8)
	2013	Both sexes	357,032.6 (353,857.8–358,035.8)	379,892.3 (375,656.5–381,076.0)	31,801.3 (31,424.0–31,950.1)	31,991.5 (31,655.3–32,090.7)	25,655.5 (17,125.2–37,047.1)	1,016.6 (679.2–1,462.3)
South Africa	1990	Both sexes	5,682,151.8 (5,666,420.2–5,700,148.2)	6,014,717.2 (5,994,831.5–6,026,629.4)	499,867.2 (498,138.1–503,100.9)	31,222.3 (31,114.2–31,303.4)	406,723.4 (272,468.7–583,883.1)	989.9 (667.3–1,418.4)
	2013	Both sexes	6,950,168.0 (6,927,801.6–6,967,705.0)	6,747,397.7 (6,728,770.0–6,765,971.4)	509,446.5 (507,553.7–510,758.4)	26,420.0 (26,341.8–26,483.9)	455,557.2 (304,850.4–655,797.0)	835.5 (559.8–1,200.8)

	Year	Sex						
Swaziland	1990	Both sexes	131,652.9 (131,314.9–131,940.1)	153,862.5 (153,553.5–154,169.9)	12,939.1 (12,902.0–12,964.4)	30,979.3 (30,898.8–31,052.3)	10,306.8 (6,883.8–14,808.1)	979.1 (655.8–1,409.2)
	2013	Both sexes	172,408.5 (171,864.2–172,841.0)	182,248.3 (181,796.2–182,652.3)	14,496.4 (14,444.8–14,535.0)	27,657.8 (27,569.6–27,733.8)	12,182.5 (8,125.6–17,516.4)	865.3 (578.0–1,245.0)
Zimbabwe	1990	Both sexes	1,540,813.8 (1,536,731.4–1,543,768.4)	1,863,981.7 (1,860,777.2–1,868,069.7)	162,319.6 (161,767.0–162,754.3)	29,871.3 (29,801.9–29,934.6)	125,300.5 (83,902.3–181,120.9)	952.5 (640.1–1,372.0)
	2013	Both sexes	2,108,926.4 (2,104,150.5–2,113,051.0)	2,393,300.9 (2,388,101.4–2,397,725.8)	205,978.6 (205,073.2–206,572.9)	30,841.6 (30,759.5–30,911.6)	161,397.4 (107,643.0–232,420.1)	987.2 (663.0–1,421.1)
Western Sub-Saharan Africa	1990	Both sexes	39,535,487.7 (39,389,009.1–39,593,152.3)	55,952,573.2 (55,863,047.5–56,072,319.8)	7,445,572.8 (7,365,220.9–7,482,216.4)	49,491.5 (49,397.5–49,569.0)	4,072,355.8 (2,757,081.4–5,773,071.0)	1,779.5 (1,207.3–2,522.1)
	2013	Both sexes	67,578,594.1 (67,485,042.9–67,677,190.7)	90,925,028.7 (90,799,139.9–91,037,378.8)	10,967,931.2 (10,845,694.1–11,021,409.1)	43,211.4 (43,146.1–43,267.4)	6,514,886.5 (4,380,919.3–9,270,522.5)	1,511.0 (1,019.0–2,150.8)
Benin	1990	Both sexes	1,003,490.2 (993,515.2–1,007,637.1)	1,561,972.5 (1,557,504.2–1,578,579.4)	226,352.8 (223,482.1–227,876.8)	54,270.9 (54,017.9–54,596.1)	115,730.5 (78,450.2–163,619.0)	2,094.2 (1,429.3–2,943.5)
	2013	Both sexes	1,923,823.4 (1,918,283.1–1,930,627.6)	2,762,803.6 (2,755,703.0–2,768,702.5)	350,170.3 (344,445.7–353,411.0)	46,838.1 (46,709.2–46,956.1)	199,898.1 (134,885.0–283,911.4)	1,738.6 (1,178.7–2,467.8)
Burkina Faso	1990	Both sexes	1,637,745.3 (1,627,374.9–1,643,764.2)	2,562,085.4 (2,556,425.4–2,570,467.7)	446,957.9 (443,054.6–448,984.7)	48,944.7 (48,777.7–49,087.2)	200,357.3 (135,649.2–282,741.8)	1,833.3 (1,244.6–2,585.8)
	2013	Both sexes	3,008,005.4 (3,000,999.8–3,017,184.9)	4,536,585.5 (4,528,457.9–4,543,539.9)	739,159.3 (729,942.6–743,467.3)	44,719.5 (44,610.3–44,817.7)	350,766.7 (236,259.5–498,594.9)	1,660.3 (1,119.0–2,351.7)

(continued on next page)

Table 2
(continued)

Location	Year	Sex	Prevalent Cases of Mild Anemia	Prevalent Cases of Moderate Anemia	Prevalent Cases of Severe Anemia	Age-Standardized Prevalence (per 100,000)	Total YLDs	Age-Standardized YLDs (per 100,000)
Cameroon	1990	Both sexes	2,148,273.8 (2,139,482.9–2,152,234.0)	2,832,292.1 (2,826,925.0–2,846,002.5)	302,233.9 (295,472.7–304,842.5)	39,656.5 (39,540.5–39,757.9)	196,372.4 (131,913.0–280,108.9)	1,332.2 (898.9–1,900.7)
	2013	Both sexes	3,712,200.4 (3,704,311.5–3,719,067.3)	4,693,449.8 (4,683,856.6–4,702,688.3)	474,327.9 (463,502.7–477,604.8)	36,418.0 (36,334.8–36,489.1)	324,303.9 (217,101.6–465,589.3)	1,215.8 (817.3–1,741.4)
Cape Verde	1990	Both sexes	59,152.3 (59,022.8–59,279.2)	79,926.2 (79,776.8–80,052.8)	8,495.5 (8,456.1–8,518.4)	37,428.9 (37,329.0–37,520.3)	5,565.9 (3,737.4–7,986.2)	1,284.5 (862.9–1,842.8)
	2013	Both sexes	71,244.9 (70,990.6–71,448.2)	78,758.2 (78,554.7–78,968.3)	7,093.2 (7,045.0–7,124.2)	30,906.5 (30,805.2–30,997.9)	5,410.4 (3,614.7–7,785.8)	1,042.3 (697.7–1,500.7)
Chad	1990	Both sexes	1,265,612.5 (1,262,472.0–1,268,407.9)	1,859,515.9 (1,856,059.8–1,862,193.3)	267,547.0 (266,307.4–268,394.9)	54,259.1 (54,135.7–54,354.0)	136,824.9 (92,602.1–193,969.7)	1,951.9 (1,321.5–2,768.5)
	2013	Both sexes	2,512,955.0 (2,508,217.7–2,516,475.3)	3,484,962.4 (3,481,038.2–3,489,370.3)	438,277.5 (434,239.1–439,831.5)	46,145.7 (46,039.3–46,237.5)	249,585.1 (168,060.2–355,683.8)	1,570.4 (1,056.4–2,243.6)
Cote d'Ivoire	1990	Both sexes	2,326,223.1 (2,314,114.3–2,330,805.6)	3,089,841.4 (3,084,532.2–3,095,408.1)	360,151.6 (356,606.6–362,849.7)	44,929.1 (44,783.3–45,020.6)	217,367.8 (146,239.6–309,431.0)	1,537.6 (1,038.8–2,179.2)
	2013	Both sexes	3,946,362.7 (3,939,229.0–3,951,968.7)	5,120,818.9 (5,113,261.2–5,128,039.2)	592,974.7 (587,927.9–596,871.4)	45,349.6 (45,264.6–45,430.6)	361,129.8 (242,419.8–515,732.1)	1,567.1 (1,055.8–2,229.9)
The Gambia	1990	Both sexes	173,164.9 (172,737.8–173,627.9)	237,681.9 (236,867.7–238,278.9)	28,752.1 (28,352.7–28,961.4)	44,513.9 (44,400.4–44,615.7)	16,928.6 (11,391.9–24,109.7)	1,536.2 (1,039.0–2,187.2)
	2013	Both sexes	316,269.5 (315,452.2–316,883.5)	426,480.9 (425,411.9–427,312.1)	46,576.7 (46,060.5–46,891.0)	38,172.8 (38,077.6–38,258.0)	29,840.8 (20,055.2–42,679.6)	1,300.9 (877.9–1,864.1)

Ghana	1990	Both sexes	2,883,315.6 (2,867,917.5–2,893,662.0)	3,978,759.5 (3,969,198.4–3,991,512.9)	491,610.1 (483,817.0–495,789.7)	48,437.4 (48,262.9–48,576.9)	284,955.9 (191,474.9–405,574.3)	1,737.1 (1,171.7–2,472.1)
	2013	Both sexes	4,464,871.4 (4,452,603.4–4,476,976.3)	5,654,548.8 (5,641,057.9–5,666,481.6)	597,041.8 (584,224.0–603,175.5)	39,618.8 (39,522.0–39,700.4)	395,770.0 (265,595.7–566,790.0)	1,379.9 (928.1–1,971.9)
Guinea	1990	Both sexes	1,115,115.5 (1,112,367.2–1,117,904.8)	1,580,914.7 (1,577,304.0–1,583,896.2)	207,966.6 (205,289.1–209,420.6)	44,856.3 (44,732.7–44,963.8)	114,436.3 (77,255.8–162,798.0)	1,596.4 (1,079.3–2,267.3)
	2013	Both sexes	2,063,617.6 (2,059,363.9–2,067,079.6)	2,831,922.3 (2,826,432.4–2,837,177.6)	347,962.9 (343,036.8–350,632.2)	41,519.4 (41,420.3–41,614.2)	203,216.8 (136,864.2–289,421.8)	1,467.7 (988.9–2,089.4)
Guinea-Bissau	1990	Both sexes	199,645.9 (199,094.1–200,283.5)	273,175.8 (272,168.9–273,868.8)	33,644.5 (33,399.0–33,828.8)	46,612.2 (46,476.1–46,738.5)	19,446.2 (13,088.2–27,674.8)	1,623.9 (1,098.5–2,308.9)
	2013	Both sexes	311,750.3 (311,092.2–312,319.8)	404,191.0 (403,464.5–405,180.7)	45,642.8 (45,370.0–45,886.0)	42,078.4 (41,994.0–42,166.3)	28,361.4 (19,058.1–40,608.6)	1,438.7 (970.1–2,054.5)
Liberia	1990	Both sexes	388,961.5 (387,750.0–389,524.7)	526,492.7 (525,779.2–527,539.4)	59,911.1 (59,458.6–60,228.9)	41,599.3 (41,520.7–41,668.6)	36,709.7 (24,723.3–52,370.3)	1,407.3 (950.8–2,008.9)
	2013	Both sexes	800,614.5 (799,083.6–801,639.2)	1,057,385.1 (1,055,914.1–1,058,648.2)	122,350.9 (121,568.2–123,005.0)	43,622.3 (43,541.4–43,690.5)	74,175.8 (49,927.8–105,715.3)	1,488.4 (1,007.9–2,120.8)
Mali	1990	Both sexes	1,635,217.2 (1,631,233.6–1,640,824.9)	2,622,107.1 (2,615,680.3–2,626,592.6)	412,636.5 (408,389.9–414,736.7)	56,888.1 (56,739.9–57,035.8)	197,571.1 (133,778.7–280,118.9)	2,215.4 (1,510.1–3,114.3)
	2013	Both sexes	2,970,336.5 (2,964,442.2–2,975,651.6)	4,600,133.5 (4,593,957.6–4,607,090.9)	661,505.4 (650,996.6–665,559.6)	51,061.1 (50,959.9–51,148.6)	340,960.6 (230,706.1–484,593.7)	1,925.0 (1,305.6–2,724.5)

(continued on next page)

Table 2
(continued)

Location	Year	Sex	Prevalent Cases of Mild Anemia	Prevalent Cases of Moderate Anemia	Prevalent Cases of Severe Anemia	Age-Standardized Prevalence (per 100,000)	Total YLDs	Age-Standardized YLDs (per 100,000)
Mauritania	1990	Both sexes	437,090.3 (435,130.5–438,363.9)	651,878.1 (650,323.7–652,918.5)	94,978.7 (94,590.5–95,252.3)	56,869.3 (56,663.7–57,000.1)	48,038.4 (32,448.0–68,215.1)	2,122.9 (1,440.5–2,995.4)
	2013	Both sexes	714,899.7 (713,012.4–716,203.3)	913,333.2 (911,724.6–914,980.1)	102,762.8 (101,958.9–103,174.1)	41,880.0 (41,788.4–41,964.5)	64,189.6 (43,103.2–91,722.5)	1,435.8 (966.5–2,045.5)
Niger	1990	Both sexes	1,431,966.4 (1,428,838.0–1,434,936.4)	2,053,472.9 (2,049,899.1–2,057,578.5)	264,513.2 (260,753.5–266,736.2)	43,828.7 (43,704.5–43,933.0)	148,586.3 (100,130.5–211,361.3)	1,534.2 (1,039.5–2,184.8)
	2013	Both sexes	3,191,938.3 (3,183,289.2–3,197,712.1)	4,604,933.5 (4,598,174.5–4,612,175.8)	580,984.2 (571,605.3–585,505.0)	41,884.0 (41,786.2–41,967.6)	332,567.0 (223,813.7–472,318.9)	1,454.7 (977.2–2,081.1)
Nigeria	1990	Both sexes	19,757,353.4 (19,607,643.9–19,807,358.1)	27,729,298.0 (27,654,491.7–27,835,401.3)	3,690,950.7 (3,615,311.5–3,722,728.9)	51,349.4 (51,168.3–51,494.8)	2,022,908.9 (1,370,837.6–2,865,970.5)	1,849.3 (1,258.4–2,622.8)
	2013	Both sexes	32,301,981.3 (32,227,249.7–32,383,902.1)	42,691,792.8 (42,590,056.8–42,780,663.6)	5,008,707.9 (4,899,840.3–5,053,751.8)	43,082.9 (42,972.7–43,172.4)	3,049,358.5 (2,056,420.3–4,342,622.1)	1,489.3 (1,005.8–2,117.2)
Sao Tome and Principe	1990	Both sexes	20,786.3 (20,734.5–20,832.7)	27,396.8 (27,337.2–27,477.1)	2,882.0 (2,816.4–2,908.2)	40,216.6 (40,109.9–40,320.8)	1,907.5 (1,279.1–2,734.7)	1,345.7 (902.9–1,924.1)
	2013	Both sexes	33,304.7 (33,227.5–33,377.3)	40,415.0 (40,335.3–40,499.0)	4,009.4 (3,926.6–4,048.9)	37,374.1 (37,278.6–37,461.2)	2,804.5 (1,882.3–4,032.1)	1,243.1 (833.9–1,781.5)
Senegal	1990	Both sexes	1,492,171.5 (1,488,896.4–1,496,807.7)	2,208,881.9 (2,203,280.2–2,212,695.0)	298,790.8 (295,886.2–300,296.4)	51,051.5 (50,932.5–51,159.7)	160,976.9 (108,874.0–228,501.7)	1,873.9 (1,268.7–2,659.8)
	2013	Both sexes	2,723,141.6 (2,716,770.1–2,727,746.0)	3,844,384.4 (3,837,846.0–3,850,356.5)	485,811.1 (481,085.2–489,249.4)	47,777.9 (47,672.2–47,865.7)	276,651.1 (186,001.5–393,735.7)	1,732.3 (1,169.1–2,458.5)

	Year	Sex						
Sierra Leone	1990	Both sexes	833,945.4 (831,340.8–835,856.9)	1,074,627.0 (1,071,854.0–1,078,084.2)	125,437.6 (122,359.6–126,685.4)	48,202.3 (48,085.5–48,309.3)	75,988.9 (51,305.2–108,313.4)	1,636.6 (1,110.1–2,324.4)
	2013	Both sexes	1,222,298.5 (1,219,209.9–1,225,080.9)	1,492,621.6 (1,488,829.4–1,496,050.5)	164,960.2 (161,588.4–166,503.9)	45,042.5 (44,913.3–45,144.2)	105,445.4 (70,870.0–150,542.5)	1,515.6 (1,020.4–2,166.4)
Togo	1990	Both sexes	725,096.6 (723,464.8–726,707.1)	1,000,864.6 (998,552.4–1,003,849.5)	121,590.7 (119,054.0–122,829.7)	45,732.7 (45,602.2–45,845.1)	71,582.5 (48,074.3–101,786.4)	1,599.7 (1,080.9–2,279.4)
	2013	Both sexes	1,288,163.2 (1,284,874.9–1,290,950.5)	1,684,683.5 (1,681,289.3–1,688,516.1)	197,525.0 (193,373.5–199,260.5)	44,162.2 (44,058.3–44,252.1)	120,392.9 (81,063.7–171,463.9)	1,543.1 (1,040.3–2,193.7)
South Sudan	1990	Both sexes	1,051,345.7 (1,048,922.0–1,053,905.4)	1,348,468.0 (1,345,389.1–1,350,605.0)	142,898.8 (142,234.3–143,419.9)	39,987.9 (39,876.7–40,085.2)	93,017.5 (62,447.8–133,264.6)	1,327.8 (894.9–1,898.2)
	2013	Both sexes	1,688,384.0 (1,683,930.7–1,691,763.1)	2,078,583.1 (2,074,293.3–2,082,367.0)	193,762.9 (192,719.3–194,601.1)	31,743.1 (31,651.0–31,814.5)	140,990.0 (94,126.6–202,333.0)	1,039.0 (695.9–1,487.3)
Sudan	1990	Both sexes	4,349,963.0 (4,340,284.9–4,358,298.3)	5,481,366.5 (5,471,676.1–5,488,896.5)	612,388.4 (610,225.0–615,256.7)	51,743.8 (51,658.7–51,818.9)	379,228.5 (254,667.2–542,773.6)	1,742.4 (1,177.5–2,482.8)
	2013	Both sexes	7,442,698.0 (7,433,356.2–7,451,250.1)	8,340,593.8 (8,329,840.9–8,350,242.2)	802,225.3 (798,474.7–804,918.7)	42,614.1 (42,559.0–42,667.0)	564,922.2 (377,719.4–813,976.9)	1,347.1 (901.2–1,935.0)

Total years of life lived with disability (YLDs) due to anemia as well as prevalent cases of mild, moderate, and severe anemia are presented for all locations, including each country, region, super-region, developed versus developing countries in aggregate, and at the global level. Age-standardized prevalence and YLD rates were calculated by aggregation of cause-specific anemia estimates for each country, age group, sex, and year and then standardizing to the global standard population table used in the Global Burden of Disease (GBD) study 2013.

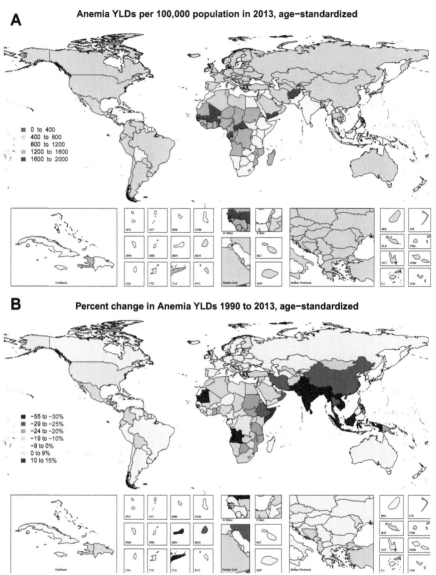

Fig. 3. Disability owing to anemia expressed as the years lived with disability (YLD) rate per 100,000 population in 2013 (*A*) and change in age-standardized YLD rate from 1990 to 2013 (*B*). The top map show the age-standardized rate of anemia disability measured in YLDs in 2013. The burden, when compared with prevalence figures, is even more concentrated in many of the countries with the highest prevalence rates of anemia, indicating a greater severity of disease. Changes from 1990 to 2013 are shown in the bottom panel. South Asia, Southeast Asia and East Asia decreased anemia burden the most. Age-standardization helps control for differences in population structure between countries and over time. ATG, Antigua and Barbuda; BRB, Barbados; COM, Comoros; DMA, Dominica; FJI, Fiji; FSM, Federated States of Micronesia; GRD, Grenada; KIR, Kiribati; MDV, Maldives; MHL, Marshall Islands; MLT, Malta; MUS, Mauritius; SGP, Singapore; SLB, Solomon Islands; SYC, Seychelles; TLS, Timor-Leste; TON, Tonga; TTO, Trinidad and Tobago; VCT, Saint Vincent and the Grenadines; WSM, Samoa.

the burden was already lower in those locations. Alarmingly, relatively little progress was seen in much of western and central sub-Saharan Africa, the same regions with the highest burden. Eight countries—Somalia, Burundi, Djibouti, Liberia, Zimbabwe, Yemen, the Czech Republic, and Moldova—all had age-standardized anemia prevalence in 2013 that were at least 1% higher than in 1990. In all of these countries, YLD rates increased even more than prevalence rates, indicating a relative worsening of anemia burden.

Age and gender patterns in global anemia prevalence and burden were striking (**Fig. 4**). Young children, especially under the age of 10, had the highest prevalence of anemia and levels were generally similar between males and females. Throughout much of adulthood, anemia prevalence was consistently higher in females than males. Improvement between 1990 and 2013 was also greater for males than females in these age groups, a phenomenon largely driven at the global level by greater improvements among males in South Asia. Convergence between the sexes occurred in older ages, roughly equilibrating around age 60 in 1990 and 75 in 2013. Age patterns were largely consistent between countries, although the magnitude varies substantially by country.

Iron deficiency was the single greatest cause of anemia globally in both 1990 and 2013. There were 552,500,091 (551,188,078–554,084,424) males and 655,860,048 (653,862,224–657,703,392) females with IDA in 2013, collectively accounting for approximately 62.6% of the global total of anemia cases (**Table 3**). This was down from 66.2% in 1990. IDA was also the greatest cause of anemia-related disability, although the proportion of total YLDs was only 59.5% in 2013, reflecting both the somewhat lower severity of IDA compared with other etiologies.

Despite the overall dominance of IDA, leading causes vary substantially by age, sex, and geography (**Fig. 5A**). For example, in females the most common causes of anemia globally in 2013 were IDA (59.2% of total), hemoglobinopathies (11.6%), gastrointestinal losses (5.3%), gynecologic conditions (5.1%), and malaria (4.9%). For males, the order was IDA (67.1%), hemoglobinopathies (9.9%), gastrointestinal losses (4.6%), and other neglected tropical diseases (4.3%). In Western and Central sub-Saharan Africa—where the highest rates of anemia occur—IDA, malaria and hemoglobinopathies collectively explain nearly 80% of anemia cases. Schistosomiasis is also an important

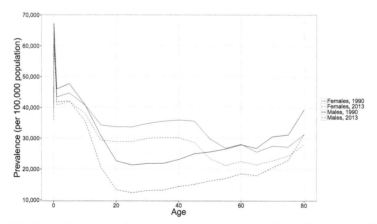

Fig. 4. Global prevalence rate of anemia by age and sex for 1990 and 2013. Global prevalence rates of anemia by age are shown in red (females) and blue (males) for both 1990 (*solid lines*) and 2013 (*dotted lines*). Anemia prevalence is highest in preschool children and consistently higher among females. Global improvements were greater for males than females from 1990 to 2013.

Table 3
Global cause pattern of anemia prevalence and disability in 1990 and 2013

Cause	Prevalent Cases in Thousands (% of Total)		Total YLDs in Thousands (% of Total)	
	1990	2013	1990	2013
Iron-deficiency anemia	1,211,369.9 (66.23)	1,208,360.1 (62.57)	40,035.5 (64.55)	36,612.3 (59.51)
Thalassemia trait	751,80.1 (4.11)	104,232.6 (5.40)	2799.6 (4.51)	3769.6 (6.13)
Malaria	57,969.1 (3.17)	80,602.4 (4.17)	2196.1 (3.54)	2935.0 (4.77)
Gastritis and duodenitis	56,836.8 (3.11)	63,222.9 (3.27)	2092.4 (3.37)	2204.4 (3.58)
Other neglected tropical diseases	62,877.1 (3.44)	59,728.3 (3.09)	2244.9 (3.62)	2048.5 (3.33)
Other hemoglobinopathies and hemolytic anemias	57,242.2 (3.13)	55,804.0 (2.89)	1566.7 (2.53)	1325.5 (2.15)
Other infectious diseases	52,324.3 (2.86)	49,771.4 (2.58)	1742.5 (2.81)	1542.4 (2.51)
Endocrine, metabolic, blood, and immune disorders	49,928.4 (2.73)	49,327.8 (2.55)	1549.8 (2.50)	1376.0 (2.24)
Sickle cell trait	29,862.3 (1.63)	43,353.9 (2.24)	1003.5 (1.62)	1396.6 (2.27)
Uterine fibroids (females only)	28,043.2 (1.53)	36,833.7 (1.91)	1106.6 (1.78)	1304.9 (2.12)
Hookworm disease	32,039.8 (1.75)	34,579.6 (1.79)	1021.8 (1.65)	1004.0 (1.63)
Peptic ulcer disease	34,671.6 (1.90)	32,726.7 (1.69)	980.6 (1.58)	974.6 (1.58)
Chronic kidney disease owing to other causes	16,459.1 (0.90)	26,007.2 (1.35)	857.2 (1.38)	1330.6 (2.16)

Schistosomiasis	14,488.1 (0.79)	20,635.1 (1.07)	485.3 (0.78)	671.0 (1.09)
Other gynecologic diseases (females only)	15,576.9 (0.85)	17,383.2 (0.90)	462.8 (0.75)	448.6 (0.73)
Chronic kidney disease owing to hypertension	10,850.3 (0.59)	14,142.6 (0.73)	587.6 (0.95)	733.8 (1.19)
Chronic kidney disease owing to glomerulonephritis	11,180.9 (0.61)	14,059.9 (0.73)	613.3 (0.99)	745.9 (1.21)
Chronic kidney disease owing to diabetes mellitus	6569.6 (0.36)	12,116.3 (0.63)	348.0 (0.56)	606.6 (0.99)
Sickle cell disorders	1801.5 (0.10)	3185.0 (0.16)	182.5 (0.29)	321.4 (0.52)
G6PD deficiency trait (females only)	1253.7 (0.07)	1983.8 (0.10)	39.5 (0.06)	48.8 (0.08)
Maternal hemorrhage (females only)	1388.0 (0.08)	1858.5 (0.10)	39.4 (0.06)	45.1 (0.07)
G6PD deficiency	519.3 (0.03)	743.5 (0.04)	24.9 (0.04)	33.8 (0.05)
Thalassemias	509.8 (0.03)	544.2 (0.03)	43.2 (0.07)	46.2 (0.08)
Total prevalence	1,828,942.2 (100.00)	1,931,202.6 (100.00)	—	—
Total YLDs	—	—	62,023.8 (100.00)	61,525.6 (100.00)

Total prevalent case numbers and total years of life lived with disability (YLDs) are listed for each of the 23 unique etiologies of anemia in both 1990 and 2013 at the global level. They are in descending order by total prevalent cases in 2013.

Abbreviations: G6PD, glucose-6-phosphate deficiency; GBD, Global Burden of Disease.

Modified from GBD 2013 Disease and Injury Incidence and Prevalence Collaborators. Global, regional, and national incidence, prevalence, and YLDs for 301 acute and chronic diseases and injuries for 188 countries, 1990-2013: a systematic analysis for the Global Burden of Disease Study 2013. Lancet 2015;386(9995):743–800.

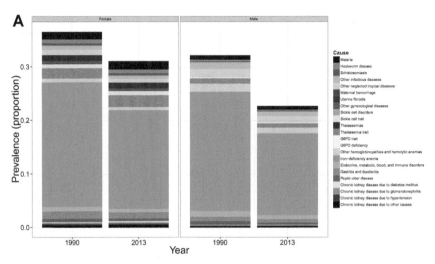

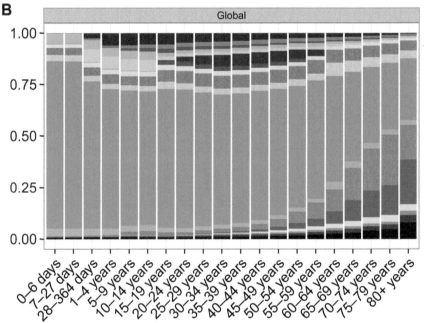

Fig. 5. Underlying cause of prevalent anemia cases by sex for 1990 and 2013 at the global level by gender (*A*) and by age (*B*). All ages anemia prevalence dropped for both sexes, though the decrease was greater in males. In both sexes, iron-deficiency anemia (IDA) was the dominant cause globally, although there were significant contributions from several other causes. In females, these include hemoglobinopathies, gynecologic conditions, gastrointestinal losses, and malaria. In males, these include hemoglobinopathies, nonmalaria infectious diseases, gastrointestinal losses, and malaria. G6PD, glucose-6-phosphate deficiency.

cause of anemia Eastern sub-Saharan Africa (8.1% of all anemia cases). Hookworm is a significant etiology in many countries of Oceania (12.2%), Tropical Latin America (8.6%), Southern sub-Saharan Africa (5.7%), and Southeast Asia (3.8%). CKD emerges as an important contributor to overall anemia burden in high-income countries (7.4%), Tropical Latin America (17.4%), Central Europe (9.8%), and Eastern Europe (10.8%).

In those under 5 years of age, anemia is mostly due to IDA (**Fig. 5**B). Hemoglobinopathies, "other" infectious diseases, and malaria (in endemic areas) are also important causes in preschool children. Throughout adulthood, the pathophysiology becomes progressively more complex. The contribution of hemoglobinopathies is relatively stable throughout adulthood in most locations. This is because heterozygous hemoglobin disorders such as sickle cell trait and thalassemia trait are the dominant component of anemia due to hemoglobinopathies in all but high-prevalence, high-mortality settings, such as Central and Western sub-Saharan Africa. Malaria peaks in importance at ages 5 to 9, but remains an important contributor to anemia burden throughout adulthood in endemic locations. Gynecologic causes, led by uterine fibroids, are important causes of anemia in females from menarche to menopause in all settings. CKD and gastrointestinal disorders increase sharply in older ages to become the most important causes of anemia in many locations.

SUMMARY AND DISCUSSION

Anemia affected 1.93 billion people in 2013 collectively causing 61.5 (41.0–88.7) million YLDs. To put this number in perspective, it is helpful to compare against other findings from the GBD 2013 study.[27] Anemia was responsible for roughly 8% of all nonfatal health loss for all diseases in 2013. Although it is lower than the total disability caused by low back and neck pain (106 million YLDs), it is roughly equivalent to the amount of health loss caused by depressive disorders (61.6 million YLDs) and is greater than disability owing to asthma, diabetes, and cardiovascular disease combined (61.3 million YLDs). It is also much more amenable to prevention and treatment than many of those conditions. The full health impact of anemia is likely even greater as these results do not include quantification of heart failure or early mortality owing to anemia, the increased risk of cognitive deficiencies associated with chronic anemia, or the disability associated with many other sequelae of severe hemoglobinopathies such as repeated infections, often painful vasoocclusive crises, and strokes.

Levels and trends in anemia burden have been uneven with respect to age, sex, and geography. Globally, anemia burden has actually improved substantially since 1990 when 33.3% of the global population was affected and anemia caused 12.4% of all disability for all conditions combined. Children have consistently had the highest burden of anemia, but have also improved less in both absolute and relative terms than adults. This change suggests at the very least that our efforts to prevent childhood anemia have been inconsistent. Improvement between 1990 and 2013 was greater for males than females, a phenomenon largely driven at the global level by larger improvements among males in South Asia. The biggest regional gains were seen in South Asia, East Asia, Southeast Asia, and Eastern sub-Saharan Africa, where many countries have national nutrition programs in place. In all of these regions, YLD rates have dropped faster than prevalence rates, which indicates that there has been an additional shift away from severe cases of anemia.

Our analysis shows that IDA is the dominant cause of anemia in most countries and populations. If we include those conditions such as hookworm, schistosomiasis, and gastrointestinal and gynecologic conditions that also manifest as IDA, its importance grows even more apparent. Despite its continued dominance, a decrease in IDA has been the primary driver of reduced global anemia burden since 1990. The improvements have been partially offset, however, by increases in anemia owing to CKDs, hemoglobinopathies, malaria, and schistosomiasis. Most of the increase in these latter conditions is related to population aging (for CKD) and population growth in endemic areas.

IDA in high-risk, high-prevalence populations is likely due to inadequate vitamin intake or absorption.[32,33] Addressing IDA by only increasing micronutrient supplementation would not be a panacea for ending anemia, however, because IDA is a final common pathway of a heterogeneous group of conditions that also includes acute or chronic hemorrhagic events and disorders of iron metabolism that may happen as a result of chronic illness or malabsorption. The WHO guidelines take some of this into account,[34] with recommendation that nutrition be optimized, including targeted supplementation of iron, vitamin A, and other micronutrients in high-risk or high prevalence groups, such as pregnant women and young children. The guidelines further recommend administration of antihelminthic medications in endemic regions.

These recommendations still fall short of addressing the complexity of anemia epidemiology, however, and others have called for a more comprehensive approach to reducing anemia burden.[35] For starters, many infectious and inflammatory conditions limit iron absorption,[36] so the underlying drivers of inflammation must be addressed. Some components of local diet such as teas (tannins) and whole grain cereals (phytates) may also retard iron uptake, so their role in the local diet should be considered and/or mitigated with agents that promote uptake such as ascorbic acid.[37] Second, our analysis shows that hemoglobinopathies are among the top 5 causes of anemia in many populations. Some subtypes may present with laboratory findings similar to IDA, but the anemia owing to these conditions will not be reversed by typical interventions for IDA.[38] Furthermore, routine supplementation for those with homozygous disease may be inappropriate because iron overload is a common complication of treatment. Third, malaria remains a crucial public health challenge in many countries of the world, especially in sub-Saharan Africa. Trials of iron supplementation in malaria endemic areas is controversial because, in isolation, it has been associated with increased parasitemia rate,[39] malarial fever,[40] and all-cause mortality.[41] These findings support at the very least implementation of malaria control and chemoprophylaxis programs to combat anemia.[42] Fourth, folic acid administration should also be considered, especially in pregnant women, to reduce anemia and prevent neural tube defects in their offspring.[43] Finally, as we see from the age pattern of anemia etiology, the prevention and treatment of CKD and gastrointestinal conditions in older persons should be a part of anemia control programs for those populations, a strategy that should focus on appropriate use of nonsteroidal antiinflammatory drugs.[44,45]

Unfortunately, 8 countries—Somalia, Burundi, Djibouti, Liberia, Zimbabwe, Yemen, the Czech Republic, and Moldova—all had age-standardized anemia prevalence in 2013 that were at least 1% higher than in 1990. In all of these countries, the YLD rates increased even more than prevalence rates, indicating a relative intensification of anemia burden. Except for the latter two, all are low-income countries that already had a high burden of anemia in 1990, have experienced internal conflict over the interim, and have received comparatively little development assistance for health for maternal, child, and newborn health, and noncommunicable diseases.[46] Addressing the anemia burden in the countries that are falling behind, and accelerating progress in other countries, will require a comprehensive program of prevention, screening and treatment that is, based on the context-specific epidemiology of anemia.

Bangladesh is an example of a country that has been especially successful in decreasing anemia burden. Anemia burden remains high there, but absolute prevalence rates changed by -43.3% and all ages YLD rates by -59.8% between 1990 and 2013. The government of Bangladesh, in cooperation with the World Bank, started a national nutrition program in 1995 called the Bangladesh Integrated Nutrition Programme, which implemented a comprehensive set of nutrition and non–nutrition-based interventions. The objective of Bangladesh Integrated Nutrition Programme was to reduce underweight and stunting rates by 50% in 5 years, an objective that was not met, but the collective benefit of its interventions are consistent with those that would be expected to be effectively reduce anemia burden. Efforts at the individual level aimed to educate mothers, encourage routine and preventive health care use, and provide multiple micronutrient supplements.[47] Parallel efforts aimed to address the high burden of diarrheal disease, expand access to safe water and sanitation, and improve food security. Such a comprehensive approach, guided by the local epidemiology, should serve as a model to all countries seeking to reduce anemia burden.

Despite broad agreements in total case numbers and YLDs between this and our previous analysis, increased data availability and enhanced analytical methods have allowed us to improve our country-specific anemia estimates. Interestingly, additional data from Turkey had little effect on the predicted magnitude of anemia burden. In contrast, our current estimates of anemia prevalence in the United Kingdom are nearly 25% higher than in GBD 2010 and they are now lower for 2013—especially in males—in both India and China. Incorporation of an increasing number of subnational locations into future GBD analyses and will be instrumental to honing our understanding of population-specific anemia epidemiology. Identification of new, existing data sources and continued inclusion of anemia surveillance in population health surveys will be crucial to this collaborative endeavor.

This analysis has several limitations. First, our calculation of anemia burden is based on hemoglobin thresholds were initially adopted by the WHO in 1968.[48] Although the thresholds have been updated over time, they remain based on statistical analysis of hemoglobin concentrations in "normal" individuals rather than a full evaluation of the risk of health loss associated with decreased hemoglobin. They also do not reflect ethnicity-specific diagnostic criteria that have been suggested by some researchers.[49] Furthermore, there is no internationally accepted threshold for diagnosing anemia in infants under 6 months of age despite the commonly held belief that very young children are the most susceptible to the detrimental effects of anemia. Second, as mentioned, we have not quantified the risk of poor growth, poor development, intellectual disability, or early mortality owing to anemia. IDA was analyzed as a specific cause of death and risk factor in GBD 2013,[23] but for other etiologies of anemia it was not possible in this framework to disentangle the role of anemia in early mortality. The full health loss associated with anemia is thus even higher than we have presented here. Third, in keeping with GBD cause of death analytical principles, we assigned each case of anemia to a single underlying cause. Owing to paucity of data, etiology-specific hemoglobin shifts were used globally, which limited our ability to account for differing treatment availability for chronic conditions. Although this approach generates estimates that accurately reflect the complexity of anemia epidemiology at the population level, it limits the direct clinical applicability of our findings. Many cases of anemia—especially severe anemia—are multifactorial, a phenomenon that must be considered when treating individuals. Fifth, also in keeping with GBD 2013 analytical principles, our estimates of uncertainty at the regional and global level assumed the uncertainty for each cause was uncorrelated. This assumption is well-supported for burden of disease analysis overall, but could be challenged in the case of underlying anemia etiologies. Correlation of uncertainty would have led to wider uncertainty intervals at the regional and global level. Sixth, while we expended great effort to collect and analyze all available data to estimate anemia burden by etiology, not all specific causes could be disaggregated. Most were assigned to our "other" categories, owing either to the rarity of the condition or insufficient data for separate modeling. Examples include anemia owing to acute and chronic hemorrhage, human immunodeficiency virus infection, AIDS, malignancy, and chemotherapy where population-specific information could be helpful in guiding anemia control efforts. Finally, owing to exclusion of those with known chronic disease from many data sources, we suspect that anemia of chronic inflammation was underestimated in some locations, especially in older ages.

Targeted anemia surveillance and intervention should be a priority in high-risk, high-burden populations such as young children and females of reproductive age. Given that anemia burden is nontrivial in all populations, there should also be a renewed focus on anemia surveillance and treatment, even in high-income settings and older persons. Treatment of individuals should be guided by consideration of population-specific anemia epidemiology, recognizing that each person may have multifactorial underpinnings to their anemia. Population-level interventions should similarly be based on context-specific factors, but also be comprehensive in nature, to maximize the likelihood of sustained success in reducing the global burden of anemia.

ACKNOWLEDGMENTS

This research has been conducted as part of the Global Burden of Diseases, Injuries, and RiskFactors Study (GBD), led by the Institute for Health Metrics and Evaluation. The GBD was partially funded by the Bill & Melinda Gates Foundation (OPP1070441); the funders had no role in the study design, data analysis, data interpretation, or writing of the report. We would like to thank all of the GBD 2013 researchers, staff, and collaborators who worked to make the project a success: Tom D. Fleming[1] (tomflem@uw.edu), Abraham Flaxman[1] (abie@uw.edu), David E. Phillips[1] (davidp6@uw.edu), Caitlyn Steiner[1] (csteiner@uw.edu), Ryan M. Barber[1] (rmbarber@uw.edu), Sarah Wulf Hanson[1] (swulf@uw.edu), Maziar Moradi-Lakeh[1] (mmoradi@uw.edu), Lucas E. Coffeng[1] (l. coffeng@erasmusmc.nl), Juanita Haagsma[1] (jhaagsma@uw.edu), Hmwe H. Kyu[1] (hmwekyu@uw.edu), Nicholas Graetz[1] (ngraetz@uw.edu), Stephen S. Lim[1] (stevelim@uw.edu), Theo Vos[1] (tvos@uw.edu), Mohsen Naghavi[1] (nagham@uw.edu), Christopher Murray[1] (cjlm@uw.edu), Naohiro Yonemoto[2] (4-1-1,Ogawahigashi, Kodaira, Tokyo, 1878551, Japan; nyonemoto@gmail.com), Jasvinder Singh[3] (2000 6th Ave S FI 3, Birmingham, AL 35233; jasvinder.md@gmail.com), Jost B. Jonas[4] (Kutzerufer 1, Mannheim 68167, Germany; Jost.Jonas@medma.uni-heidelberg.de), Itamar S. Santos[5] (Cidade Universitária, Av. Lineu Prestes 2565, 05508-000 Sao Paulo Brazil; itamarss@usp.br), Isabela M. Bensenor[5] (Hospital Universitario, Av Lineu Prestes, 2565, 05508-000 Sao Paulo Brazil; isabensenor@gmail.com), Paulo A. Lotufo[5] (University of São Paulo, Faculdade de Medicina / Hospital Universitario, Av Lineu Prestes, 2565, 05508-

---

[1] Institute for Health Metrics and Evaluation, University of Washington, Seattle, WA, USA.

[2] National Center of Neurology and Psychiatry, Kodira, Tokyo, Japan.

[3] University of Alabama at Birmingham, Birmingham, AL, USA.

[4] Department of Ophthalmology, Medical Faculty Mannheim, Ruprecht-Karls-University Heidelberg, Germany.

[5] University of Sao Paulo, Sao Paulo, Brazil.

000 Sao Paulo Brazil; palotufo@usp.br), Saleem M. Rana[6] (54-A, HBFC Faisal Town, Lahore 54700, Pakistan; smrmep@gmail.com), Bradford D. Gessner[7] (21 bd. Pasteur, 75015 Paris, France; bgessner@aamp.org), Kingsley N. Ukwaja[8] (Dept of Internal Medicine, Federal Teaching Hospital, A 343 Abakaliki, Nigeria; ukwajakingsley@yahoo.co. uk), Frédéric B. Piel[9] (Department of Zoology, University of Oxford, The Tinbergen Building, South Parks Road, Oxford OX1 3PS, UK; fred.piel@zoo.ox.ac.uk), Yousef S. Khader[10] (Ar Ramtha, Irbid 22110, Jordan; yskhader@just.edu.jo), Neeraj Bhala[11,12] (Queen Elizabeth Medical Centre, Birmingham B15 2TH, UK; neeraj.bhala@uhb.nhs. uk), Carl A. T. Antonio[13] (Lara Hall, 625 Pedro Gil Street, Ermita, Manila, 1000 Metro Manila, Philippines; ctantoniomd@gmail.com), Amanda G. Thrift[14] (Epidemiology & Prevention Unit Stroke and Ageing Research Ctr, Department of Medicine, Southern Clinical School, Monash University, Level 1/43–51, Kanooka Grove, Clayton, Victoria 3168, Australia; amanda.thrift@monash.edu), Walter Mendoza[15] (Av. Guardia Civil 1231, Lima 27, Peru; mendoza@unfpa.org), Maysaa El Sayed Zaki[16] (Rabaea street, Mansoura 35514, Egypt; may_s65@hotmail.com), Anders Larsson[17] (Akademiska sjukhuset, Ing.40, 5 tr, 751 85 Uppsala, Sweden; anders.larsson@akademiska.se), Devina Nand[18] (Dinem House, 88 Amy Street, Toorak, Suva, Fiji; dr.devinanand@gmail.com), Reza Malekzadeh[19,20] (Digestive Disease Research Inst, Shariati Hospital, Jamshidiyeh, Tehran, 14117-13135, Iran; malek@tums.ac.ir), Yongmei Li[21] (Anolinx LLC, 428 E. Winchester St, Salt Lake City, UT 84107; yongmeil@hotmail.com), Kim Yun Jin[22] (Southern University College, 81300 Skudai, Johor, Malaysia; yjkim@sc.edu.my), Teresa Shamah Levy[23] (Av. Universidad # 655, Col. Sta. Ma. Ahuacatitlán, Cuernavaca, Morelos, Mexico 62100 C.P; tshamah@insp.mx).

[6] Department of Public Health, University of the Punjab, Lahore, Pakistan, Punjab, India.

[7] Agence de Medecine Preventive, Paris, France.

[8] Department of Internal Medicine Federal Teaching Hospital, Abakaliki, Ebonyi State, Nigeria.

[9] University of Oxford, Oxford, UK.

[10] Jordan University of Science and Technology, Irbid, Jordin.

[11] Queen Elizabeth Hospital Birmingham, Birmingham, UK.

[12] University of Otago Medical School, Wellington, New Zealand.

[13] Department of Health Policy and Administration, College of Public Health, University of the Philippines Manila.

[14] Department of Medicine, Monash University, Melbourne, VIC, Australia.

[15] United Nations Population Fund (UNFPA), Lima, Peru.

[16] Mansoura Faculty of Medicine, Mansoura, Egypt.

[17] Uppsala University, Uppsala, Sweden.

[18] Ministry of Health Fiji, Suva, Republic of Fiji.

[19] Digestive Diseases Research Center, Shariati Hospital, Tehran University of Medical Sciences, Tehran, Iran.

[20] Shiraz University of Medical Sciences, Shiraz, Iran.

[21] Anolinx, LLC, Salt Lake City, UT, USA.

[22] Southern University College, Johor, Malaysia.

[23] National Public Health Institute, Cuernavaca, Morelos, Mexico.

REFERENCES

1. Haas JD, Fairchild MW. Summary and conclusions of the International Conference on Iron Deficiency and Behavioral Development, October 10-12, 1988. Am J Clin Nutr 1989;50(3):703–5.
2. Edgerton VR, Ohira Y, Hettiarachchi J, et al. Elevation of hemoglobin and work tolerance in iron-deficient subjects. J Nutr Sci Vitaminol (Tokyo) 1981;27(2):77–86.
3. Sachdev H, Gera T, Nestel P. Effect of iron supplementation on mental and motor development in children: systematic review of randomised controlled trials. Public Health Nutr 2005;8(2):117–32.
4. McCann JC, Ames BN. An overview of evidence for a causal relation between iron deficiency during development and deficits in cognitive or behavioral function. Am J Clin Nutr 2007;85(4):931–45.
5. Beard JL, Connor JR. Iron status and neural functioning. Annu Rev Nutr 2003;23:41–58.
6. Mireku MO, Davidson LL, Koura GK, et al. Prenatal hemoglobin levels and early cognitive and motor functions of one-year-old children. Pediatrics 2015;136(1):e76–83.
7. Schorr T, Hediger M. Anemia and iron-deficiency anemia: compilation of data on pregnancy outcome. Am J Clin Nutr 1994;59(Suppl):492S–501S.
8. Rasmussen KM. Is there a causal relationship between iron deficiency or iron-deficiency anemia and weight at birth, length of gestation and perinatal mortality? J Nutr 2001;131(2):590S–603S.
9. Brabin BJ, Hakimi M, Pelletier D. An analysis of anemia and pregnancy-related maternal mortality. J Nutr 2001;131(2):604S–15S.
10. Brabin BJ, Premji Z, Verhoeff F. An analysis of anemia and child mortality. J Nutr 2001;131(2):636S–48S.
11. Hershko C, Karsai A, Eylon L, et al. The effect of chronic iron deficiency on some biochemical functions of the human hemopoietic tissue. Blood 1970;36(3):321–9.
12. Anand IS. Anemia and chronic heart failure implications and treatment options. J Am Coll Cardiol 2008;52(7):501–11.
13. Thein M, Ershler WB, Artz AS, et al. Diminished quality of life and physical function in community-dwelling elderly with anemia. Medicine (Baltimore) 2009;88(2):107–14.
14. Sabbatini P. The relationship between anemia and quality of life in cancer patients. Oncologist 2000;5(Suppl 2):19–23.
15. Musallam KM, Tamim HM, Richards T, et al. Preoperative anaemia and postoperative outcomes in non-cardiac surgery: a retrospective cohort study. Lancet 2011;378(9800):1396–407.
16. Martinsson A, Andersson C, Andell P, et al. Anemia in the general population: prevalence, clinical correlates and prognostic impact. Eur J Epidemiol 2014;29(7):489–98.
17. Brotanek JM, Halterman JS, Auinger P, et al. Iron deficiency, prolonged bottle-feeding, and racial/ethnic disparities in young children. Arch Pediatr Adolesc Med 2005;159(11):1038–42.
18. Cusick SE, Mei Z, Freedman DS, et al. Unexplained decline in the prevalence of anemia among US children and women between 1988–1994 and 1999–2002. Am J Clin Nutr 2008;88(6):1611–7.
19. Stevens GA, Finucane MM, De-Regil LM, et al. Global, regional, and national trends in haemoglobin concentration and prevalence of total and severe anaemia

in children and pregnant and non-pregnant women for 1995–2011: a systematic analysis of population-representative data. Lancet Glob Health 2013;1(1): e16–25.

20. Beghé C, Wilson A, Ershler WB. Prevalence and outcomes of anemia in geriatrics: a systematic review of the literature. Am J Med 2004;116(Suppl 7A):3S–10S.

21. Guralnik JM, Eisenstaedt RS, Ferrucci L, et al. Prevalence of anemia in persons 65 years and older in the United States: evidence for a high rate of unexplained anemia. Blood 2004;104(8):2263–8.

22. Kassebaum NJ, Jasrasaria R, Naghavi M, et al. A systematic analysis of global anemia burden from 1990 to 2010. Blood 2014;123(5):615–24.

23. Global Burden of Disease Study 2013 Mortality and Cause of Death Collaborators. Global, regional, and national age–sex specific all-cause and cause-specific mortality for 240 causes of death, 1990–2013: a systematic analysis for the Global Burden of Disease Study 2013. Lancet 2015;385(9963):117–71.

24. Mathers C, Rastogi T. WHO | global burden of iron deficiency anaemia in the year 2000. Geneva, Switzerland: World Health Organization; 2002.

25. WHO. Haemoglobin concentrations for the diagnosis of anaemia and assessment of severity. Geneva (Switzerland): World Health Organization; 2011.

26. Salomon JA, Vos T, Hogan DR, et al. Common values in assessing health outcomes from disease and injury: disability weights measurement study for the Global Burden of Disease Study 2010. Lancet 2012;380(9859):2129–43.

27. Global Burden of Disease Study 2013 Collaborators. Global, regional, and national incidence, prevalence, and years lived with disability for 301 acute and chronic diseases and injuries in 188 countries, 1990–2013: a systematic analysis for the Global Burden of Disease Study 2013. Lancet 2015;386(9995):743–800.

28. Centers for Disease Control and Prevention (CDC). Iron deficiency–United States, 1999-2000. MMWR Morb Mortal Wkly Rep 2002;51(40):897–9.

29. Looker AC, Dallman PR, Carroll MD, et al. Prevalence of iron deficiency in the united states. JAMA 1997;277(12):973–6.

30. Pearson K. Mathematical contributions to the theory of evolution. VII. On the correlation of characters not quantitatively measurable. Philos Trans R Soc Math Phys Eng Sci 1900;195(262–273):1–405. Available at: https://archive.org/details/philtrans05420907.

31. Bishop YM, Fienberg SE, Holland PW. Discrete multivariate analysis theory and practice. New York: Springer New York; 2007.

32. Ahmed F. Anaemia in Bangladesh: a review of prevalence and aetiology. Public Health Nutr 2000;3(4):385–93.

33. Pasricha S-R, Black J, Muthayya S, et al. Determinants of anemia among young children in rural India. Pediatrics 2010;126(1):e140–9.

34. WHO. Essential nutrition actions: improving maternal, newborn, infant and young child health and nutrition. WHO. Available at: www.who.int/nutrition/publications/infantfeeding/essential_nutrition_actions/en/. Accessed September 18, 2013.

35. Pasricha S-R, Drakesmith H, Black J, et al. Control of iron deficiency anemia in low- and middle-income countries. Blood 2013;121(14):2607–17.

36. Ganz T, Nemeth E. Hepcidin and disorders of iron metabolism. Annu Rev Med 2011;62(1):347–60.

37. Siegenberg D, Baynes RD, Bothwell TH, et al. Ascorbic acid prevents the dose-dependent inhibitory effects of polyphenols and phytates on nonheme-iron absorption. Am J Clin Nutr 1991;53(2):537–41.

38. Sungthong R, Mo-suwan L, Chongsuvivatwong V, et al. Once weekly is superior to daily iron supplementation on height gain but not on hematological improvement among schoolchildren in Thailand. J Nutr 2002;132(3):418–22.
39. Oppenheimer SJ, Gibson FD, Macfarlane SB, et al. Iron supplementation increases prevalence and effects of malaria: Report on clinical studies in Papua New Guinea. Trans R Soc Trop Med Hyg 1986;80(4):603–12.
40. Smith AW, Hendrickse RG, Harrison C, et al. The effects on malaria of treatment of iron-deficiency anaemia with oral iron in Gambian children. Ann Trop Paediatr 1989;9(1):17–23.
41. Sazawal S, Black RE, Ramsan M, et al. Effects of routine prophylactic supplementation with iron and folic acid on admission to hospital and mortality in preschool children in a high malaria transmission setting: community-based, randomised, placebo-controlled trial. Lancet 2006;367(9505):133–43.
42. Menendez C, Kahigwa E, Hirt R, et al. Randomised placebo-controlled trial of iron supplementation and malaria chemoprophylaxis for prevention of severe anaemia and malaria in Tanzanian infants. Lancet 1997;350(9081):844–50.
43. Christian P, Shrestha J, LeClerq SC, et al. Supplementation with micronutrients in addition to iron and folic acid does not further improve the hematologic status of pregnant women in rural Nepal. J Nutr 2003;133(11):3492–8.
44. Hooper L, Brown TJ, Elliott R, et al. The effectiveness of five strategies for the prevention of gastrointestinal toxicity induced by non-steroidal anti-inflammatory drugs: systematic review. BMJ 2004;329(7472):948.
45. Gooch K, Culleton BF, Manns BJ, et al. NSAID use and progression of chronic kidney disease. Am J Med 2007;120(3):280.e1–7.
46. Financing global health 2014: shifts in funding as the MDG era closes. Available at: www.healthdata.org/policy-report/financing-global-health-2014-shifts-funding-mdg-era-closes. Accessed July 1, 2015.
47. The Bangladesh integrated nutrition project effectiveness and lessons. Bangladesh development series – paper no.8. The World Bank: Dhaka, Bangladesh; 2005. Available at: http://siteresources.worldbank.org/NUTRITION/Resources/BNGBINP8.pdf.
48. WHO Scientific Group on Nutritional Anaemias. Nutritional anaemias: report of a WHO scientific group [meeting held in Geneva from 13 to 17 March 1967]. 1968.
49. Beutler E, Waalen J. The definition of anemia: what is the lower limit of normal of the blood hemoglobin concentration? Blood 2006;107(5):1747–50.

Iron Deficiency Anemia

Problems in Diagnosis and Prevention at the Population Level

Sant-Rayn Pasricha, MPH, PhD, FRACP, FRCPA*, Hal Drakesmith, BSc, PhD

KEYWORDS

- Iron • Hepcidin • Anemia • Public health • Children • Infection • Malaria

KEY POINTS

- Anemia remains a highly prevalent global health problem, affecting 43% of children younger than 5 years, 38% of pregnant women, and 29% of nonpregnant women worldwide.
- Current public health strategies to alleviate this burden include iron supplementation, home fortification with multiple micronutrient powders, and/or universal fortification of staple foods.
- Evidence that iron interventions benefit health outcomes is strongest in pregnant and nonpregnant women and weakest in young children.
- Emerging evidence indicates that iron interventions, especially in children, increase the risk of infection (especially from malaria and diarrhea) in areas of high transmission.
- Stratification of iron interventions toward children most in need, for example, using novel biomarkers, such as hepcidin, may facilitate more rational, safer, and effective interventions in the population for the future.

EPIDEMIOLOGY OF ANEMIA

There have been several recent estimates of the prevalence of anemia across the world. Overall, these studies indicate that the prevalence of anemia has marginally reduced. Although, with growth in the global population, the absolute number of anemic individuals continues to increase. Stevens and colleagues[1] studied the trends in hemoglobin (Hb) concentrations for each country between 1995 and 2011 using an ongoing systematic review of 257 national surveys, peer-reviewed scientific reports of national and subnational surveys held on the World Health Organization (WHO) Vitamins and Mineral Nutrition Information System, and data from national and

Disclosure statement: The authors have nothing to disclose.
MRC Human Immunology Unit, MRC Weatherall Institute of Molecular Medicine, John Radcliffe Hospital, University of Oxford, Oxford OX3 9DS, UK
* Corresponding author.
E-mail address: sant-rayn.pasricha@imm.ox.ac.uk

Hematol Oncol Clin N Am 30 (2016) 309–325
http://dx.doi.org/10.1016/j.hoc.2015.11.003   hemonc.theclinics.com

international agencies. Data were specifically considered for children younger than 5 years and pregnant and nonpregnant women, adjusted for altitude and smoking, and were reported in the original resources. The investigators estimated that in 2011, the global mean Hb concentration and anemia prevalence in children was 111 g/L and 43% respectively, in pregnant women 114 g/L and 38% respectively, and in nonpregnant women 126 g/L and 29% respectively.

These estimates reflect a probable improvement in Hb concentrations and anemia prevalence since 1995. However, enormous disparity persists, reflecting differences in economic development and infection burden. For example, the prevalence of anemia in Central and West African children exceeds 70%, and the prevalence also exceeds 50% in East Africa and in South Asia; the prevalence is only 11% in high-income countries. Similar patterns are seen among pregnant and nonpregnant women. Overall, Stevens and coworkers[1] estimated that about 273 million children, 496 million nonpregnant women, and 32 million pregnant women were anemic in 2011. The investigators also estimated that, although most anemia was amenable to iron in settings where few other causes of anemia exist (eg, Latin America, high-income countries), this decreases to less than half in settings where malaria infection is endemic.[1] In mid-2015, the WHO republished global estimates for the prevalence of anemia, confirming approximately 800 million women and children were anemic worldwide in 2011 (**Figs. 1–3**).[2]

A second estimate of the global prevalence of anemia, which subsequently estimated the disease burden of anemia, was published in 2014 by Kassebaum and colleagues.[3] Using data from more than 400 references, the investigators modeled the global prevalence of anemia in 187 countries and across both sexes and 20 age groups and then modeled cause-specific attribution to anemia due to 17 key diseases. The investigators then estimated the total years lived with disability (YLDs) using global burden of disease methodology. The investigators reported that 32.6% of the world's population were anemic in 2010 and that about 50% of cases of anemia overall were attributable to iron deficiency. In contrast to the Stevens analysis, the prevalence of anemia attributable to iron deficiency was smaller (not higher) in high-income countries where other causes (eg, hemoglobinopathies, renal impairment) were

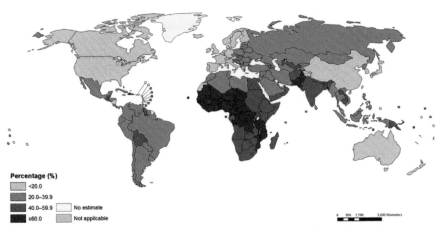

Fig. 1. Prevalence of anemia in children aged 6 to 59 months, 2011. (*From* World Health Organization. The global anaemia prevalence in 2011. Geneva (Switzerland): World Health Organization; 2015; with permission.)

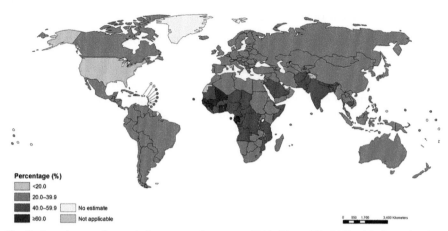

Fig. 2. Prevalence of anemia in pregnant women, 2011. (*From* World Health Organization. The global anaemia prevalence in 2011. Geneva (Switzerland): World Health Organization; 2015; with permission.)

considered more important. Malaria was responsible for a quarter of cases of anemia in sub-Saharan Africa. The investigators identified a similar distribution of anemia among populations (ie, most prevalent in young children and pregnant women). The investigators estimated that anemia accounts for about 68 million YLDs, almost 9% of the total for all conditions, underlining the potential importance of anemia as a global health problem; even though the individual disability weights assigned to mild and moderate anemia are relatively small, the enormous prevalence of this condition makes it a global health priority. The results of this study should be considered with some reserve, however, as the investigators used thresholds for defining anemia in children younger than 5 years (Hb <120 g/L) inconsistent with clinical recommendations (Hb <110 g/L), likely overestimating the prevalence (and burden) of anemia in this group.[3,4]

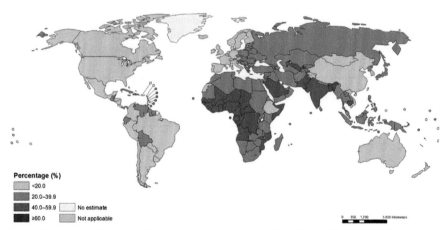

Fig. 3. Prevalence of anemia in nonpregnant women, 2011. (*From* World Health Organization. The global anaemia prevalence in 2011. Geneva (Switzerland): World Health Organization; 2015; with permission.)

FRAMEWORK FOR ANEMIA CONTROL

Reduction of the global burden of anemia is generally considered within the scope of public health nutrition, and solutions have focused on micronutrient interventions incorporating iron. Public health approaches must be implementable on a large scale by health workers without specialized training and at low cost per individual recipient. Modern public health interventions must be able to be justified on risk-benefit and health economic analyses, whereby costs incorporate the price not just the unit costs of iron but also the broader implementation program. Several solutions are presently available for providing iron in the public health context. These solutions include iron supplementation, home fortification with multiple micronutrient powders, and central food fortification (**Table 1**).[5]

Iron supplements (medicinal iron) are an established and effective approach for giving iron to women (including pregnant women) and are cheap to manufacture and distribute. However, this intervention has been difficult to implement in children because of the limited ability of children to swallow tablets; liquid supplements or dispersible tablets are required. An alternative approach for delivery of iron in children is home-based fortification with multiple micronutrient powders (MMPs, often also abbreviated as MNPs). These powders comprise lipid-encapsulated iron together with other micronutrients (at least vitamin A and zinc and often also several other micronutrients). These doses are provided in individual sachets that are then applied on the child's food after serving.[6] The two approaches seem to have comparable adherence and effects on Hb.[7] The key benefit for MMPs may be in their ease of delivery. However, despite escalating implementation in programs in many countries, there are surprisingly few data directly comparing iron supplements with MMPs or confirming the benefits of MMPs on functional health outcomes beyond improvements in nutritional biomarkers.[7]

Fortification of food with iron centrally (eg, at point of manufacture) is mandated in many countries. Fortification of staple foods, including wheat, maize, and rice, can improve iron intake and has been shown to restitute iron stores.[8] Long-term population studies indicate these interventions can reduce the burden of iron deficiency and anemia in the short to medium term,[9] although some studies question their efficacy in the longer term. Fortification can occur centrally, for example, at the point where flour is milled and packaged or more peripherally at the level of local distribution points. Key limitations of fortification as a solution to iron deficiency anemia in developing countries include the possibility that iron may not reach groups at highest risk of undernutrition unless special efforts are made to target programs, whereas groups at lower risk

Table 1	
Public health strategies for controlling anemia	
Children	**Women**
Iron supplements	Iron supplements
• Daily	• Daily
• Intermittent	• Intermittent
Multiple micronutrient powders	Multiple micronutrient tablets
Central staple-food fortification	
Improve dietary diversity	
Deworming	
Delayed cord clamping	Birth spacing
Prevent infection (especially malaria)	

of iron deficiency (eg, men) may consume the equivalent amounts of the fortified food. Monitoring and evaluation of these programs should, therefore, incorporate not just assessment of the impact of the interventions on iron deficiency but also on the risk of iron overload in susceptible groups (for example, populations with high burdens of hemoglobinopathies where iron absorption may be enhanced).[10]

OTHER MEASURES TO ADDRESS IRON DEFICIENCY ANEMIA
Delayed Cord Clamping

Following birth, placental transfer of blood to the newborn continues through the cord post partum. Delayed cord clamping (1–3 minutes after delivery rather than immediately after delivery) enables improved placental transfusion and has been shown to improve infant iron stores at 6 months of age,[11] and recent evidence indicates that this strategy improves long-term child fine-motor and social (but not overall cognitive) development.[12] The WHO recommends delayed cord clamping for all uncomplicated deliveries.[13] However, delayed cord clamping is also associated with an increased risk of neonatal hyperbilirubinemia,[11] a condition that can result in long-term neurologic sequelae.

Malaria Control

An adverse effect from malaria on iron absorption now seems well established. Studies measuring iron absorption during and following convalescence from acute infection with malaria in women and children have shown that, during infection, there are elevations in hepcidin associated with a reduction in iron absorption, with improvement in iron absorption once the infection is treated. For example, Cercamondi and colleagues[14] showed that, in Beninese women with asymptomatic *Plasmodium falciparum* infection, treatment increased the mean dietary iron absorption from 10% to 18%, associated with a marked decrease in serum hepcidin. Doherty and colleagues[15] showed that toddlers infected with malaria have much poorer iron incorporation into red cells (8%) than those without malaria (28%). Epidemiologically, marked increases in the prevalence of iron deficiency, iron deficiency anemia, and anemia in Gambian children from the beginning to end of the malaria season (iron deficiency: 18% to 31%; iron deficiency anemia 14% to 25%; anemia 56% to 69%) have been observed, suggesting a seasonal effect on iron deficiency potentially mediated by infection.[16]

A second study has supported these findings from a different perspective: Frosch and colleagues[17] studied the prevalence of iron deficiency in children younger than 5 years living in 2 Kenyan villages before and after a 12-month documented period of interruption of malaria transmission achieved by widespread indoor residual insecticide spraying and introduction of artemisinin combination therapy for malaria. The prevalence of iron deficiency decreased from 36% to 26% and anemia from 54% to 32%; regression analyses confirmed these changes were larger than would be expected for changes in age alone. Thus, malaria is likely to contribute to the burden of iron deficiency anemia in developing countries by elevating hepcidin and preventing iron absorption, and control of malaria may independently alleviate iron deficiency. Conclusive data on the effect of malaria control on the burden of iron deficiency and iron deficiency anemia are not yet available; however, malaria chemoprevention (for example, using intermittent preventative therapy) has similar effects on the prevalence of anemia as iron supplementation.[18] Other infectious diseases producing a systemic inflammatory response (eg, diarrhea, pneumonia) may contribute to the burden of iron deficiency through a similar mechanism (raising hepcidin and preventing iron absorption); but this has not yet been measured.

Antihelminthic Therapy

Hookworm infection is an important cause of iron deficiency.[19] Deworming is generally safe and cheap, reduces the burden of anemia, and should be included as part of anemia-control programs where hookworm is prevalent.[20]

Iron Enrichment of Cooked Foods

Several approaches have been trialed to improve the iron content of cooked foods through leaching of iron from the vessel or an added component. Iron can enter the food when prepared in an acidic environment. For example, an Ethiopian study found that cooking food in iron pots improved iron content in the food and improved iron indices and Hb in children.[21] More recently, efforts to fortify cooked foods using an iron fish added to food under preparation (together with acidification) have been attempted. Published reports from this approach indicate a short-term benefit on Hb and iron stores that does not persist beyond 3 months of use.[22]

Benefits from Iron on Functional Health Outcomes

Data indicate that iron supplementation consistently improves Hb and iron stores and reduces the risk of anemia and iron deficiency in women and children. However, the functional benefits from iron on health outcomes have been less extensively reported in randomized controlled trials. In pregnancy, iron supplements increase birthweight and reduce the risk of low birth weight.[23,24] Studies in Nepal[25] and China[26] have found that children of mothers randomized to iron interventions have reduced short- and long-term mortality. Two studies have reported on the effects of iron on long-term child development, with one trial identifying a beneficial effect from iron,[27] whereas a second trial found no difference.[28] The presence of an effect may depend on the underlying burden of iron deficiency in the population.

In nonpregnant women, meta-analyses indicate that iron supplementation improves both peak and submaximal exercise performance, particularly in women undergoing training and with iron deficiency.[29] In women presenting with fatigue and ferritin levels less than 50 ug/L, oral[30] iron treatment improves fatigue scores, although evidence of benefit on psychological symptoms and cognition in adults is ambiguous.

In children, although there are extensive observational data linking anemia and iron deficiency in young children (younger than 2 years) to impaired functional outcomes including poorer cognitive (mental and psychomotor) development, meta-analyses of available trials have not identified evidence of benefit from iron supplementation on this critical outcome[31–33]; 2 long-term follow-up studies (in Nepal[34] and Thailand[35]) are now available, which similarly fail to show any effect from iron supplementation in young childhood on long-term cognitive outcomes. The overall quality of evidence for the effects of iron on cognitive development in preschool children is low, and further studies are urgently needed to identify whether a benefit exists, the magnitude of any effect, and whether baseline iron and anemia status predict a favorable response to iron.[36] In older (school aged) children, iron supplementation improves child cognitive scores, including IQ in anemic children.[37] It is important to note that, although impaired growth has been postulated as an effect from iron deficiency, interventional studies of iron supplements have identified evidence that iron supplements actually seem to reduce linear growth and weight gain, particularly in iron-replete children.[31]

In malaria-endemic settings, a rationale for iron supplementation has been to reduce the risk of severe anemia, a life-threatening complication of infection, especially with malaria; however, current evidence indicates that severe anemia is *not* predominantly due to iron deficiency but rather inflammation and red cell destruction.[38] Trials administering iron to children in malaria-endemic settings have never identified a reduction in hospitalization due to severe anemia, and reductions in severe anemia due to iron are 50% smaller than reductions in severe anemia achievable by malaria chemoprophylaxis; furthermore, coadministration of iron together with antimalarials does not reduce severe anemia beyond just giving antimalarials alone.[39] Thus, there is presently inadequate evidence to establish the functional benefits of iron supplementation in young children, including in children in malaria-endemic settings.

Risks of Iron Supplementation

Infection

The potential risk of iron supplementation on infection has been long postulated, and human trials and experimental studies have consistently reported an increase in infection when organisms are provided excess iron.[40] For example, historic trials in Somali Nomads identified a 5-fold increase in infection risk when treated with iron compared with a control, with infections resulting from a range of bacterial and parasitic microorganisms.[41]

Microorganisms require iron, and the discovery of the hepcidin-ferroportin axis during the previous 15 years provides confirmatory evidence of the likely protective role, the iron-withholding response.[42] Systemic iron homeostasis is orchestrated by hepcidin, a predominantly hepatic-derived hormone, which is expressed in response to iron (in order to suppress iron absorption and recycling by preventing iron egress into the serum from the duodenum and macrophage respectively). Importantly, hepcidin also comprises a component of and is elevated directly by the innate immune response (especially interleukin [IL]-6[43] and IL-22[44]); it is, therefore, elevated in a range of infections, including malaria; bacterial infections, including typhoid[45] and tuberculosis; and viral infections, including influenza A virus[40] and human immunodeficiency virus.[46] These findings demonstrates a clear physiologic drive to reduce serum iron (induce hypoferremia) during infection, which can be potentially overwhelmed by high doses of administered iron.[40]

Data from more recent randomized controlled trials seem to indicate an increased risk from iron and iron-containing interventions on 3 key infections (malaria, diarrhea, and acute respiratory infection), which are highly prevalent among children in low-income countries. Mechanistic data support a direct interaction between iron interventions and malarial and bacterial infection.

Clinical trials data

In 2006, the *Lancet* published the results of the 2 largest randomized controlled trials of iron supplementation in young children ever in Pemba, Tanzania (a sub-Saharan African malaria-endemic setting)[47] and Nepal (a South Asian non–malaria-endemic setting).[48] These trials together randomized almost 34,000 children aged 1 to 35 months to iron and folate (12.5 mg unless younger than 12 months of age, in which case 6.25 mg), with or without zinc, versus about 16,600 whom were assigned to placebo and were powered to detect an effect (a hypothesized benefit) from iron on mortality and serious morbidity. The two trials were both stopped early by the Data Safety Monitoring Board (DSMB) for different reasons. The Nepal study was ceased because the DSMB identified no evidence of a difference in morbidity between the groups and determined the power to identify an effect on mortality would be inadequate. The study found no effect from iron on overall or cause-specific mortality and no significant effect from iron on the incidence of diarrhea or pneumonia.

Conversely, the Pemba study was stopped for a different reason: Here, the DSMB was concerned about a significant increase in serious events among children randomized to iron, necessitating early cessation of the trial. The investigators reported that children in the iron folate group experienced a 12% increased risk of serious adverse events (defined as mortality or hospitalization) and were 11% more likely to be admitted to hospital, with a trend toward increased mortality. Children receiving iron had a 16% increased risk of serious adverse events due to clinical malaria and a 22% increased risk of cerebral malaria. There was also a 28% increase in hospitalization and 61% increase in death from nonmalarial infections. A substudy suggested that the increased risk was observed in children who were randomized to iron but were baseline iron replete, whereas a protective effect from iron on infection was seen in children with baseline iron deficiency anemia. However, these definitions were based on zinc protoporphyrin (ZPP) measurements, which are inaccurate in sub-Saharan African settings and which can represent not just iron deficiency but also inflammation; thus, the underlying iron status predicting these responses is uncertain.[49] Key concerns with the applicability and implications of this trial have been that malaria control measures were not implemented as part of the study and coverage of prevention measures was considered fairly poor (eg, insecticide-treated net coverage was less than 40% in the main trial and 50% in the substudy). However, this is likely to reflect the situation in many sub-Saharan African settings, where bed net coverage exceeds 50% in only 4 of 23 countries evaluated.[50]

Three further subsequent clinical trials have been undertaken to try to further assess the risk of infection from iron interventions in low-income settings. Each of these was considerably smaller than the initial two studies. These interventions did not use iron supplementation per se but instead deployed home fortification using iron-containing MMPs. In Ghana, Zlotkin and colleagues[51] cluster randomized almost 2000 children to iron-containing or noncontaining MMPs, with coadministration of insecticide-treated bed nets as well as malaria treatment when needed. The trial was powered for superiority of placebo to be able to detect a 15% increase in malaria rate with iron. The investigators found a lower unadjusted rate of malaria in children randomized to iron-containing MMPs, which was no longer observed once analyses were adjusted for baseline anemia and malarial incidence. However, the investigators observed a significant 23% increase in hospitalization rate among children receiving iron, although cause-specific morbidity was not different between groups.

Two nonblinded trials of MMPs containing iron were undertaken in Pakistan. Soofi and colleagues[52] cluster randomized 2746 children to no intervention or MMPs containing iron with or without zinc for 12 months from 6 to 18 months of age. The investigators observed an increase in rate of bloody diarrhea and severe diarrhea (reported by parents) as well as the proportion of days with diarrhea. The investigators also observed an increase in respiratory infection (evidenced by reported rapid breathing or chest indrawing) in children receiving one of the MMPs. A second smaller trial in Pakistan, unblinded and providing iron-containing MMPs to young children, again reported an increase in diarrhea incidence among children randomized to intervention.[53] Critically, lack of blinding of these studies makes data based on parental reporting of symptoms difficult to interpret.

Mechanistic evidence for increased risk from iron interventions on malaria

In Malawian preschool children, an observational cohort study found that those with baseline iron deficiency had a lower incidence of malaria parasitemia (hazard ratio [HR] 0.55) and clinical malaria (HR 0.49) over 12 months.[54] A similar cohort study in

Tanzania found that children younger than 3 years with iron deficiency had a 23% reduction in subsequent clinical malaria, 38% reduction in severe malaria, 60% reduction in all-cause mortality, and 66% reduction in malaria-specific mortality.[55] These data indicate that iron deficiency seems to protect against malaria; they conflict with the more generally prevailing view that to optimize health, iron deficiency should be averted.

Effects of iron depletion on malaria parasite growth in vitro have been long observed. For example, in vitro studies using a range of iron chelators and human trials of the iron chelator desferrioxamine reduce plasmodial infection.[56] Recent experimental studies have shown that *Plasmodium falciparum* infects iron-deficient erythroblasts less efficiently and that reticulocytes generated during erythropoietic recovery from iron deficiency anemia are at increased susceptibility to merozoite invasion.[57] These data support the hypothesis that restitution of erythropoiesis during treatment of iron deficiency exacerbates the risk of malaria.

Other potential pathways have been hypothesized to mediate the effect of iron on malaria risk. For example, large doses of iron may exceed plasma iron-binding capacity, resulting in a spike in non–transferrin-bound iron (NTBI), which may increase reactive oxygen species and cell damage, potentially enhancing endothelial damage and promoting parasitic adhesion as well as perhaps supporting bacterial infection.[58] However, the role of NTBI infection in exacerbating malaria infection has not been confirmed experimentally or in humans. Importantly, because of the facilitative role of iron deficiency on iron absorption, NTBI is increased when iron is administered to an iron-deficient, compared with replete, individual.[59]

Together, these mechanisms suggest a diabolical paradox: iron administration may in fact be at greatest risk of promoting infection among iron-deficient (and especially iron-deficient anemic) individuals, the very same group whom might benefit most from receiving iron.

Experimental evidence for increased risk from iron interventions on diarrhea

There has been considerable recent interest on the effects of iron interventions on the intestinal microbiome. Two studies undertaken in sub-Saharan African children where sanitation was poor and potentially harmful bacteria already comprised a sizable proportion of the intestinal microflora have found evidence that food fortification with iron (both at low doses and higher doses using MMPs) causes a shift toward pathogenic bacteria. In Côte d'Ivoire, in 6- to 14-year old children, iron-fortified biscuits containing a relatively low concentration of poorly bioavailable iron increased enterobacteria, reduced lactobacilli, and increased intestinal inflammation as measured by fecal calprotectin.[60] Subsequently, using 16s pyrosequencing, Jaeggi and colleagues[61] characterized the intestinal microbiomes of Kenyan infants participating in 2 randomized controlled trials of low-dose iron (2.5 mg) in micronutrient powders versus control or high-dose iron in MMPs (12.5 mg) versus control. In both trials, although most of the intestinal bacteria at baseline were nonpathogenic, a high proportion of potentially pathogenic bacteria were also observed. Among children receiving iron, there was a significant increase in potentially pathogenic enterobacteria, including *Escherichia* and *Shigella* and *Clostridium*. In the high dose iron trial, there was a trend toward an increase in clinical diarrhea among children receiving iron. Importantly, iron-containing MMPs increased fecal calprotectin, a biomarker of intestinal inflammation. Notably, however, in a trial among older children in South Africa, where there was a lower prevalence of pathogenic bacteria at baseline, iron provision of high-dose iron in the form of 50-mg tablets did not increase the risk of diarrhea, increase intestinal inflammation, or alter enteric flora.[62] Thus, the clinical observations of increased risk of diarrhea from iron may be attributable to increases in intestinal burden of pathogenic bacteria, which may be particularly frequent among children where carriage of such bacteria is already endemic.

Other risks of iron supplementation

In adults, iron supplementation with ferrous sulfate is associated with gastrointestinal side effects, including abdominal discomfort, nausea, and constipation (as well as stool discoloration).[63] These side effects can be ameliorated by reducing the dose or frequency of doses or taking the iron with food rather than in between meals. The incidence of these adverse effects in young children is less well defined, as reporting of side effects is less feasible. However, a systematic review identified an increase in the risk of vomiting among children receiving iron.[31]

In children, there is evidence that iron supplementation can reduce growth rate.[31] The mechanism for this is unclear; potential explanations include increased risk of infection, reduced appetite due to gastrointestinal adverse effects, or impairment in dietary zinc (which is important for linear growth) absorption or utilization due to interference by iron. Indeed, meta-analysis has confirmed that coadministration of iron and zinc is less effective at improving zinc concentrations compared with zinc supplementation alone.[31]

Ferrous salt preparations can be lethal in overdose, especially in children: the dose that is lethal to 50% of experimental animals for ferrous sulfate is 255 to 350 mg/kg.[64] In the United States, 30.2% of deaths due to accidental overdose in children between 1983 and 1991 were caused by iron preparations.[65] Iron supplementation programs (for example, to pregnant or nonpregnant women) could potentially distribute hundreds of thousands of courses of iron nationally, with potentially limited time for education at the level of interaction between health worker and consumer regarding safe storage and potential risks. Furthermore, packaging may not be secure; in many settings, supplements are not provided in individual blisters but are in bottles or even paper envelopes, from which they could be accessed and consumed by children. Data on risk of unintentional poisoning from iron in low-income settings are unavailable, but the risk is unlikely to be remote. Several alternative iron formulations are considered nontoxic in overdose, such as carbonyl iron and iron polymaltose complex.

MEASUREMENT OF IRON STATUS IN THE PUBLIC HEALTH CONTEXT

Assessment of the iron status in a population is necessary to identify the burden of iron deficiency and, hence, the likely need for and potential impact of an iron intervention and to monitor the effectiveness of these interventions. The most widely used biomarker of iron status in population surveys is Hb, generally reported as the percentage of the population with anemia. However, although end-stage iron deficiency can result in anemia, iron stores are usually depleted before anemia occurs; conversely, there are many other causes of anemia relevant to the public health contexts that are not attributable to iron deficiency. Anemia has a low sensitivity and specificity for iron deficiency.[66]

Measurement of specific iron indices is more challenging for both practical and biological reasons. Traditional iron indices include ferritin, soluble transferrin receptor (sTfR), the sTfR-log (ferritin) index, serum iron, and transferrin saturation. These indices all require collection of serum or plasma, which requires access to a centrifuge in the field or collection of samples as dried blood spots, followed by analysis on a biochemistry analyzer. These indices each reliably detect iron deficiency in individuals without comorbidities but are prone to distortion in complex patients and populations, impairing their interpretability.

Serum ferritin is widely available and perhaps the most commonly used iron index. It has been identified as the test, together with Hb, which most reliably defines a response from an iron intervention in a population.[67] However, ferritin is also an acute phase protein and is, thus, distorted by even small levels of inflammation. Thus, in low-income countries, and especially among children, ferritin levels cannot be easily interpreted. There are considerable efforts being made to identify the best way in which to account for inflammation at the population level when interpreting ferritin levels to define the prevalence of iron deficiency. Surveys should probably measure at least one inflammatory biomarker to enable adjustment for inflammation. Potential approaches include adjusting ferritin thresholds among inflamed individuals, excluding inflamed individuals from the analysis, or using regression techniques (either externally defined or defined within the individual dataset) to adjust ferritin for biomarkers in a continuous fashion.[68] Epidemiologic design of the survey should be optimized to minimize sampling from potentially inflamed individuals (for example, studying populations during a season of lower infection transmission or excluding acutely unwell participants from the survey). A comprehensive effort is presently underway to systematically define the optimal thresholds for ferritin to diagnose iron deficiency, incorporating a consideration of the effect of inflammation.[69]

sTfR has been available for more than a decade and is available in many clinical laboratories. It is an indicator of tissue iron deficiency and reflects the increased expression of sTfR by erythroblasts and tissues when cellular iron requirements are enhanced. Although originally considered impervious to inflammation, recent evidence suggests it is indeed distorted (elevated) by inflammation. It is also a direct biomarker of erythropoiesis (indeed, has been trialed clinically for this use in patients undergoing chemotherapy[70] and with thalassemia[71]) and is, thus, distorted in individuals with suppressed or enhanced red cell production (for example, recovery from bleeding, hemolytic anemia, malaria). Its value in sub-Saharan settings where malaria is endemic resulting in fluctuations in erythroid activity is unclear, but it is likely to overestimate the burden of iron deficiency.[49] Furthermore, its widespread deployment has been limited by lack of a standardized reference material, which has resulted in different manufacturer assays returning different (although correlated) results for the same sample.

The sTfR to $\log_{10}$ ferritin ratio incorporates indices of both storage iron and tissue iron need and has been considered a superior index of iron deficiency to either index alone.[72] However, it has not been validated against gold standards in African or pediatric community populations, and elevations in sTfR and differences between assays may distort interpretation of the index.

ZPP reflects aberrant incorporation of zinc into protoporphyrin instead of iron, when iron is unavailable for heme synthesis. It is elevated in iron deficiency as well as other conditions producing anemia, such as inflammation and hemoglobinopathy as well as lead poisoning. It can be measured in the field using a portable hematofluorometer, which has made it a commonly used method for determining iron deficiency in studies in low-income settings. For example, it was used to define iron deficiency in the Pemba study. The multitude of reasons it can be elevated make it of uncertain value in low-income settings, especially in children. For example, the authors found ZPP to have an area under the receiver operating characteristic curve (AUC-ROC) for detecting iron deficiency in Gambian children of 0.74 and to be even less valuable in distinguishing between iron deficiency and anemia of inflammation (AUC-ROC 0.63).[49]

Reticulocyte Hb estimates the iron available for erythropoiesis over the previous 3 to 4 days and has been shown to be a useful index of iron deficiency in adults and children. It also provides a useful early index of response to iron supplementation. However, it is only available on selected hematology analyzers, and its value in the public health context remains uncertain. Serum iron and transferrin saturation are widely used indices of iron transport. They are useful indices of iron availability for erythropoiesis but do not accurately reflect body iron stores within the normal range and are distorted (reduced) by inflammation. Estimation of the prevalence of iron deficiency from these indices in populations where inflammation is common is difficult.

In population surveys, the WHO presently recommends measurement of Hb, serum ferritin, sTfR if possible, and ideally at least one marker of inflammation to enable adjustment for inflammation. The WHO also recommends that surveys for iron status be undertaken during seasons of lower risk of inflammation.[73]

Measurement of hepcidin in the serum, plasma, or urine can now be performed using several enzyme-linked immunosorbent assay or mass spectrometry platforms. Hepcidin is the master orchestrator of systemic iron homeostasis and directly regulates intestinal iron absorption and macrophage iron recycling through its actions on the sole cellular iron exporter, ferroportin. Hepcidin is transcriptionally regulated by iron (via the BMP6/SMAD and the Tfr2/HFE pathways), inflammation (via the STAT3 pathway),[74] and erythropoiesis (perhaps via the recently discovered erythroid hormone, erythroferrone).[75] Thus, measurement of hepcidin could synthesize the net input provided by these signals and provide a critically valuable index to assess iron need at an individual or population level. Measurement of hepcidin can accurately estimate oral iron absorption and incorporation into erythrocytes, and studies in children[76] and in women[77] indicate it can identify iron deficiency. Hepcidin measurement in African children identifies a subpopulation who are likely to be in greatest need for iron supplementation.[49] The clinical value of hepcidin as an index of iron deficiency is under active clinical investigation.

FUTURE DIRECTIONS

Only marginal progress has been made in alleviating the global burden of anemia over the past 2 decades. Modern understanding of the biology of iron regulation provides critical new insights that inform measurement, prevention, and treatment of the condition.

New iron formulations are being developed that improve on the side-effect profile of iron salts. For example, iron nanoparticles (iron hydroxide adipate tartrate [IHAT]) have been developed that mimic the ferritin molecule, may make iron unavailable to gut microbiota, but are highly bioavailable and effectively absorbed making them useful clinically.[78] Further clinical trials are necessary to establish their role in humans.

In pregnancy and among nonpregnant women, as well as in school-aged children, there is convincing evidence that iron supplementation provides functional health benefits. The role of iron supplementation for anemia control as a public health (rather than clinical) intervention for young children living in low-income countries is, however, increasingly uncertain, chiefly because of the lack of high-quality evidence regarding the benefits of iron when compared with the stronger evidence that iron can cause harm. Further studies are necessary to define the benefits (ie, on child development, well-being, and overall health) as well as harms associated with iron supplementation in children in low-income settings. The one-size-fits-all (universal supplementation) approach to public health iron interventions may require revision given the likelihood that iron-deficient children experience both the greatest benefit and risk from iron interventions. Selection of children for intervention using presupplementation screening, for example, with hepcidin may be an interesting approach. Ultimately, policy should be guided by analysis of the comparative benefits (on well-being and child development) and risks (from infection) from iron interventions.

Although the WHO recommends iron interventions in malaria-endemic settings be implemented together with strategies to 'prevent, diagnose and treat malaria',[5] the specific nature of these interventions remains uncertain. Malaria chemoprevention is an exciting strategy for reducing the burden of clinical malaria and has been recommended (although infrequently implemented) for prevention of seasonal malaria. Newer combination drug regimens offer sustained efficacy and are relatively safe to administer and may offer an opportunity for safe implementation of iron cointerventions. However, it is also important to determine whether the gains from alleviating iron deficiency can be achieved simply by restoring iron absorption through control of infection alone; this could provide further impetus to restore implement infection control measures.

REFERENCES

1. Stevens GA, Finucane MM, De-Regil LM, et al. Global, regional, and national trends in haemoglobin concentration and prevalence of total and severe anaemia in children and pregnant and non-pregnant women for 1995-2011: a systematic analysis of population-representative data. Lancet Glob Health 2013;1(1):e16–25.
2. World Health Organization. The global prevalence of anaemia in 2011. Geneva (Switzerland): World Health Organization; 2015.
3. Kassebaum NJ, Jasrasaria R, Naghavi M, et al. A systematic analysis of global anemia burden from 1990 to 2010. Blood 2013;123(5):615–24.
4. Pasricha SR. Anemia: a comprehensive global estimate. Blood 2014;123(5): 611–2.
5. World Health Organization. Essential nutrition actions: improving maternal, newborn, infant and young child health and nutrition. Geneva (Switzerland): World Health Organization; 2013.
6. Pasricha SR, Drakesmith H, Black J, et al. Control of iron deficiency anemia in low and middle-income countries. Blood 2013;121(14):2607–17.
7. De-Regil LM, Suchdev PS, Vist GE, et al. Home fortification of foods with multiple micronutrient powders for health and nutrition in children under two years of age. Cochrane Database Syst Rev 2011;(9):CD008959.
8. Allen L, de Benoist B, Dary O, et al. Guidelines on food fortification with micronutrients. Geneva (Switzerland): World Health Organization; Food and Agricultural Organization of the United Nations; 2006.
9. Garcia-Casal MN, Layrisse M. Iron fortification of flours in Venezuela. Nutr Rev 2002;60(7 Pt 2):S26–9.
10. Jones E, Pasricha SR, Allen A, et al. Hepcidin is suppressed by erythropoiesis in hemoglobin E beta-thalassemia and beta-thalassemia trait. Blood 2015;125(5): 873–80.
11. McDonald SJ, Middleton P. Effect of timing of umbilical cord clamping of term infants on maternal and neonatal outcomes. Cochrane Database Syst Rev 2008;(2):CD004074.
12. Andersson O, Lindquist B, Lindgren M, et al. Effect of delayed cord clamping on neurodevelopment at 4 years of age: a randomized clinical trial. JAMA Pediatr 2015;169(7):631–8.

13. World Health Organization. Optimal timing of cord clamping for the prevention of iron deficiency anaemia in infants. e-Library of Evidence for Nutrition Actions (eLENA); 2014. Accessed June 1, 2015. Available at: http://www.who.int/elena/titles/cord_clamping/en/Geneva.

14. Cercamondi CI, Egli IM, Ahouandjinou E, et al. Afebrile Plasmodium falciparum parasitemia decreases absorption of fortification iron but does not affect systemic iron utilization: a double stable-isotope study in young Beninese women. Am J Clin Nutr 2010;92(6):1385–92.

15. Doherty CP, Cox SE, Fulford AJ, et al. Iron incorporation and post-malaria anaemia. PLoS One 2008;3(5):e2133.

16. Atkinson SH, Armitage AE, Khandwala S, et al. Combinatorial effects of malaria season, iron deficiency, and inflammation determine plasma hepcidin concentration in African children. Blood 2014;123(21):3221–9.

17. Frosch AE, Ondigo BN, Ayodo GA, et al. Decline in childhood iron deficiency after interruption of malaria transmission in highland Kenya. Am J Clin Nutr 2014; 100(3):968–73.

18. Meremikwu MM, Donegan S, Sinclair D, et al. Intermittent preventive treatment for malaria in children living in areas with seasonal transmission. Cochrane Database Syst Rev 2012;(2):CD003756.

19. Pasricha SR, Caruana SR, Phuc TQ, et al. Anemia, iron deficiency, meat consumption, and hookworm infection in women of reproductive age in northwest Vietnam. Am J Trop Med Hyg 2008;78(3):375–81.

20. Gulani A, Nagpal J, Osmond C, et al. Effect of administration of intestinal anthelmintic drugs on haemoglobin: systematic review of randomised controlled trials. BMJ 2007;334(7603):1095.

21. Adish AA, Esrey SA, Gyorkos TW, et al. Effect of consumption of food cooked in iron pots on iron status and growth of young children: a randomised trial. Lancet 1999;353(9154):712–6.

22. Charles CV, Dewey CE, Daniell WE, et al. Iron-deficiency anaemia in rural Cambodia: community trial of a novel iron supplementation technique. Eur J Public Health 2011;21(1):43–8.

23. Haider BA, Olofin I, Wang M, et al. Anaemia, prenatal iron use, and risk of adverse pregnancy outcomes: systematic review and meta-analysis. BMJ 2013;346:f3443.

24. Pena-Rosas JP, De-Regil LM, Dowswell T, et al. Daily oral iron supplementation during pregnancy. Cochrane Database Syst Rev 2012;(12):CD004736.

25. Christian P, Stewart CP, LeClerq SC, et al. Antenatal and postnatal iron supplementation and childhood mortality in rural Nepal: a prospective follow-up in a randomized, controlled community trial. Am J Epidemiol 2009;170(9):1127–36.

26. Zeng L, Dibley MJ, Cheng Y, et al. Impact of micronutrient supplementation during pregnancy on birth weight, duration of gestation, and perinatal mortality in rural western China: double blind cluster randomised controlled trial. BMJ 2008;337:a2001.

27. Christian P, Murray-Kolb LE, Khatry SK, et al. Prenatal micronutrient supplementation and intellectual and motor function in early school-aged children in Nepal. JAMA 2010;304(24):2716–23.

28. Parsons AG, Zhou SJ, Spurrier NJ, et al. Effect of iron supplementation during pregnancy on the behaviour of children at early school age: long-term follow-up of a randomised controlled trial. Br J Nutr 2008;99(5):1133–9.

29. Pasricha SR, Low M, Thompson J, et al. Iron supplementation benefits physical performance in women of reproductive age: a systematic review and meta-analysis. J Nutr 2014;144(6):906–14.

30. Verdon F, Burnand B, Stubi CL, et al. Iron supplementation for unexplained fatigue in non-anaemic women: double blind randomised placebo controlled trial. BMJ 2003;326(7399):1124.
31. Pasricha S-R, Hayes E, Kalumba K, et al. Effect of daily iron supplementation on health in children aged 4—23 months: a systematic review and meta-analysis of randomised controlled trials. Lancet Glob Health 2013;1(2):e77–86.
32. Sachdev H, Gera T, Nestel P. Effect of iron supplementation on mental and motor development in children: systematic review of randomised controlled trials. Public Health Nutr 2005;8(2):117–32.
33. Wang B, Zhan S, Gong T, et al. Iron therapy for improving psychomotor development and cognitive function in children under the age of three with iron deficiency anaemia. Cochrane Database Syst Rev 2013;(6):CD001444.
34. Murray-Kolb LE, Khatry SK, Katz J, et al. Preschool micronutrient supplementation effects on intellectual and motor function in school-aged Nepalese children. Arch Pediatr Adolesc Med 2012;166(5):404–10.
35. Pongcharoen T, DiGirolamo AM, Ramakrishnan U, et al. Long-term effects of iron and zinc supplementation during infancy on cognitive function at 9 y of age in northeast Thai children: a follow-up study. Am J Clin Nutr 2011;93(3):636–43.
36. Murray-Kolb L. Iron supplementation in early life and child health. Lancet Glob Health 2013;1(2):e56–7.
37. Low M, Farrell A, Biggs BA, et al. Effects of daily iron supplementation in primary-school-aged children: systematic review and meta-analysis of randomized controlled trials. CMAJ 2013;185(17):E791–802.
38. Calis JC, Phiri KS, Faragher EB, et al. Severe anemia in Malawian children. N Engl J Med 2008;358(9):888–99.
39. Menendez C, Kahigwa E, Hirt R, et al. Randomised placebo-controlled trial of iron supplementation and malaria chemoprophylaxis for prevention of severe anaemia and malaria in Tanzanian infants. Lancet 1997;350(9081):844–50.
40. Drakesmith H, Prentice AM. Hepcidin and the iron-infection axis. Science 2012; 338(6108):768–72.
41. Murray MJ, Murray AB, Murray MB, et al. The adverse effect of iron repletion on the course of certain infections. Br Med J 1978;2(6145):1113–5.
42. Prentice AM, Verhoef H, Cerami C. Iron fortification and malaria risk in children. JAMA 2013;310(9):914–5.
43. Nemeth E, Valore EV, Territo M, et al. Hepcidin, a putative mediator of anemia of inflammation, is a type II acute-phase protein. Blood 2003;101(7):2461–3.
44. Armitage AE, Eddowes LA, Gileadi U, et al. Hepcidin regulation by innate immune and infectious stimuli. Blood 2011;118(15):4129–39.
45. Darton TC, Blohmke CJ, Giannoulatou E, et al. Rapidly escalating hepcidin and associated serum iron starvation are features of the acute response to typhoid infection in humans. PLoS Negl Trop Dis 2015;9(9):e0004029.
46. Armitage AE, Stacey AR, Giannoulatou E, et al. Distinct patterns of hepcidin and iron regulation during HIV-1, HBV, and HCV infections. Proc Natl Acad Sci U S A 2014;111(33):12187–92.
47. Sazawal S, Black RE, Ramsan M, et al. Effects of routine prophylactic supplementation with iron and folic acid on admission to hospital and mortality in preschool children in a high malaria transmission setting: community-based, randomised, placebo-controlled trial. Lancet 2006; 367(9505):133–43.
48. Tielsch JM, Khatry SK, Stoltzfus RJ, et al. Effect of routine prophylactic supplementation with iron and folic acid on preschool child mortality in southern

Nepal: community-based, cluster-randomised, placebo-controlled trial. Lancet 2006;367(9505):144–52.

49. Pasricha SR, Atkinson SH, Armitage AE, et al. Expression of the iron hormone hepcidin distinguishes different types of anemia in African children. Sci Transl Med 2014;6(235):235re233.

50. Vanderelst D, Speybroeck N. An adjusted bed net coverage indicator with estimations for 23 African countries. Malar J 2013;12:457.

51. Zlotkin S, Newton S, Aimone AM, et al. Effect of iron fortification on malaria incidence in infants and young children in Ghana: a randomized trial. JAMA 2013; 310(9):938–47.

52. Soofi S, Cousens S, Iqbal SP, et al. Effect of provision of daily zinc and iron with several micronutrients on growth and morbidity among young children in Pakistan: a cluster-randomised trial. Lancet 2013;382(9886):29–40.

53. Yousafzai AK, Rasheed MA, Rizvi A, et al. Effect of integrated responsive stimulation and nutrition interventions in the Lady Health Worker programme in Pakistan on child development, growth, and health outcomes: a cluster-randomised factorial effectiveness trial. Lancet 2014;384(9950): 1282–93.

54. Jonker FA, Calis JC, van Hensbroek MB, et al. Iron status predicts malaria risk in Malawian preschool children. PLoS One 2012;7(8):e42670.

55. Gwamaka M, Kurtis JD, Sorensen BE, et al. Iron deficiency protects against severe Plasmodium falciparum malaria and death in young children. Clin Infect Dis 2012;54(8):1137–44.

56. Hershko C, Gordeuk VR, Thuma PE, et al. The antimalarial effect of iron chelators: studies in animal models and in humans with mild falciparum malaria. J Inorg Biochem 1992;47(3–4):267–77.

57. Clark MA, Goheen MM, Fulford A, et al. Host iron status and iron supplementation mediate susceptibility to erythrocytic stage Plasmodium falciparum. Nat Commun 2014;5:4446.

58. Hershko C. Mechanism of iron toxicity. Food Nutr Bull 2007;28(4 Suppl):S500–9.

59. Brittenham GM, Andersson M, Egli I, et al. Circulating non-transferrin-bound iron after oral administration of supplemental and fortification doses of iron to healthy women: a randomized study. Am J Clin Nutr 2014;100(3):813–20.

60. Zimmermann MB, Chassard C, Rohner F, et al. The effects of iron fortification on the gut microbiota in African children: a randomized controlled trial in Cote d'Ivoire. Am J Clin Nutr 2010;92(6):1406–15.

61. Jaeggi T, Kortman GA, Moretti D, et al. Iron fortification adversely affects the gut microbiome, increases pathogen abundance and induces intestinal inflammation in Kenyan infants. Gut 2015;64(5):731–42.

62. Dostal A, Baumgartner J, Riesen N, et al. Effects of iron supplementation on dominant bacterial groups in the gut, faecal SCFA and gut inflammation: a randomised, placebo-controlled intervention trial in South African children. Br J Nutr 2014;112(4):547–56.

63. Pasricha SR, Flecknoe-Brown SC, Allen KJ, et al. Diagnosis and management of iron deficiency anaemia: a clinical update. Med J Aust 2010;193(9):525–32.

64. Toblli JE, Cao G, Olivieri L, et al. Comparative study of gastrointestinal tract and liver toxicity of ferrous sulfate, iron amino chelate and iron polymaltose complex in normal rats. Pharmacology 2008;82(2):127–37.

65. Litovitz T, Manoguerra A. Comparison of pediatric poisoning hazards: an analysis of 3.8 million exposure incidents. A report from the American Association of Poison Control Centers. Pediatrics 1992;89(6 Pt 1):999–1006.

66. White KC. Anemia is a poor predictor of iron deficiency among toddlers in the United States: for heme the bell tolls. Pediatrics 2005;115(2):315–20.
67. Mei Z, Cogswell ME, Parvanta I, et al. Hemoglobin and ferritin are currently the most efficient indicators of population response to iron interventions: an analysis of nine randomized controlled trials. J Nutr 2005;135(8):1974–80.
68. Raiten DJ, Ashour FA, Ross AC, et al. Inflammation and Nutritional Science for Programs/Policies and Interpretation of Research Evidence (INSPIRE). J Nutr 2015;145(5):1039S–108S.
69. Garcia-Casal MN, Peña-Rosas JP, Pasricha S-R. Rethinking ferritin cutoffs for iron deficiency and overload. Lancet Haematol 2014;1(2):e92–4.
70. Pasricha SR, Rooney P, Schneider H. Soluble transferrin receptor and depth of bone marrow suppression following high dose chemotherapy. Support Care Cancer 2009;17(7):847–50.
71. Pasricha SR, Frazer DM, Bowden DK, et al. Transfusion suppresses erythropoiesis and increases hepcidin in adult patients with beta-thalassemia major: a longitudinal study. Blood 2013;122(1):124–33.
72. Suominen P, Punnonen K, Rajamaki A, et al. Serum transferrin receptor and transferrin receptor-ferritin index identify healthy subjects with subclinical iron deficits. Blood 1998;92(8):2934–9.
73. World Health Organization, Centers for Disease Control and Prevention. Assessing the iron status of populations: including literature reviews. Report of a Joint World Health Organization/Centers for Disease Control and Prevention technical consultation on the assessment of iron status at the population level, Geneva, Switzerland, 6–8 April 2004. Geneva (Switzerland): World Health Organization/ Centers for Disease Control and Prevention; 2007.
74. Ganz T. Systemic iron homeostasis. Physiol Rev 2013;93(4):1721–41.
75. Kautz L, Jung G, Valore EV, et al. Identification of erythroferrone as an erythroid regulator of iron metabolism. Nat Genet 2014;46(7):678–84.
76. Choi HS, Song SH, Lee JH, et al. Serum hepcidin levels and iron parameters in children with iron deficiency. Korean J Hematol 2012;47(4):286–92.
77. Pasricha SR, McQuilten Z, Westerman M, et al. Serum hepcidin as a diagnostic test of iron deficiency in premenopausal female blood donors. Haematologica 2011;96(8):1099–105.
78. Pereira DI, Bruggraber SF, Faria N, et al. Nanoparticulate iron (III) oxo-hydroxide delivers safe iron that is well absorbed and utilised in humans. Nanomedicine 2014;10(8):1877–86.

The Present and Future Global Burden of the Inherited Disorders of Hemoglobin

Frédéric B. Piel, PhD

KEYWORDS

- Genetic disease • Sickle cell disease • Thalassemias • Public health
- Newborn screening • Malaria selection • Consanguinity • Human migrations

KEY POINTS

- The global burden of the inherited disorders of hemoglobin is increasing and this is finally starting to be recognized.
- Global, regional, and national newborn and population estimates need to be regularly updated to account for health and demographic changes, and this relies on reliable contemporary epidemiologic data.
- The highest burden of the inherited disorders of hemoglobin is and will remain in sub-Saharan Africa for sickle cell disease and in Southeast Asia for the thalassemias, and better prevention and management policies are urgently needed.

INTRODUCTION

The inherited disorders of hemoglobin represent the most common monogenic diseases. It has been estimated that around 7% of humans are carrying one of the mutations responsible for these disorders.[1] Although they have been extensively studied at the molecular and cellular level, epidemiologic data to assess the health burden of these disorders are often limited, particularly in regions of high prevalence, which are mostly found in tropical areas.[2] These neglected disorders are becoming an increasing health burden in low-, middle-, and high-income countries.[3] After a short description of the inherited disorders of hemoglobin, this article summarizes progress made toward better awareness and recognition of these disorders as a global health problem before presenting the main factors that influence their present and future burden, and discussing the strengths and limitations of existing estimates.

Department of Zoology, University of Oxford, South Parks Road, Oxford OX1 3PS, UK
E-mail address: fred.piel@zoo.ox.ac.uk

Hematol Oncol Clin N Am 30 (2016) 327–341
http://dx.doi.org/10.1016/j.hoc.2015.11.004
0889-8588/16/$ – see front matter © 2016 Elsevier Inc. All rights reserved.

INHERITED DISORDERS OF HEMOGLOBIN

These disorders are classified into two main groups: the structural variants of hemoglobin and the thalassemias, which both follow an autosomal-recessive pattern of inheritance. Maps showing the distribution of each disorder are shown in **Fig. 1**.

Structural Hemoglobin Variants

More than 1200 structural variants resulting mostly from single amino acid substitutions in the α- or β-globin chains have been identified.[4] Most of them have a limited geographic distribution and reached a low frequency. Nevertheless, the three polymorphisms described next are common and clinically significant.

Hemoglobin S

Hemoglobin S (HbS), also called sickle hemoglobin, is a structural variant of normal adult hemoglobin (HbA) caused by an amino acid substitution at position 6 of the β-globin chain (HBB c.20A > T; p.Glu6Val). Carriers or heterozygotes (HbAS) are almost always asymptomatic, whereas homozygotes (HbSS) suffer from sickle cell anemia, which often leads to acute and chronic complications including vaso-occlusive crisis, acute chest crisis, or hemolytic crisis.[5] Because of its high level of protection against *Plasmodium falciparum* malaria, HbS was initially largely restricted to Africa, the Middle East, and parts of India.[6] Nowadays, this variant is found in almost every country, but particularly in the Americas, the Caribbean, and Europe following human diasporas (see **Fig. 1**A).[7]

Hemoglobin C

HbC is another structural variant of HbA caused by an amino acid substitution (HBB c.19G > A; p.Glu6Lys) occurring at the same position as HbS. Although carriers

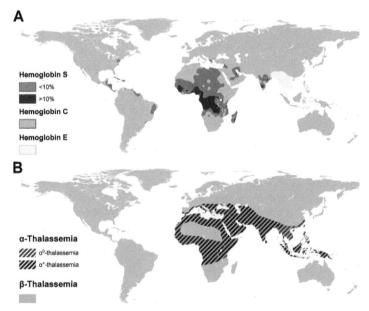

Fig. 1. Maps of the distribution of the inherited disorders of hemoglobin. (*A*) Structural hemoglobin variants. (*B*) Thalassemias. (*Adapted from* Refs.[7–9,61])

(HbAC) are asymptomatic, the inheritance of HbC from both parents (HbCC) causes clinically mild hemolytic anemia. In HbCC, red blood cells have a reduced solubility, which can lead to crystal formation. HbC is mainly of clinical significance when inherited in combination with HbS or with β-thalassemia. HbSC disease causes chronic hemolytic anemia and intermittent sickle cell crises, although slightly less severe or frequent than in HbSS. HbC-β thalassemia leads to moderate hemolytic anemia with splenomegaly. HbC was prevalent only in Western Africa but carriers are now found much more widely (see **Fig. 1**A).[8]

Hemoglobin E

HbE is a structural variant of normal hemoglobin (HBB c.79G > A; p.Glu26Lys) affecting the production rate of HbA. Heterozygotes with HbAE are asymptomatic, whereas homozygotes can present some mild clinical features similar to individuals with β-thalassemia trait. Globally, compound individuals with HbE and β-thalassemia represent the highest burden with a wide range of clinical severity. The most severely affected individuals are transfusion-dependent. HbE reaches frequencies up to 60% in parts of Thailand, Laos, and Cambodia, and is highly prevalent in India, Sri Lanka, and Malaysia (see **Fig. 1**A).

Thalassemias

The most common forms of thalassemias affect the rate of production of either the α- or β-globin chains that form the subunits of adult hemoglobin, leading to α- and β-thalassemia, respectively. Thalassemias are caused by a large variety of mutations and deletions, causing severity proportional to the inability to synthesize globin chains. Genotypically, both α- and β-thalassemias are classified into minor, intermediate, and major forms. Phenotypically, there is a continuum of severity ranging from asymptomatic to lethal. The geographic distribution of α- and β-thalassemias, which corresponds to the "thalassemia belt" (an area extending from the Mediterranean area through the Middle East and India, to Southeast Asia) is believed to be largely overlapping (see **Fig. 1**B). They are now also commonly found in many other parts of the world.[9]

α-Thalassemia

More than one hundred genetic variants of α-thalassemia have been identified.[4] Clinically relevant forms of α-thalassemia usually involve either the deletion of both pairs of α-globin genes on both chromosome resulting in hemoglobin Bart hydrops fetalis syndrome; or the coinheritance of one deleted or inactivated pair on one chromosome (termed α^0-thalassemia) and a partial production of α-globin chains on the other chromosome (termed α^+-thalassemia), caused by deletional or nondeletional variants, and causing HbH disease.[10] Furthermore, mild variants of α-thalassemia act as genetic modifiers of β-thalassemia and HbS. A recent study conducted in Sri Lanka confirmed that substantial variations in the prevalence of α-thalassemia variants can occur over relatively short distances.[11,12] Because most couples at risk for conceiving fetuses with hemoglobin Bart hydrops fetalis are not currently identified, determining the frequency of the different genetic variants observed in communities and identifying couples who are at risk is urgently needed.

β-Thalassemia

Approximately 250 variants of β-thalassemia identified at the molecular level have so far been shown to reduce the production of β-globin chains. Although most of these are single-nucleotide substitutions, reaching a low frequency within a limited geographic area, a handful of common variants is usually responsible for most of the clinical cases observed in any given region. Patients with the most severe forms of β-thalassemia require regular blood transfusions (typically every 3 weeks) and iron chelation to survive. Stem cell transplantation is the only curative treatment currently available and has been successfully performed in a large number of cases with severe β-thalassemia in high-income countries, but also more recently in some low- and middle-income countries. Screening programs for the prevention and control of β-thalassemia implemented in the 1970s, and often combined with prenatal or premarital diagnosis, have resulted in marked reductions in the birth rate of affected children in Greece, Cyprus, and Italy. Despite high levels of consanguinity, similar results have been reported in several countries in the Middle East following the implementation of large-scale education and counseling programs. However, facilities for simple screening are still lacking in many low- and middle-income countries.

GLOBAL HEALTH BURDEN
Awareness and Recognition

There is a concerning absence of official recognition of the inherited disorders of hemoglobin as a priority in public health at national, regional, and global scales.[13] Despite being the most common group of monogenic disorders in human populations, few countries have implemented large-scale prevention and management programs for the inherited disorders of hemoglobin and those programs are usually not in place in countries the most affected. This is probably best illustrated by the absence of any national program for sickle cell disease in African countries, whereas universal newborn screening has been implemented in high-income countries, such as the United Kingdom and the United States.[14] We next describe three institutions that have major roles in creating awareness about the inherited disorders of hemoglobin, before listing several initiatives led by the clinical and academic communities to create global and regional networks.

World Health Organization

The World Health Organization (WHO; http://www.who.int/en/) adopted two resolutions recognizing the importance of the inherited hemoglobin disorders. In May 2006, the 59th World Health Assembly's resolution on sickle cell disease (WHA59.20) recognized that "sickle cell anemia is one of the world's foremost genetic diseases, that it has severe physical, psychological and social consequences for those affected and their families, and that in its homozygote form it is one of the most lethal genetic diseases" and urged Member States to develop and strengthen efforts to prevent and manage sickle cell anemia.[15] This first resolution was further highlighted shortly after at the 118th meeting of the WHO Executive Board by a second one on the thalassemias and other hemoglobinopathies raising concerns about the impact of these disorders on global mortality and morbidity, especially in developing countries, and calling on affected countries and the Secretariat of WHO to strengthen their response to these conditions.[16] In May 2010, the 63rd World Health Assembly adopted an additional resolution on the prevention and management of birth defects, including sickle cell disease and the thalassemias. Through these resolutions, the WHO committed to (1) increase awareness among the international community of the global burden of these disorders, (2) promote equitable access to health services, (3) provide technical support to countries for the prevention and management of these disorders, and (4) promote and support research to improve the quality of life of those affected. In practice, however, the leading role of the WHO to achieve these goals seems to have been quite limited.

Global Burden of Diseases, Injuries, and Risk Factors Study
The Global Burden of Diseases, Injuries, and Risk Factors Study (GBD)[17] is a comprehensive regional and global assessment of mortality (in terms of years of life lost) and disability (in terms of years lived with a disability) from major diseases, injuries, and risk factors (See Kassebaum NJ: The Global Burden of Anemia, in this issue). GBD 2013 produced estimates for 323 diseases and injuries, 67 risk factors, and 1500 sequelae for 188 countries. Disability-adjusted life-years (DALYs) is used as an overall measure of years of life lost and years lived with a disability. The first GBD was published in 1990, which is now used as a reference point for later iterations. GBD 2010 was the first GBD to include the inherited disorders of hemoglobin. Future iterations are expected to be generated on an annual basis. One of the main findings of the GBD is the shift in global health burden from infectious (or communicable) diseases to chronic (or noncommunicable) diseases. GBD 2010 ranked sickle cell disorders 70th (up from 74th in 1990) and the thalassemias 68th (down from 65th in 1990) in terms of DALYs across all ages, respectively. These disorders ranked 17th and 24th, respectively, in the 1- to 4-years age group, reflecting their substantial impact on mortality and morbidity in children younger than 5. GBD 2010 estimated that sickle cell disorders and thalassemias were resulting in 28,640 (confidence interval, 16,756–40,869) and 17,860 (confidence interval, 15,071–20,430) deaths per year, respectively. Although these rankings and estimates are often based on limited epidemiologic data and need refining, they help to show the global health burden associated with the inherited disorders of hemoglobin. Data from GBD 2013 confirm that, whereas the global burden of communicable diseases is decreasing, the inherited disorders of hemoglobin present an increasing burden (http://ghdx.healthdata.org/global-burden-disease-study-2013-gbd-2013-data-downloads).

Thalassaemia International Federation
Thalassaemia International Federation (TIF)[18] is a patient-driven organization working in official relations with the WHO since 1996 and with more than 100 national thalassemia associations within 57 countries. Its primary mission is to work toward equal access to quality health care for every patient with a thalassemia syndrome across the world. TIF's aims to achieve this largely overlap with those of the WHO. In addition to organizing regular global and regional conferences involving clinicians, academics, and patients and patient societies, TIF participates in the formulation and/or amendment of policies in many areas related to the inherited disorders of hemoglobin and actively contributes in adapting these policies to the national level.

Global Sickle Cell Disease Network, Caribbean Association for Researchers in Sickle Cell Disease and Thalassemia, and Sickle Cell Disease Research Network in Central Africa
The Global Sickle Cell Disease Network[19] brings together leading researchers and clinicians in sickle cell disease from high-, middle-, and low-income countries to lead a real change in terms of awareness, research, prevention, and treatment that will not only have a positive impact on children born with sickle cell disease, but also on whole communities and regions. In parallel, several regional networks have been created including, in 2006, the Caribbean Association for Researchers in Sickle Cell Disease and Thalassemia, which brings together 11 countries in the Caribbean region, and in 2010, the Sickle Cell Disease Research Network in Central Africa—Réseau d'Etudes de la Drépanocytose en Afrique Centrale, in which eight Central African countries are involved. Similar networks in West Africa, the Middle East, and India are currently being set up. Such networks aim at stimulating South-South collaborative research projects within regions affected, while promoting awareness and improving prevention

and management of the inherited disorders of hemoglobin. Through such networks, policies, methods, and protocols can be standardized, which facilitates epidemiologic studies aiming to assess the burden of these disorders.

Factors Affecting the Health Burden of the Inherited Disorders of Hemoglobin

Malaria selection

The inherited disorders of hemoglobin represent a textbook example of natural selection and balanced polymorphism. It is now well established that they reached high frequencies across large geographic areas because of the protection conferred by heterozygote forms against P falciparum malaria.[20,21] The improved fitness of those individuals compensates the loss of severely affected homozygotes, allowing the frequency of these disorders to increase. This hypothesis, now commonly called the malaria hypothesis, was first formulated by Haldane[22] in 1949 for the thalassemias and Allison[23] in 1954 for sickle cell disease because of a striking overlap in the geographic distribution of malaria and these disorders. Clear evidence from clinical studies and mechanistic studies conducted in vitro and ex vivo has now added strong support to this hypothesis. Although the mechanisms for malaria protection have been elucidated for some inherited disorders of hemoglobin, controversies remain for others.[24] Recent clinical[25] and theoretic[26] studies have highlighted the importance of epistatic interactions in explaining the frequency and geographic distribution of the inherited disorders of hemoglobin. It is worth keeping in mind that despite considerable efforts to eliminate malaria, this selection mechanism is still ongoing in malarious regions.[27] In nonmalarious regions, whether the mutations have been selected for previously or introduced through population migrations, kinetic models of the spread of genetic disease suggest that declines in the frequency of these disorders are likely to occur very slowly over multiple generations.[28] Studies on sickle cell disease conducted over a couple of decades in Jamaica also showed that substantial improvements in the survival of homozygotes can interfere with the expected decline in allele frequency.[29,30]

Consanguinity

In many parts of the world, marriages between close biologic kin are preferred for a range of cultural, ethnical, socioeconomic, and religious reasons. Such marriages are categorized as consanguineous when they occur between persons biologically related as second cousins (F $\geq$0.0156). This is common practice among one-fifth of the world population mostly residing in the Middle East, West Asia, and North Africa, and among emigrants from these communities now residing in North America, Europe, and Australia.[31] From a genetic perspective, consanguinity contributes to increasing the frequency of deleterious recessive mutations.[32] Although consanguinity certainly contributes to increasing the global burden of the inherited disorders of hemoglobin,[33] it is difficult to measure and likely to vary substantially within most countries. Current prevalence data are quite limited and inaccurate, and do not allow to precisely account for the effect of consanguinity on burden estimates.[32]

Population growth

The number of individuals affected by the inherited disorders of hemoglobin is proportional to the overall human population. Based on a total population of 7.3 billion individuals in 2015 and an estimate of 7% carrying one of the mutations underlying these disorders, half a billion individuals either suffer from one inherited disorder of hemoglobin or face the risk of having a child affected. With a world population expected to reach almost 10 billion in 2050 and much faster population growth in tropical and subtropical regions, demography alone provides strong evidence for the increasing burden of this group of disorders. Recent estimates purely based on demographic projections suggested that the annual number of births affected by sickle cell anemia would increase by 33% between 2010 and 2050.[34]

Epidemiologic transition

The epidemiologic transition theory assumes that a shift from high birth and death rates to low birth and death rates along with the economic development is also accompanied by a relative increase in the impact of chronic noninfectious diseases in terms of mortality and morbidity (**Fig. 2**).[35] Through substantial improvements in hygiene, nutrition, public health policies, and infrastructures, partly driven by the Millennium Development Goals, impressive reductions in overall infant and childhood mortality have been observed.[36,37] As a result, newborns with a severe inherited disorder of hemoglobin who would have previously died undiagnosed are now more likely to survive. As shown in high-income countries, early diagnosis can help prevent serious long-term complications.[38,39] Nevertheless, such a diagnosis is only meaningful if it is accompanied by access to health care and regular follow-up.

Human migrations

The mobility of human beings worldwide has reached an unprecedented level. With changes in the modes and speed of international transportation, constraints previously imposed by natural barriers and long distances have greatly reduced. The number of international migrants increased from 92.6 million in 1960, to 165.2 million in 2000, and estimates suggest that the global number of migrants potentially carrying the sickle cell mutation increased from about 1.6 million in 1960 to 3.6 million in 2000.[40] As best illustrated by the example of the Americas, international migrations can have a long-term effect on public health through the introduction of deleterious genes into populations in which they were previously absent. The presence of the sickle cell mutation is a reminder of the legacies of the slave trade from the African continent to North and South America and the Caribbean islands and of more recent immigration from Mediterranean countries (including Greece and Italy),[41,42] whereas large immigration from southeast Asian countries to California and other parts of the United States in recent decades has led to increasing numbers of patients affected by severe forms of thalassemias.[43] Similar trends are observed in Western Europe.[44] Population movements also affect the distribution of inherited disorders of hemoglobin within countries, with previously isolated populations increasingly interacting and large numbers of migrants moving from rural to urban areas,[45] and the complexity of genotypes that can be observed, because newly introduced variants can interact with local ones to create more or less severe phenotypes.[46]

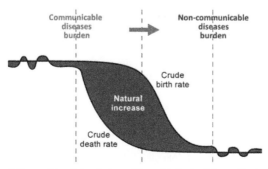

Fig. 2. Schematic of the epidemiologic transition. (*Adapted from* Rockett IRH. Population and health: an introduction to epidemiology. Popul Bull 1999;54(4):3–44.)

Population stratification

A range of factors, including socioeconomic, genetic, ethnic, cultural, or religious considerations, can lead to a local population being divided into subgroups, which affects reproductive behaviors.[47] Population stratification is particularly obvious in earlier generations of immigrant populations following international migrations or in large urban centers where populations presenting different frequencies of genetic traits might converge but not necessarily mix.[48] Similarly to consanguinity, such behaviors can contribute to increasing the probability of having children affected by inherited disorders of hemoglobin compared with random mating.[32] Population stratification should therefore be accounted for when calculating estimates of populations affected and the health burden of inherited disorders of hemoglobin.

Current Health Burden

Most current efforts to assess the burden of the inherited disorders of hemoglobin are based on the remarkable work conducted by Livingstone,[49] who assembled a global database of the frequencies of hemoglobin variants, thalassemias, glucose-6-phosphate dehydrogenase deficiency, and ovalocytosis in human populations during more than two decades, from the 1960s to the middle of the 1980s.

Newborn estimates

In the 1990s, Bernadette Modell updated Livingstone's work on hemoglobin variants and gathered additional data on the thalassemias from research reviews, country visits, and members of the former WHO Working Group on Hemoglobin Disorders into an almanac. This work led to the publication of global, regional, and national estimates of annual affected births and pregnant carriers for all major inherited disorders of hemoglobin in addition to a range of other indicators of annual service needs.[33] Some of the national estimates produced were based on a limited number of small surveys and did not reflect or account for the striking spatial heterogeneities observed in micromapping surveys. Nevertheless, despite these limitations, these are the only estimates of the overall health burden posed by the inherited disorders of hemoglobin. Regional estimates are presented in **Table 1**.

Recently, we combined an evidence-base dataset on sickle cell disease based on a systematic review of the published literature with demographic data into a modern geostatistical modeling framework to account for spatial heterogeneities and provide precision measures. We estimated the global number of HbAS and HbSS births in 2010 to be 5,476,000 (interquartile range, 5,291,000–5,679,000) and 312,000 (294,000–330,000), respectively.[7] These estimates were calculated using Hardy-Weinberg assumptions and do not account for deviations from this model, caused for example, by consanguinity or population structure. Further work suggests that correcting for these factors could lead to substantially higher estimates.[50] A region-by-region comparison of our estimates with Modell's is shown in **Table 2**. Significant differences were frequently observed at the national level, highlighting the need for detailed and reliable epidemiologic data. Although a similar methodology has also been applied to estimate the number of births affected by HbC[8] or populations carrying Duffy negativity[51] and severe variants of glucose-6-phosphate dehydrogenase deficiency deficiency,[52] similar work is still lacking for α- and β-thalassemia.

Population estimates

Although newborn estimates certainly allow to some extent to measure the magnitude of the burden of the inherited disorders of hemoglobin and spatiotemporal changes, estimates across all ages are required to define overall public health policies.

Table 1
Global and regional estimates of newborns affected by severe forms of the inherited disorders of hemoglobin, based on demographic data from 2003

WHO Region	Population (×1000)	Births/Year (×1000)	Structural Hb Variants					Thalassemia					Total
			Sickle Cell Disorders			HbC	HbE	α-Thalassemia		β-Thalassemia			
			SS	S/C	S/bThal	CC	EE	HbH Disease	Hb Bart Hydrops	β Major	HbE/βTh	HbC/βTh	
AFRO	586,363	22,895.0	184,812	52,298	7367	14,227	0	11	0	1517	2	2717	262,951
AMRO	852,769	16,608.9	4432	2283	1381	366	233	484	17	347	76	368	9989
EMRO	573,249	16,798.5	7389	62	6639	99	101	2	0	11,566	158	113	26,129
EURO	879,419	10,458.8	376	127	274	28	16	0	0	1310	10	18	2159
SEARO	1,564,232	38,139.0	25,768	0	270	0	56,254	2599	1017	7556	14,155	0	107,619
WPRO	1,761,269	23,914	9	1	3	0	29,623	6479	4152	2869	4735	0	47,873
World	6,217,301	128,814	222,785	54,771	15,934	14,719	86,228	9576	5187	25,164	19,137	3216	456,720

Adapted from Modell B, Darlison M. Global epidemiology of haemoglobin disorders and derived service indicators. Bull World Health Organ 2008;86:480–7. Available online at: http://www.modell-almanac.net/; with permission.

Table 2
Annual estimates of newborns with sickle cell anemia within each WHO region from Piel and colleagues,[7] 2013, compared with those of Modell and Darlison,[33] 2008

	Mean	Median	IQR		M&D	
AFRO	239,547	238,083	224,003	253,047	184,812	a
AMRO	13,708	13,104	11,126	15,606	4432	a
EMRO	10,007	8239	6012	11,951	7389	—
EURO	3653	3271	2408	4366	376	a
SEARO	44,132	42,597	35,022	50,750	25,768	a
WPRO	4	9	2	33	9	—

Abbreviations: IQR, interquartile range; M&D, Modell and Darlison.
 [a] Significant differences (P<.05).
 Data from Piel FB, Patil AP, Howes RE, et al. Global epidemiology of sickle haemoglobin in neonates: a contemporary geostatistical model-based map and population estimates. Lancet 2013;381(9861):142–51; and Modell B, Darlison M. Global epidemiology of haemoglobin disorders and derived service indicators. Bull World Health Organ 2008;86:480–7.

Generating such estimates relies on the availability of mortality data and survival curves, which are currently nonexistent in areas of high prevalence and high burden.[53] The challenges associated with calculating such estimates, even in high-income countries, have recently been highlighted in the context of sickle cell disease in the United States.[54] The GBD 2013 has started to produce estimates of the prevalence, mortality, and DALYs associated with the inherited disorders of hemoglobin, which will be very important to increase the focus on their prevention and management. Beyond this project, it is essential to conduct specific epidemiologic studies on the inherited disorders of hemoglobin to validate the GBD results and to monitor achievements.

Future Health Burden

Although the burden of the inherited disorders of hemoglobin is increasing and this global issue is finally being recognized, there are relatively few data aimed at quantifying this increase. Assessing the future health burden of diseases primarily relies on the quality of past and present epidemiologic data. Existing data on the prevalence of the inherited disorders of hemoglobin are often limited and patchy, which is reflected by large uncertainties in national estimates and, to some extent, by discrepancies between estimates from different sources. As shown for sickle cell disease,[34] the combination of detailed evidence-based newborn estimates with high-resolution demographic projections allows to quantify the expected increase in births affected and to test the impact of different intervention scenarios. Until more reliable contemporary estimates are available for the thalassemias, any estimates of their future burden should be considered with great caution. Generating and assembling epidemiologic data at national, regional, and global levels is a crucial element to defining sustainable policies for the prevention and management of the inherited disorders of hemoglobin. A range of health policies can be implemented to prevent or manage these disorders and there is now some good evidence from a range of countries to draw important conclusions about their long-term impact.

Preventing affected births

Until cures that can be used at large scale in low- and middle-income settings become available, the only way to substantially reduce the future burden of the inherited disorders of hemoglobin is through the prevention of affected births. The underlying idea is that, if patients and carriers are aware of their status, they can make informed choices about their partner when they reach reproductive stages. The implementation of public education, population screening, genetic counseling, and antenatal diagnosis in the 1970s in Cyprus, Greece, and Sicily has successfully reduced the number of patients affected by severe thalassemia.[55,56] Similar measures, sometimes supported by legal measures, have been reported more recently in various countries in the Middle East.[57] Successful examples of the impact of these interventions on sickle cell disease are more limited, which could be partly explained by the remarkable heterogeneity in the severity of this disease.[58]

Managing affected births

Although most newborns affected by severe forms of the inherited disorders of hemoglobin in low- and middle-income are still very likely to die in early childhood, substantial improvements in their survival have been achieved in high-income countries, in particular in the United States and in the United Kingdom, through early diagnosis followed by for sickle cell disease, the use of penicillin prophylaxis to prevent infections (eg, *Streptococcus pneumonia*, *Haemophilus influenzae*, *Salmonella* spp, and *Escherichia Coli*), transcranial Doppler ultrasound, followed by life-long blood transfusion to prevent strokes, and access to pain killers, including opioids, to reduce the impact of acute pain crises; and for the thalassemias the use of lifelong blood transfusion and the availability of efficient iron chelators. Despite these advances, the life expectancy of patients with the inherited disorders of hemoglobin is still often 30 years less than the average life expectancy and the costs of health care for children and adults with these disorders are extremely high.[59] Progress in low- and middle-income countries has been much more limited particularly across sub-Saharan Africa for sickle cell disease and across Southeast Asia for severe thalassemias.[2,60]

Carrier detection

Finally, whether carriers, including individuals with sickle cell trait (HbAS) or those with thalassemia minor (also called silent carriers), should be part of any health policy about the prevention and management of the inherited disorders of hemoglobin is still an open debate within the clinical and academic communities.[56] Although it is obvious that they do not represent a health burden in the short-term, the future burden of these disorders depends on them and on their reproductive behaviors. The impact of large population movements and increased admixture will contribute to dilute the mutations responsible for these disorders within a larger part of the population worldwide, which will have important consequences in terms of the needs for precise and reliable identification techniques.

SUMMARY

A global success in the prevention and management of the increasing health burden of inherited disorders of hemoglobin depends on progress made, in terms of (1) access to health care; (2) reliable diagnosis and screening (premarital, neonatal, and/or postnatal); and (3) awareness, education, and genetic counseling in low- and middle-income countries, particularly in sub-Saharan Africa for sickle cell disease and in Southeast Asia for severe thalassemias. Now that the burden of these disorders is finally being recognized, this relies on the development of specific interventions tailored to these settings, rather than on the replication of those implemented in high-income countries, and on the support of health organizations and funding agencies. At all stages of this process, it is crucial to continue gathering epidemiologic data to assess spatial and temporal changes, and to measure progress made.

ACKNOWLEDGMENTS

The author thanks Carina Hockham for comments on an earlier version of the article.

REFERENCES

1. Weatherall D, Akinyanju O, Fucharoen S, et al. Inherited disorders of hemoglobin. In: Jamison DT, Breman JG, Measham AR, et al, editors. Disease control priorities in developing countries. 2nd edition. Washington, DC: World Bank; 2006. p. 663–80.
2. Weatherall DJ. The challenge of haemoglobinopathies in resource-poor countries. Br J Haematol 2011;154(6):736–44.
3. Weatherall DJ. The inherited diseases of hemoglobin are an emerging global health burden. Blood 2010;115(22):4331–6.
4. Giardine B, Borg J, Viennas E, et al. Updates of the HbVar database of human hemoglobin variants and thalassemia mutations. Nucleic Acids Res 2014; 42(Database issue):D1063–9.
5. Rees DC, Williams TN, Gladwin MT. Sickle-cell disease. Lancet 2010;376(9757): 2018–31.
6. Piel FB, Patil AP, Howes RE, et al. Global distribution of the sickle cell gene and geographical confirmation of the malaria hypothesis. Nat Commun 2010; 1:104.
7. Piel FB, Patil AP, Howes RE, et al. Global epidemiology of sickle haemoglobin in neonates: a contemporary geostatistical model-based map and population estimates. Lancet 2013;381(9861):142–51.
8. Piel FB, Howes RE, Patil AP, et al. The distribution of haemoglobin C and its prevalence in newborns in Africa. Sci Rep 2013;3:1671.
9. Weatherall DJ, Clegg JB. The thalassaemia syndromes. 4th edition. Oxford (United Kingdom); Malden (MA): Blackwell Science; 2001.
10. Piel FB, Weatherall DJ. The α-thalassemias. N Engl J Med 2014;371(20):1908–16.
11. Weatherall DJ. The importance of micromapping the gene frequencies for the common inherited disorders of haemoglobin. Br J Haematol 2010;149(5): 635–7.
12. Suresh S, Fisher C, Ayyub H, et al. Alpha thalassaemia and extended alpha globin genes in Sri Lanka. Blood Cells Mol Dis 2013;50(2):93–8.
13. Weatherall D. The inherited disorders of haemoglobin: an increasingly neglected global health burden. Indian J Med Res 2011;134:493–7.
14. Streetly A, Latinovic R, Hall K, et al. Implementation of universal newborn bloodspot screening for sickle cell disease and other clinically significant haemoglobinopathies in England: screening results for 2005-7. J Clin Pathol 2009;62(1): 26–30.
15. World Health Organization. Sickle-cell anaemia (WHA59.20). Fifty-ninth world health assembly resolutions and decisions. Geneva (Switzerland): WHO; 2006.
16. WHO Executive Board. Resolution on thalassaemia and other haemoglobinopathies (EB118.R1), 118th session. Geneva (Switzerland): WHO; 2008.
17. Global Burden of Diseases IaRF. Available at: http://www.healthdata.org/gbd. Accessed June 30, 2015.
18. Thalassemia International Federation. Available at: http://www.thalassaemia.org. cy/. Accessed June 30, 2015.

19. Global Sickle Cell Disease Network. Available at: http://globalsicklecelldisease. org/. Accessed June 30, 2015.
20. Kwiatkowski DP. How malaria has affected the human genome and what human genetics can teach us about malaria. Am J Hum Genet 2005;77(2):171–92.
21. Hedrick PW. Population genetics of malaria resistance in humans. Heredity (Edinb) 2011;107(4):283–304.
22. Haldane JBS. The rate of mutation of human genes. Hereditas 1949;35(S1): 267–73.
23. Allison AC. Protection afforded by sickle-cell trait against subtertian malareal infection. Br Med J 1954;1(4857):290–4.
24. Williams TN, Weatherall DJ. World distribution, population genetics, and health burden of the hemoglobinopathies. Cold Spring Harb Perspect Med 2012;2(9): a011692.
25. Williams TN, Mwangi TW, Wambua S, et al. Negative epistasis between the malaria-protective effects of alpha+-thalassemia and the sickle cell trait. Nat Genet 2005;37(11):1253–7.
26. Penman BS, Pybus OG, Weatherall DJ, et al. Epistatic interactions between genetic disorders of hemoglobin can explain why the sickle-cell gene is uncommon in the Mediterranean. Proc Natl Acad Sci U S A 2009;106(50):21242–6.
27. Elguero E, Delicat-Loembet LM, Rougeron V, et al. Malaria continues to select for sickle cell trait in central Africa. Proc Natl Acad Sci U S A 2015;112(22): 7051–4.
28. Veytsman B. Environment change, geographic migration and sickle cell anaemia. Evol Ecol 1997;11(5):519–29.
29. Hanchard NA, Hambleton I, Harding RM, et al. The frequency of the sickle allele in Jamaica has not declined over the last 22 years. Br J Haematol 2005;130(6): 939–42.
30. Hanchard NA, Hambleton I, Harding RM, et al. Predicted declines in sickle allele frequency in Jamaica using empirical data. Am J Hematol 2006;81(11): 817–23.
31. Hamamy H. Consanguineous marriages: preconception consultation in primary health care settings. J Community Genet 2012;3(3):185–92.
32. Bittles AH, Black ML. Consanguinity, human evolution, and complex diseases. Proc Natl Acad Sci U S A 2010;107(Suppl 1):1779–86.
33. Modell B, Darlison M. Global epidemiology of haemoglobin disorders and derived service indicators. Bull World Health Organ 2008;86:480–7.
34. Piel FB, Hay SI, Gupta S, et al. Global burden of sickle cell anaemia in children under five, 2010-2050: modelling based on demographics, excess mortality, and interventions. PLoS Med 2013;10(7):e1001484.
35. Omran AR. The epidemiologic transition: a theory of the epidemiology of population change. 1971. Milbank Q 2005;83(4):731–57.
36. Rajaratnam JK, Marcus JR, Flaxman AD, et al. Neonatal, postneonatal, childhood, and under-5 mortality for 187 countries, 1970-2010: a systematic analysis of progress towards millennium development goal 4. Lancet 2010;375(9730): 1988–2008.
37. GBD 2013 Mortality and Causes of Death Collaborators. Global, regional, and national age–sex specific all-cause and cause-specific mortality for 240 causes of death, 1990–2013: a systematic analysis for the Global Burden of Disease Study 2013. Lancet 2015;385(9963):117–71.
38. Gaston MH, Verter JI, Woods G, et al. Prophylaxis with oral penicillin in children with sickle cell anemia. N Engl J Med 1986;314(25):1593–9.

39. Adams RJ, McKie VC, Hsu L, et al. Prevention of a first stroke by transfusions in children with sickle cell anemia and abnormal results on transcranial Doppler ultrasonography. N Engl J Med 1998;339(1):5–11.
40. Piel FB, Tatem AJ, Huang Z, et al. Global migration and the changing distribution of sickle haemoglobin: a quantitative study of temporal trends between 1960 and 2000. Lancet Glob Health 2014;2(2):e80–9.
41. Schroeder WA, Munger ES, Powars DR. Sickle cell anaemia, genetic variations, and the slave trade to the United States. J Afr Hist 1990;31(2):163–80.
42. Pante-de-Sousa G, Mousinho-Ribeiro RDC, Santos EJMD, et al. Origin of the hemoglobin S gene in a Northern Brazilian population: the combined effects of slave trade and internal migrations. Genet Mol Biol 1998;21:427–30.
43. Vichinsky EP, MacKlin EA, Waye JS, et al. Changes in the epidemiology of thalassemia in North America: a new minority disease. Pediatrics 2005;116(6): e818–25.
44. Aguilar Martinez P, Angastiniotis M, Eleftheriou A, et al. Haemoglobinopathies in Europe: health & migration policy perspectives. Orphanet J Rare Dis 2014; 9:97.
45. Mohammed AO, Attalla B, Bashir FMK, et al. Relationship of the sickle cell gene to the ethnic and geographic groups populating the Sudan. Community Genet 2006;9(2):113–20.
46. McBride KL, Snow K, Kubik KS, et al. Hb Dartmouth [α66(E15)Leu → Pro (α2) (CTG → CCG)]: a novel α2-globin gene mutation associated with severe neonatal anemia when inherited in trans with Southeast Asian α-thalassemia-1. Hemoglobin 2001;25(4):375–82.
47. Garnier-Géré P, Chikhi L. Population subdivision, Hardy–Weinberg equilibrium and the Wahlund effect. Chichester: John Wiley & Sons, Ltd; 2001.
48. Overall AD, Ahmad M, Thomas MG, et al. An analysis of consanguinity and social structure within the UK Asian population using microsatellite data. Ann Hum Genet 2003;67(Pt 6):525–37.
49. Livingstone FB. Frequencies of hemoglobin variants: thalassemia, the glucose-6-phosphate dehydrogenase deficiency, G6PD variants, and ovalocytosis in human populations. New York: Oxford University Press; 1985.
50. Piel FB, Adamkiewitzc TV, Amendah DD, et al. Observed and expected frequencies of structural haemoglobin variants in newborn screening programmes in Africa and the Middle East. Genetics in Medicine 2015. [Epub ahead of print].
51. Howes RE, Patil AP, Piel FB, et al. The global distribution of the Duffy blood group. Nat Commun 2011;2:266.
52. Howes RE, Piel FB, Patil AP, et al. G6PD deficiency prevalence and estimates of affected populations in malaria endemic countries: a geostatistical model-based map. PLoS Med 2012;9(11):e1001339.
53. Grosse SD, Odame I, Atrash HK, et al. Sickle cell disease in Africa: a neglected cause of early childhood mortality. Am J Prev Med 2011;41(6 Suppl 4): S398–405.
54. Hassell KL. Population estimates of sickle cell disease in the U.S. Am J Prev Med 2010;38(4 Suppl):S512–21.
55. Angastiniotis MA, Hadjiminas MG. Prevention of thalassaemia in Cyprus. Lancet 1981;1(8216):369–71.
56. Cao A, Kan YW. The prevention of thalassemia. Cold Spring Harb Perspect Med 2013;3(2):a011775.
57. Al Arrayed S, Al Hajeri A. Newborn screening services in Bahrain between 1985 and 2010. Adv Hematol 2012;2012:4.

58. Steinberg MH. Predicting clinical severity in sickle cell anaemia. Br J Haematol 2005;129(4):465–81.
59. Kauf TL, Coates TD, Huazhi L, et al. The cost of health care for children and adults with sickle cell disease. Am J Hematol 2009;84(6):323–7.
60. Colah R, Gorakshakar A, Nadkarni A. Global burden, distribution and prevention of β-thalassemias and hemoglobin E disorders. Expert Rev Hematol 2010;3(1): 103–17.
61. Weatherall DJ. Phenotype—genotype relationships in monogenic disease: lessons from the thalassaemias. Nat Rev Genet 2001;2(4):245–55.

Sickle Cell Disease in Sub-Saharan Africa

Thomas N. Williams, MBBS, DCH, DTM&H, MRCP, PhD[a,b],*

KEYWORDS

- Sickle cell disease • Children • Public health • Bacteremia • Sub-Saharan Africa

KEY POINTS

- Sickle cell disease is a common and growing health problem in many parts of sub-Saharan Africa (SSA), where at least 240,000 affected children are born with the condition every year.
- Sickle cell disease is widely neglected on the continent, where an estimated 50% to 90% of those born with the condition die undiagnosed before their fifth birthdays.
- An unknown, but probably large, proportion of these deaths are almost certainly attributable to 2 main conditions: malaria and invasive bacterial infections.
- With economic and public health advancements in many parts of the region, survival of affected children is likely to improve, which will lead to a growing need for appropriate medical services.
- A greater emphasis on basic and applied research in the area of sickle cell disease in SSA could lead to substantial improvements to the lives and livelihoods of millions of affected people and their families.

INTRODUCTION

Sickle hemoglobin (HbS) is a structural variant of normal adult hemoglobin (HbA; $\alpha_2\beta_2$) in which the normal beta-globin subunit is replaced by a mutant form of the molecule (β^S) in which the glutamic acid residue normally present at position 6 is replaced by a valine residue, the result of a single nucleotide polymorphism (thymine to adenine; rs334) at position 17 of the HBB gene.[1] This abnormal HbS polymerizes reversibly under low oxygen tension, and alterations to the shape, rheological properties, and membrane properties of the red blood cells that result from these

Disclosure: The author has nothing to disclose.
[a] Department of Medicine, Imperial College of Science, Technology and Medicine, St Mary's Hospital, Praed Street, London W21N, UK; [b] Department of Epidemiology and Demography, KEMRI/Wellcome Trust Research Programme, PO Box 230, Kilifi, Kenya
* Corresponding author. Imperial College of Science Technology and Medicine, St Mary's Hospital, London W21N, UK.
E-mail address: tom.williams@imperial.ac.uk

Hematol Oncol Clin N Am 30 (2016) 343–358
http://dx.doi.org/10.1016/j.hoc.2015.11.005
0889-8588/16/$ – see front matter © 2016 Elsevier Inc. All rights reserved.

hemonc.theclinics.com

polymerization events are central to the pathophysiology of the resultant disease.[2] The term sickle cell disease (SCD) refers to a heterogeneous group of conditions in which HbS predominates. The most common form of SCD results from the homozygous inheritance of the β^S mutation, a condition most commonly referred to as either HbSS or sickle cell anemia (SCA). Although SCA is responsible for at least 70% of SCD globally,[3] SCD can also result from compound heterozygosity for HbS in association with a wide range of other *HBB* mutations, including the mutation that results in the production of another structural variant, hemoglobin β^C (HbSC) and one of the many β-thalassemia mutations that lead to the reduced production of normal beta-globin (HbS/β-thalassemia).[4] Although the geographic range of HbS extends throughout most of sub-Saharan Africa (SSA) north of the Zambezi river, both HbC and β-thalassemia are confined to more limited parts of West Africa and to the historic trade routes of North Africa. As a result, HbSS is by far the most significant form of SCD in SSA, and the form of SCD about which most is known. HbSS is therefore the main focus of this article.

ORIGINS OF THE SICKLE MUTATION

Haplotype analysis suggests that the rs334 allele that encodes for β^s has arisen, and been independently amplified to its current population frequencies, on at least 2 and likely more occasions.[5,6] Despite being detrimental in its homozygous form (HbSS) the rs334 allele has reached high population frequencies throughout much of SSA to the extent that through much of the continent more than 15% of the population are heterozygotes (HbAS; sickle cell trait), and notably more than twice that in small surveys from selected populations.[7] That such high heterozygote frequencies might result from selection for HbAS through a survival advantage against malaria was first suggested more than 6 decades ago[8] and, despite some early skepticism, this hypothesis has since been confirmed beyond any reasonable doubt (reviewed in Ref.[9]). In a recent meta-analysis of available data from 44 studies conducted throughout the continent, Taylor and colleagues[10] estimated that children with HbAS are more than 90% less likely to develop severe and complicated *Plasmodium falciparum* malaria, the form of malaria associated with the most deaths, than normal children with HbAA. This conclusion has recently been reaffirmed in the most substantial study of its kind conducted to date, involving almost 12,000 children with severe malaria and more than 17,000 controls recruited from 12 sites throughout the malaria-endemic world, in which the odds ratio (OR) for severe malaria among HbAS children was 0.14 and was associated with a significance level rarely seen in such studies ($P = 1.6 \times 10^{-225}$).[11] Moreover, the effect of HbAS is not limited to the most severe forms of malaria but also extends to protection against uncomplicated forms of the disease,[10] with the result that HbAS confers even wider health benefits and survival advantages by protecting against the longer-term consequences of uncomplicated malaria, such as chronic anemia,[12] malnutrition,[12,13] and invasive bacterial infections.[14,15]

The precise mechanism by which HbS protects against malaria remains a subject of some speculation. Early work suggested that erythrocytes containing HbS might be less supportive of *P falciparum* growth and multiplication than normal red cells under low oxygen tension,[16–19] but more recently it has been suggested that HbS might protect against malaria by mediating the reduced display of the parasite-encoded protein *P falciparum* erythrocyte membrane protein-1 (PfEMP1) on the surface of malaria-infected erythrocytes.[20,21] The adherence of *P falciparum*–infected red blood cells to capillary endothelium has been implicated in both the pathogenesis of severe malaria and in the evasion of parasite-infected red blood cells from immunologic removal by the spleen, and so it has been speculated that reduced PfEMP1 display might result in both fewer pathologic consequences and improved clearance of infected red cells during malaria infections.[20] In addition, it has also been suggested that parasite-infected HbS-containing erythrocytes may be removed more rapidly from circulation through innate or acquired immune-mediated processes[16,22–24]; a process that might also result in their premature destruction by the spleen.[16,25]

SICKLE CELL DISEASE IN SUB-SAHARAN AFRICA

The corollary of positive selection for HbAS through a survival advantage against malaria is that a small but variable proportion of children in malaria-endemic parts of SSA are born with either HbSS or with compound heterozygosity for both HbS and a second mutation that, together with HbS, results in SCD, the most notable being HbSC and HbS/β-thalassemia. Historically, SCD has nevertheless been profoundly neglected in the African context and even today the knowledge of a range of basic facts regarding the condition within the region is decades behind that for regions where SCD is considerably less common.

Despite the publication of a growing number of reports on the prevalence and distribution of the sickle cell trait in Africa toward the middle of the last century, SCD was rarely recognized by physicians on the continent even 40 years after the condition was first described in the United States.[26] This remarkable observation even led some clinicians to question whether the mode of inheritance of SCD might be different in the African context.[27] Even now, in the absence of newborn screening across much of the continent, there are no accurate, up-to-date figures regarding the survival rates for SCD in SSA, but, by analyzing population data on the age-specific prevalence of SCA, an indirect measure of the loss through death of patients with this condition, it was recently concluded that mortality among children less than 5 years old born with SCA in SSA remains unacceptably high at between 50% and 90%.[28] These figures are in stark contrast to those from the north, where in recent years many countries have adopted universal screening for SCD and where most now provide comprehensive care for affected individuals. As a result, mortality is now rare among children born with SCD in Europe, the United States, and the Caribbean, where most affected children live to their 40s and 50s.[29–31]

Because official statistics are so poor, even basic facts such as the number of births of children with SCD in Africa can only be estimated using indirect approaches. For example, we recently used a geostatistical model that combined data on the population frequencies of HbAS from the published and unpublished literature, and birth rates and population densities based on United Nations figures, to estimate birth rates for SCA (which accounts for approximately 70% of SCD) for every country in the world. We concluded that 312,000 (294,000–330,000) children were born with SCA globally in 2010, that almost 80% of these children were born in SSA, and that half were born in just 3 countries: Nigeria, the Democratic Republic of Congo, and India[32] (**Fig. 1**). Nevertheless, the veracity of these estimates is undermined by the paucity of data on which they are based, and given the high rates of consanguinity in many parts of the region the true numbers could be substantially larger. In combination, the high number of affected births and the high rate of early mortality mean that SCD is probably responsible for more than 6% of all child deaths in many parts of SSA.[3]

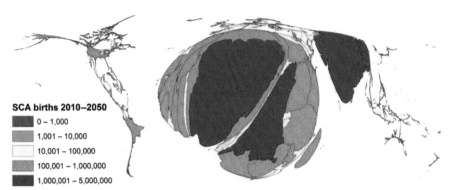

SCA births 2010–2050
- 0 – 1,000
- 1,001 – 10,000
- 10,001 – 100,000
- 100,001 – 1,000,000
- 1,000,001 – 5,000,000

Fig. 1. The global distribution of SCD, with the size of countries scaled to the number of annual births. (*From* Piel FB, Hay SI, Gupta S, et al. Global burden of sickle cell anaemia in children under five, 2010–2050: modelling based on demographics, excess mortality, and interventions. PLoS Med 2013;10(7):e100148.)

THE NATURAL HISTORY OF SICKLE CELL DISEASE IN AFRICA

When the very high birth and death rates for children with SCD in Africa are considered, it is notable how poorly the natural history of the condition has been documented on the continent. Despite almost 80% of SCD births occurring in SSA (see **Fig. 1**), academic research from the continent lags far behind that from the north. Less than 7% of all articles published on the subject since 1940 have included the word Africa, and, even now, research output on SCD from Africa is at a similar level to that of the north from more than 60 years ago (**Fig. 2**). Until recently, there were no programs for newborn screening, and no comprehensive studies of the natural history of SCD in Africa have been undertaken. As a result, the common causes of death among children with SCD on the continent have remained a matter of speculation, although it is likely that a substantial proportion of deaths have been attributable to just 2 conditions: malaria and invasive bacterial infections.

MALARIA

Although it has frequently been assumed that malaria is a common cause for death in African patients with SCD, few reliable data are available on which to base this conclusion.

In light of the protective effects of HbS against malaria, which seems to be directly proportional to the intracellular concentrations of HbS in heterozygotes,[33] it might be expected that homozygotes would be even more protected. However, there are also reasons why malaria might cause more problems in patients with SCD than in normal people. For example, the marked reticulocytosis seen in such patients might increase the efficiency of infection by P falciparum parasites, which show a preference for the youngest, most metabolically active red blood cells.[34] Moreover, the characteristic hyposplenia seen in patients with SCA could lead to reduced clearance of infected red blood cells. With steady state hemoglobin concentrations that are typically in the rage of 6 to 8 g/dL, patients with SCA might also be vulnerable to the sudden onset of catastrophic anemia brought on by the hemolysis or ineffective erythropoiesis that is commonly associated with malaria infections,[35] and it seems likely that the tissue hypoxia and inflammatory processes that typically accompany malaria infection might be potent triggers of sequestration crises. Nevertheless, clinical

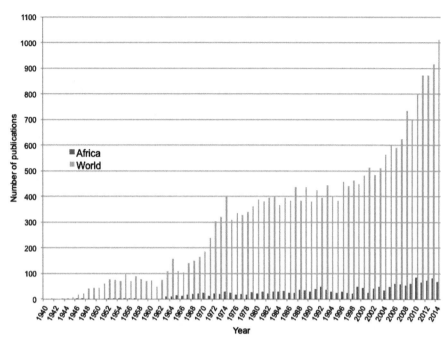

Fig. 2. Number of publications per year mentioning "sickle" for the world and for Africa, as detected by a PubMed search using the terms "sickle" (global articles) and "sickle AND Africa" (articles from Africa). The numbers returned are maximum estimates because they also include articles on sickle cell trait.

data relating to the relative risk of malaria and its consequences in patients with SCD are confusing.

Although malaria did not feature strongly in early descriptions of the natural history of SCD,[36,37] it was implicated as a significant problem in several later reports.[38–44] Nevertheless, although such reports confirmed that children with SCD can have malaria infections, they shed no light on the relative risks or consequences of the disease compared with normal children. Moreover, given the perception that malaria can be dangerous in patients with SCD, malaria prophylaxis is prescribed in most SCD clinics in malaria-endemic areas, making data from prospective cohort studies difficult to interpret. Through a birth cohort study conducted in western Kenya, in which participants were tested retrospectively for SCD on completion of the study (reducing the bias of prophylactic treatment) it was shown that, although all-cause mortality was significantly higher among children with SCD than control children, the incidence rates of both severe malaria anemia and high-density *P falciparum* infections were lower in children with SCD than in normal children.[45] This finding suggests that children with SCD might have a degree of resistance to *P falciparum* infections but does not exclude the possibility that malaria infection might have been a precipitating event in some or all of those who died.

Intervention studies potentially offer a more robust approach to investigating the importance of malaria as a health problem in patients with SCD. Several placebo-controlled trials of antimalarial prophylaxis have been conducted in patients with SCD, including 2 considered sufficiently robust to be included in a recent Cochrane Review.[46] The investigators concluded that malaria prophylaxis reduces the risks of sickle cell crises, blood transfusions, and hospital admissions, and results in increased mean hemoglobin levels, all of which suggest that malaria is an important cause of ill health among children with SCD in many parts of Africa and that such children should be protected from the disease.

Although the literature on the relationship between malaria and SCD remains confusing, the following describes the most likely situation. SCD is associated with protection against the acquisition of P falciparum infections, to a degree that may even be higher than the protection that is associated with HbAS. However, this protection is not complete, and when patients with SCD do become infected by malaria parasites the consequences can be catastrophic, through the precipitation of crises and the rapid development of severe anemia. With this in mind, it seems highly likely that, by diagnosing SCD through screening in early life and protecting affected children from malaria, the survival of children living with SCD in areas of high malaria transmission will be significantly improved. However, important questions still remain about the most appropriate strategies for malaria prevention. For example, should all malaria-exposed patients be prescribed prophylaxis throughout life, or is it possible that, at lower levels of malaria transmission, the risks of treatment might outweigh the risks of infection? With increasing resistance to antimalarial drugs and side effects from the long-term use of some, which antimalarial drugs offer the best balance between risk and benefit? Might alternative approaches, such as intermittent presumptive treatment of malaria or transmission avoidance through methods such as impregnated bed nets or indoor residual spraying of houses, be more appropriate in areas of lower transmission? Definitive clinical trials are needed to address these important questions.

BACTEREMIA

Invasive bacterial infections are a second group of conditions that make a significant but unknown contribution to the high early mortality seen in African children with SCD. Children with SCD manifest several immunologic abnormalities, including decreased splenic function, reduced serum opsonin activity, and abnormal neutrophil function, and it has long been known that children with SCA in the north are at considerable risk of invasive bacterial infections, particularly those caused by capsulated organisms such as Streptococcus pneumoniae, Haemophilus influenzae, and non-Typhi Salmonella species.[47–52] Early studies conducted in the north showed that the risk of invasive pneumococcal disease during early life was up to 50-fold higher in children with SCD compared with normal children, and the subsequent implementation of strategies such as pneumococcal vaccination and penicillin prophylaxis led to the virtual elimination of this excess risk in multiple populations in subsequent years.[47–52]

Despite being well documented in the north, data regarding the risks of bacteremia among patients with SCD in Africa have been slow to accumulate and subject to controversy. S pneumoniae was the most common organism isolated from children with SCD in an early study conducted in the Congo[15] but subsequent studies conducted in Uganda and Nigeria[53–57] suggested that other organisms, particularly Staphylococcus aureus, Escherichia coli, Klebsiella spp, and non-Typhi Salmonella, may be more important in the African context. In these studies, both S pneumoniae and H influenzae were found infrequently,[53–58] leading some commentators to question the potential benefits of antimicrobial prophylaxis in African patients with SCD.[55,57,59] Nevertheless, most of these studies were open to misinterpretation, because serious bacterial infections have their peak incidence in very early childhood, whereas most of the African studies were conducted in older children who survived their early years to present with symptoms of SCD. Furthermore, organisms like S pneumoniae and H influenzae are considerably more fastidious and difficult to grow than some of these other organisms, and culture sensitivity may therefore have biased the distribution of the pathogens observed in some of these studies.

Despite this early confusion, it has now been shown beyond all doubt that, just like children with SCD born in the north, children born with SCD in Africa are at substantial risk of severe infections in early life and that the highest risks relate to the same pathogenic organisms: S pneumoniae, H influenzae, and non-Typhi Salmonella species.[60] Taking as a starting point more than 1700 children who were diagnosed with bacteremia through the surveillance of all admissions to a general pediatric facility, it was shown through retrospective genotyping for SCD that young children with the condition were at very high risk of bacteremia from these top 3 organisms (1.2–5.0 episodes/100 person years), a risk that was similar to that reported from developed countries (1.5–11.6 episodes/100 person years) during the era before the introduction of antibiotic prophylaxis or pneumococcal vaccines.[47–52] A subsequent meta-analysis of available case-control studies conducted in African children showed that the risk of all-cause invasive bacterial infections was 19 times higher in children with SCD compared with normal children, 36 times higher for S pneumoniae, and 13-times higher for H influenzae type b.[61] Collectively these observations suggest that invasive bacterial diseases make a significant contribution to the high mortality associated with SCA in African children.

THE FUTURE OF SICKLE CELL DISEASE IN SUB-SAHARAN AFRICA

Despite the historically low priority that SCD has had throughout much of SSA, there are promising signs that the situation is now beginning to improve. SCD has recently been recognized as an important but neglected problem by several key agencies, including the United Nations[62] and the World Health Organization,[63] and a growing number of research groups and governments are taking an increasingly active interest in the detection and management of the condition (see **Fig. 2**). Moreover, in recent years, pilot projects of newborn screening have been reported from several centers,[64–66] which suggest that, in principle, early detection is within the reach of many countries in the region. Because the highest rates of mortality are likely to occur in the first few years of life, establishing such services in areas with the highest prevalence of SCD will be key to reducing the current levels of mortality in affected patients, and in many parts of Africa might also have a substantial effect on child mortality overall.[3] The gradual introduction of newborn screening for SCD in the United States and many parts of Europe in the last 40 years, coupled with the provision of a basic package of care (including vaccination for common bacterial infections and penicillin prophylaxis until at least 5 years of age), has led to a situation in which most children born with SCD in the north can now expect to live until their 40s and 50s.[29–31] However, as discussed later, to assume that similar advances could be achieved in most parts of Africa without substantial education programs, the careful fostering of political will, and significant financial investment, would be simplistic.

BOTTLENECKS IN THE CARE OF SICKLE CELL DISEASE IN SUB-SAHARAN AFRICA

Unlike the north, where newborn screening programs for SCD and a wide range of other genetic conditions have been implemented for many years, in most parts of SSA the infrastructure for screening is not available. Moreover, in many African communities, SCD is associated with significant stigmatization to which the mothers of affected children can be particularly vulnerable.[67–69] Screening for the condition can precipitate disharmony, which at times includes domestic violence and the break-down of marriages.[67–69] Careful consideration of such issues should therefore be a prerequisite to the implementation of newborn screening programs within the region. Even beyond the anthropologic issues, establishing such programs is not trivial and involves the development of efficient methods for the transport of samples from testing sites (such as mother and child health clinics) to well-resourced reference lab-oratories with reliable facilities for the storage and testing of samples, and efficient methods for the tracing, follow-up, and confirmatory testing of affected babies. An effective system requires computer-based record keeping, a sufficient number of well-trained staff to conduct all functions, reliable power supply, and other elements that make the cost implications of screening substantial. Careful cost-benefit analyses and considerable advocacy will be required before African governments begin to establish such programs at a national scale. Nevertheless, several countries in the re-gion are heading in the right direction. For example, in partnership with the govern-ment of Brazil, Ghana is moving toward a national newborn screening program for SCD, and discussions regarding a national strategy for SCD are also underway in Tanzania.[70]

Even without newborn screening, with progressive epidemiologic and demo-graphic transition, and the roll-out of an increasing range of newborn vaccines (including those for *S pneumoniae* and *H influenzae*) in many countries within the re-gion, it is inevitable that an increasing number of children born with SCD in SSA will survive and require appropriate treatment. The implications of this emerging epidemic for health systems in SSA may be considerable. As SCD transitions from a condition that is fatal in early life to a chronic condition needing lifelong care, health services will come under increasing pressure to provide appropriate preventive and curative services. Moreover, this transition will come with substantial implications for families of affected children, who will face increasing pressures from issues that will include the considerable financial and emotional costs that can result from med-ical fees, to the inability to maintain income-generating activities on account of the high levels of child-care that will be required.[67] Blood transfusion services are one area that will face increasing pressure: patients with SCD are significant recipients of emergency transfusions and with longer-term survival and increased use of trans-fusion therapy they will not only be the recipients of a growing proportion of available supplies but also, with repeated transfusions, will be vulnerable to transfusion-acquired infections and to alloimmunization.[71] Without appropriate monitoring through transcranial Doppler (TCD) ultrasonography coupled with lack of access to chronic blood transfusion or hydroxyurea therapy in the event of an abnormal TCD result, an increasing proportion of African patients with SCD will develop acute and chronic cerebrovascular events, with significant impacts on their quality of life.[72] In addition, without appropriate monitoring and treatment, patients with SCD will also have an increased burden of many of the other chronic consequences of the condi-tion, including mental health issues and depression,[73,74] chronic pulmonary disease, renal failure, chronic bone diseases, and ocular complications.[2] Given the virtual absence of data regarding the age-specific incidence of any of these complications from studies conducted anywhere in Africa, it is impossible to predict the precise burden of any of these sequelae going forward; however, the logic of simple arithmetic suggests that, in the absence of specific treatments, these chronic compli-cations of SCD will have major implications for African societies and health systems in the years ahead.

FUTURE PRIORITIES FOR SICKLE CELL DISEASE IN AFRICA

Given the demands that the growing number of patients living with SCD will increasingly place on African health systems in future, it is essential that clinicians, researchers, health ministries, and international organizations begin to consider the priority questions with increasing urgency. Describing the number of patients affected and estimating survival and complication rates with greater precision must be early priorities for research in the next few years. Although recent estimates provide an excellent starting point,[75,76] much of the data on which the estimates were based are out of date, and are too sparse to be sufficiently useful at a local level. Better estimates from larger-scale contemporary studies would be more meaningful to the health planners whose responsibly it is to make decisions regarding priorities for health spending and the allocation of scarce resources. These planners will also benefit from cost-economic estimates regarding various approaches to diagnosis and treatment. Further, it is likely that such data would be most influential if the end users, particularly national ministries of health, were engaged from the outset. As described earlier, the current need for quality-controlled, centralized diagnostic services is beyond the reach of many countries in SSA and the development of reliable, cheap, point-of-care methods for the diagnosis of SCD that could also be used for newborn screening could revolutionize the management of patients with SCD in Africa, and would also benefit studies designed to refine estimates of its distribution. Several such devices are under development and show considerable promise. In addition, a clear understanding of the sociologic and anthropologic issues surrounding SCD in different societies[67–69] will be important going forward, and may influence decisions about local policies with regard to diagnosis and treatment.

SPECIFIC TREATMENTS FOR SICKLE CELL DISEASE IN SUB-SAHARAN AFRICA

Beyond the standard treatments that will continue to be needed for the prevention of malaria and bacterial infections, the long-term consequences of SCD[2] will place an increasing burden on African societies without the widespread implementation of disease-modifying therapies. For the time being, hydroxyurea (also known as hydroxycarbamide), the only disease-modifying agent that is currently licensed for the treatment of SCD in the north, represents perhaps the only current viable option for Africa in this regard. Nevertheless, despite its well-documented benefits among both adults and children in the north,[77–79] legitimate questions surround the potential risks and benefits of hydroxyurea for the treatment of patients with SCD in Africa. Hydroxyurea is an oral medication with excellent bioavailability, but is associated with variable pharmacokinetics and pharmacodynamics.[80] Although its therapeutic mechanisms in SCD are incompletely understood, they seem to relate to several actions, including the promotion of fetal hemoglobin production and reductions in the inflammatory response.[81] As a potent inhibitor of ribonucleotide reductase, hydroxyurea is both cytotoxic and myelosuppressive,[82] and treatment is associated with reversible reductions in the production of all blood cell lineages. This predictable effect of hydroxyurea relates to its therapeutic benefit, and, for each specific patient on treatment, the daily dose must be titrated against these reductions until the maximum tolerated dose is reached.[83] Although hydroxyurea is increasingly being used in the ad-hoc management of patients with SCA in many parts of SSA,[84] no consensus management guidelines have yet been established and no prospective clinical trials have yet been performed to ensure that the treatment is equally safe and effective in the African context.[84] Given that the safe use of hydroxyurea requires titration of dosing and frequent laboratory monitoring to evaluate potential hematological toxicities, it is critical to prospectively evaluate hydroxyurea in various settings across SSA in order to establish local dosing and monitoring guidelines. In many parts of SSA, capacity for this kind of monitoring is limited, and the costs lead to questions of affordability.[85] Moreover, the infectious disease exposure (including bacterial diseases and malaria) and reduced nutritional status of children living with SCA in many parts of SSA present additional challenges for the initiation and maintenance of hydroxyurea therapy. Nevertheless, if hydroxyurea was proved to be both safe and effective for children with SCA in SSA, it could realistically emerge as the main disease-modifying therapeutic intervention to help improve the health of children born with SCA on the continent. Several clinical trials are currently underway in various parts of SSA Africa that, it is hoped, will begin to answer this question, including one ambitious trial (Realizing Effectiveness Across Continents with Hydroxyurea [REACH]) that is studying the safety and effectiveness of hydroxyurea in Angola, the Demographic Republic of Congo, Uganda, and Kenya (NCT01966731; https://clinicaltrials.gov/ct2/show/record/NCT01966731).[86]

The only other option with obvious potential for modifying the course of SCD among patients in Africa is transfusion therapy. Transfusion therapy has played a pivotal role in the management of SCD in the north, most notably in the primary prevention of strokes in patients with abnormal TCD velocities[87,88] and through improved oxygenation in patients presenting with the acute chest syndrome (ACS).[89] Transfusion therapy may also be more effective than other treatments in reducing the incidence of both painful crises and ACS.[90,91] Nevertheless, despite these well-recognized benefits, transfusion therapy can result in iron overload, and should therefore be used in conjunction with iron monitoring and chelation therapy. Moreover, regular transfusions come with the additional risk of alloimmunization (an even greater risk in SSA, in which most blood for transfusion is not leucodepleted); transfusion-acquired infections; issues related to venous access, such as thrombosis and line-related sepsis; and loss of work and schooling.[92] Even in the north, the total economic costs of transfusion therapy far exceed those of treatment with hydroxyurea,[93,94] and it is therefore reserved for a limited number of specific indications. Together, these considerations make transfusion therapy unrealistic for most patients living in Africa.

In addition, the only curative treatment that is currently available for SCD is allogeneic hematopoietic stem-cell transplantation (HSCT).[95] Successful HSCT can result in disease-free survival and stabilization of neurologic lesions. However, even in the north, the variable and unpredictable severity of SCD mean that HSCT is reserved for the most severely affected patients,[96] and the fine balance between the risks and benefits of treatment, including long-term toxicities such as infertility and endocrinopathies[97] and a failure rate of 10% to 15%,[95] make the decision to proceed to HSCT complex. Although HSCT has been advocated by some experts as a viable option for African patients with SCD,[98] given the issues of benefit versus harm, the limited facilities and infrastructure for HSCT in the region, and the likely costs, investment in HSCT does not seem an immediate priority.

SUMMARY

Given the enormous current and future burden of SCD in SSA, and the contribution that it makes to total child mortality, the condition has historically been neglected. In recent years some progress has been made in reversing this situation; however, substantial investments are required to move SCD up the agenda to its rightful place as a priority disease for African governments going forward. Some key areas for future work include better and more up-to-date descriptions of the burden of SCD at a local scale and studies of the natural history of SCD among patients in SSA who are on routine treatment, with a particular emphasis on describing the incidence of the acute and chronic complications of the disease in the African context. Although widespread programs for the early diagnosis and treatment of SCD in SSA could yield substantial benefits for patients and their families, a great deal more needs to be known about the local anthropologic and social attitudes to SCD, and steps need to be taken to mitigate against any adverse consequences for affected populations. Health care planners need to be convinced of the benefits of a greater focus on SCD through cost-economic analyses of various approaches to diagnosis and treatment. Beyond descriptions of the disease, there is a clear need for clinical trials designed to address a wide range of issues, including optimal approaches to the prevention of bacterial infections and malaria, strategies in the area of blood transfusion and blood safety, and trials of disease-modifying treatments, including hydroxyurea. Underlying all of these must be the principle that not all of the lessons that have been learnt about SCD from studies conducted in the north during the last 60 years are appropriate or applicable to Africa. Forward-planning will best be informed by extensive research on all aspects of SCD in the African context.

REFERENCES

1. Murayama M. Structure of sickle cell hemoglobin and molecular mechanism of the sickling phenomenon. Clin Chem 1967;13(7):578–88.
2. Rees DC, Williams TN, Gladwin MT. Sickle-cell disease. Lancet 2010;376(9757): 2018–31.
3. Modell B, Darlison M. Global epidemiology of haemoglobin disorders and derived service indicators. Bull World Health Organ 2008;86(6):480–7.
4. Weatherall DJ, Clegg JB. The thalassaemia syndromes. 3rd edition. Oxford (United Kingdom): Blackwell Scientific Publications; 2002.
5. Kulozik AE, Wainscoat JS, Serjeant GR, et al. Geographical survey of beta S-globin gene haplotypes: evidence for an independent Asian origin of the sickle-cell mutation. Am J Hum Genet 1986;39(2):239–44.
6. Flint J, Harding RM, Boyce AJ, et al. The population genetics of the haemoglobinopathies. Baillieres Clin Haematol 1998;11(1):1–51.
7. Piel FB, Patil AP, Howes RE, et al. Global distribution of the sickle cell gene and geographical confirmation of the malaria hypothesis. Nat Commun 2010;1(8):104.
8. Allison AC. Protection afforded by sickle cell trait against subtertian malarial infection. Br Med J 1954;1:290–5.
9. Williams TN. Human red blood cell polymorphisms and malaria. Curr Opin Microbiol 2006;9(4):388–94.
10. Taylor SM, Parobek CM, Fairhurst RM. Haemoglobinopathies and the clinical epidemiology of malaria: a systematic review and meta-analysis. Lancet Infect Dis 2012;12(6):457–68.
11. The Malaria Genomic Epidemiology Network. Reappraisal of known malaria resistance loci in a large multicenter study. Nat Genet 2014;46(11):1197–204.
12. Kreuels B, Kreuzberg C, Kobbe R, et al. Differing effects of HbS and HbC traits on uncomplicated falciparum malaria, anemia, and child growth. Blood 2010; 115(22):4551–8.
13. Nyakeriga AM, Troye-Blomberg M, Chemtai AK, et al. Malaria and nutritional status in children living on the coast of Kenya. Am J Clin Nutr 2004;80(6):1604–10.
14. Scott JA, Berkley JA, Mwangi I, et al. Relation between falciparum malaria and bacteraemia in Kenyan children: a population-based, case-control study and a longitudinal study. Lancet 2011;378(9799):1316–23.

15. Eeckels R, Gatti F, Renoirte AM. Abnormal distribution of haemoglobin genotypes in Negro children with severe bacterial infections. Nature 1967;216(113):382.
16. Friedman MJ. Erythrocytic mechanism of sickle cell resistance to malaria. Proc Natl Acad Sci U S A 1978;75(4):1994–7.
17. Friedman MJ, Roth EF, Nagel RL, et al. The role of hemoglobins C, S, and Nbalt in the inhibition of malaria parasite development in vitro. Am J Trop Med Hyg 1979; 28(5):777–80.
18. Pasvol G, Weatherall DJ, Wilson RJ. Cellular mechanism for the protective effect of haemoglobin S against P. falciparum malaria. Nature 1978;274(5672):701–3.
19. Fairhurst RM, Fujioka H, Hayton K, et al. Aberrant development of Plasmodium falciparum in hemoglobin CC red cells: implications for the malaria protective effect of the homozygous state. Blood 2003;101(8):3309–15.
20. Cholera R, Brittain NJ, Gillrie MR, et al. Impaired cytoadherence of Plasmodium falciparum-infected erythrocytes containing sickle hemoglobin. Proc Natl Acad Sci U S A 2008;105(3):991–6.
21. Fairhurst RM, Baruch DI, Brittain NJ, et al. Abnormal display of PfEMP-1 on erythrocytes carrying haemoglobin C may protect against malaria. Nature 2005; 435(7045):1117–21.
22. Ayi K, Turrini F, Piga A, et al. Enhanced phagocytosis of ring-parasitized mutant erythrocytes. A common mechanism that may explain protection against falciparum malaria in sickle trait and beta-thalassemia trait. Blood 2004;104:3364–71.
23. Luzzatto L, Nwachuku-Jarrett ES, Reddy S. Increased sickling of parasitised erythrocytes as mechanism of resistance against malaria in the sickle-cell trait. Lancet 1970;1(7642):319–21.
24. Roth EF Jr, Friedman M, Ueda Y, et al. Sickling rates of human AS red cells infected in vitro with Plasmodium falciparum malaria. Science 1978;202(4368):650–2.
25. Shear HL, Roth EF Jr, Fabry ME, et al. Transgenic mice expressing human sickle hemoglobin are partially resistant to rodent malaria. Blood 1993;81(1):222–6.
26. Herrick JB. Peculiar elongated and sickle-shaped red blood corpuscles in a case of severe anemia. Arch Intern Med 1910;6(5):517–21.
27. Lehmann H, Raper AB. Maintenance of high sickling rate in an African community. Br Med J 1956;2(4988):333–6.
28. Grosse SD, Odame I, Atrash HK, et al. Sickle cell disease in Africa: a neglected cause of early child mortality. Am J Prev Med 2011;41(6 Suppl 4):S398–405.
29. Telfer P, Coen P, Chakravorty S, et al. Clinical outcomes in children with sickle cell disease living in England: a neonatal cohort in East London. Haematologica 2007;92(7):905–12.
30. Quinn CT, Rogers ZR, McCavit TL, et al. Improved survival of children and adolescents with sickle cell disease. Blood 2010;115(17):3447–52.
31. Wierenga KJ, Hambleton IR, Lewis NA. Survival estimates for patients with homozygous sickle-cell disease in Jamaica: a clinic-based population study. Lancet 2001;357(9257):680–3.
32. Piel FB, Patil AP, Howes RE, et al. Global epidemiology of sickle haemoglobin in neonates: a contemporary geostatistical model-based map and population estimates. Lancet 2012;381(9861):142–51.
33. Williams TN, Mwangi TW, Wambua S, et al. Negative epistasis between the malaria-protective effects of a+-thalassemia and the sickle cell trait. Nat Genet 2005;37:1253–7.
34. Pasvol G, Weatherall D, Wilson RJM. The increased susceptibility of young red cells to invasion by the malaria parasite Plasmodium falciparum. Br J Haematol 1980;45:285–95.

35. Lamikanra AA, Brown D, Potocnik A, et al. Malarial anemia: of mice and men. Blood 2007;110(1):18–28.
36. Trowell HC, Raper AB, Welbourn HF. The natural history of homozygous sickle-cell anaemia in Central Africa. Q J Med 1957;26(104):401–22.
37. Lambotte-Legrand J, Lambotte-Legrand C. Le prognostic de l'anemie drepano-cytaire au Congo Belge (a propos de 300 case et de 150 deces). Ann Soc Belg Med Trop 1955;35:53–7.
38. Adeloye A, Luzzatto L, Edington GM. Severe malarial infection in a patient with sickle-cell anaemia. Br Med J 1971;2(759):445–6.
39. Konotey-Ahulu FI. Malaria and sickle-cell disease. Br Med J 1971;2(763):710–1.
40. Seymour A. Malaria and sickle cell disease. Br Med J 1971;2(763):711.
41. Pichanick AM. Severe malarial infection. Br Med J 1971;3(766):114.
42. Ambe JP, Fatunde JO, Sodeinde OO. Associated morbidities in children with sickle-cell anaemia presenting with severe anaemia in a malarious area. Trop Doct 2001;31(1):26–7.
43. Ibidapo MO, Akinyanju OO. Acute sickle cell syndromes in Nigerian adults. Clin Lab Haematol 2000;22(3):151–5.
44. Okuonghae HO, Nwankwo MU, Offor E. Malarial parasitaemia in febrile children with sickle cell anaemia. J Trop Pediatr 1992;38(2):83–5.
45. Aidoo M, Terlouw DJ, Kolczak MS, et al. Protective effects of the sickle cell gene against malaria morbidity and mortality. Lancet 2002;359(9314):1311–2.
46. Oniyangi O, Omari AA. Malaria chemoprophylaxis in sickle cell disease. Cochrane Database Syst Rev 2006;(4):CD003489.
47. Wollstein M, Kreidel KV. Sickle cell anemia. Am J Dis Child 1928;36:998–1011.
48. Robinson MG, Watson RJ. Pneumococcal meningitis in sickle-cell anemia. N Engl J Med 1966;274(18):1006–8.
49. Barrett-Connor E. Bacterial infection and sickle cell anemia. An analysis of 250 infections in 166 patients and a review of the literature. Medicine (Baltimore) 1971;50(2):97–112.
50. Lobel JS, Bove KE. Clinicopathologic characteristics of septicemia in sickle cell disease. Am J Dis Child 1982;136(6):543–7.
51. Powars D, Overturf G, Turner E. Is there an increased risk of *Haemophilus influenzae* septicemia in children with sickle cell anemia? Pediatrics 1983;71(6):927–31.
52. Diggs LW. Bone and joint lesions in sickle-cell disease. Clin Orthop 1967;52:119–43.
53. Akinyanju O, Johnson AO. Acute illness in Nigerian children with sickle cell anaemia. Ann Trop Paediatr 1987;7(3):181–6.
54. Okuonghae HO, Nwankwo MU, Offor EC. Pattern of bacteraemia in febrile children with sickle cell anaemia. Ann Trop Paediatr 1993;13(1):55–64.
55. Akuse RM. Variation in the pattern of bacterial infection in patients with sickle cell disease requiring admission. J Trop Pediatr 1996;42(6):318–23.
56. Aken'ova YA, Bakare RA, Okunade MA. Septicaemia in sickle cell anaemia patients: the Ibadan experience. Cent Afr J Med 1998;44(4):102–4.
57. Kizito ME, Mworozi E, Ndugwa C, et al. Bacteraemia in homozygous sickle cell disease in Africa: is pneumococcal prophylaxis justified? Arch Dis Child 2007;92(1):21–3.
58. Makani J, Mgaya J, Balandya E, et al. Bacteraemia in sickle cell anaemia is associated with low haemoglobin: a report of 890 admissions to a tertiary hospital in Tanzania. Br J Haematol 2015. [Epub ahead of print].

59. Serjeant GR. Mortality from sickle cell disease in Africa. BMJ 2005;330(7489): 432–3.
60. Williams TN, Uyoga S, Macharia A, et al. Bacteraemia in Kenyan children with sickle-cell anaemia: a retrospective cohort and case-control study. Lancet 2009;374(9698):1364–70.
61. Ramakrishnan M, Moisi JC, Klugman KP, et al. Increased risk of invasive bacterial infections in African people with sickle-cell disease: a systematic review and meta-analysis. Lancet Infect Dis 2010;10(5):329–37.
62. United Nations press office. Press conference on raising awareness of sickle-cell anaemia. 2009. Available at: http://www.un.org/News/briefings/docs/2009/090619_Anaemia.doc.htm. Accessed December 15, 2015.
63. World Health Organization Regional Office for Africa. Sickle-cell disease: a strategy for the WHO African Region. Report of the Regional Director. AFR/RC60/8, 22 June 2010. 2010.
64. Tshilolo L, Aissi LM, Lukusa D, et al. Neonatal screening for sickle cell anaemia in the Democratic Republic of the Congo: experience from a pioneer project on 31 204 newborns. J Clin Pathol 2009;62(1):35–8.
65. Kafando E, Nacoulma E, Ouattara Y, et al. Neonatal haemoglobinopathy screening in Burkina Faso. J Clin Pathol 2009;62(1):39–41.
66. McGann PT, Ferris MG, Ramamurthy U, et al. A prospective newborn screening and treatment program for sickle cell anemia in Luanda, Angola. Am J Hematol 2013;88(12):984–9.
67. Marsh VM, Kamuya DM, Molyneux SS. 'All her children are born that way': gendered experiences of stigma in families affected by sickle cell disorder in rural Kenya. Ethn Health 2011;16(4–5):343–59.
68. Assimadi JK, Gbadoe AD, Nyadanu M. The impact on families of sickle cell disease in Togo. Arch Pediatr 2000;7(6):615–20 [in French].
69. Bamisaiye A, Bakare CG, Olatawura MO. Some social-psychologic dimensions of sickle cell anemia among Nigerians. Clin Pediatr (Phila) 1974;13(1): 56–9.
70. Makani J, Soka D, Rwezaula S, et al. Health policy for sickle cell disease in Africa: experience from Tanzania on interventions to reduce under-five mortality. Trop Med Int Health 2015;20(2):184–7.
71. Dzik WS, Kyeyune D, Otekat G, et al. Transfusion medicine in sub-Saharan Africa: conference summary. Transfus Med Rev 2015;29(3):195–204.
72. Ohene-Frempong K, Weiner SJ, Sleeper LA, et al. Cerebrovascular accidents in sickle cell disease: rates and risk factors. Blood 1998;91(1):288–94.
73. Lukoo RN, Ngiyulu RM, Mananga GL, et al. Depression in children suffering from sickle cell anemia. J Pediatr Hematol Oncol 2015;37(1):20–4.
74. Ohaeri JU, Shokunbi WA, Akinlade KS, et al. The psychosocial problems of sickle cell disease sufferers and their methods of coping. Soc Sci Med 1995;40(7): 955–60.
75. Piel FB, Hay SI, Gupta S, et al. Global burden of sickle cell anaemia in children under five, 2010-2050: modelling based on demographics, excess mortality, and interventions. PLoS Med 2013;10(7):e1001484.
76. Piel FB, Tatem AJ, Huang Z, et al. Global migration and the changing distribution of sickle haemoglobin: a quantitative study of temporal trends between 1960 and 2000. Lancet Glob Health 2014;2(2):e80–9.
77. Charache S, Terrin ML, Moore RD, et al. Effect of hydroxyurea on the frequency of painful crises in sickle cell anemia. Investigators of the Multicenter Study of Hydroxyurea in Sickle Cell Anemia. N Engl J Med 1995;332(20):1317–22.

78. Kinney TR, Helms RW, O'Branski EE, et al. Safety of hydroxyurea in children with sickle cell anemia: results of the HUG-KIDS study, a phase I/II trial. Pediatric Hydroxyurea Group. Blood 1999;94(5):1550–4.

79. Wang WC, Ware RE, Miller ST, et al. Hydroxycarbamide in very young children with sickle-cell anaemia: a multicentre, randomised, controlled trial (BABY HUG). Lancet 2011;377(9778):1663–72.

80. Ware RE, Despotovic JM, Mortier NA, et al. Pharmacokinetics, pharmacodynamics, and pharmacogenetics of hydroxyurea treatment for children with sickle cell anemia. Blood 2011;118(18):4985–91.

81. Platt OS, Orkin SH, Dover G, et al. Hydroxyurea enhances fetal hemoglobin production in sickle cell anemia. J Clin Invest 1984;74(2):652–6.

82. Lewis WH, Wright JA. Altered ribonucleotide reductase activity in mammalian tissue culture cells resistant to hydroxyurea. Biochem Biophys Res Commun 1974; 60(3):926–33.

83. Ware RE. How I use hydroxyurea to treat young patients with sickle cell anemia. Blood 2010;115(26):5300–11.

84. Mulaku M, Opiyo N, Karumbi J, et al. Evidence review of hydroxyurea for the prevention of sickle cell complications in low-income countries. Arch Dis Child 2013; 98(11):908–14.

85. Galadanci NA, Abdullahi SU, Tabari MA, et al. Primary stroke prevention in Nigerian children with sickle cell disease (SPIN): challenges of conducting a feasibility trial. Pediatr Blood Cancer 2015;62(3):395–401.

86. Available at: https://clinicaltrials.gov/ct2/show/record/NCT01966731. Accessed July 23, 2015.

87. Adams RJ, McKie VC, Hsu L, et al. Prevention of a first stroke by transfusions in children with sickle cell anemia and abnormal results on transcranial Doppler ultrasonography. N Engl J Med 1998;339(1):5–11.

88. Adams RJ, Brambilla D, Optimizing Primary Stroke Prevention in Sickle Cell Anemia (STOP 2) Trial Investigators. Discontinuing prophylactic transfusions used to prevent stroke in sickle cell disease. N Engl J Med 2005;353(26):2769–78.

89. Vichinsky EP, Neumayr LD, Earles AN, et al. Causes and outcomes of the acute chest syndrome in sickle cell disease. National Acute Chest Syndrome Study Group. N Engl J Med 2000;342(25):1855–65.

90. Miller ST, Wright E, Abboud M, et al. Impact of chronic transfusion on incidence of pain and acute chest syndrome during the Stroke Prevention Trial (STOP) in sickle-cell anemia. J Pediatr 2001;139(6):785–9.

91. Alvarez O, Yovetich NA, Scott JP, et al. Pain and other non-neurological adverse events in children with sickle cell anemia and previous stroke who received hydroxyurea and phlebotomy or chronic transfusions and chelation: results from the SWiTCH clinical trial. Am J Hematol 2013;88(11):932–8.

92. Chou ST. Transfusion therapy for sickle cell disease: a balancing act. Hematol Am Soc Hematol Educ Program 2013;2013:439–46.

93. Wayne AS, Schoenike SE, Pegelow CH. Financial analysis of chronic transfusion for stroke prevention in sickle cell disease. Blood 2000;96(7):2369–72.

94. Wang WC, Oyeku SO, Luo Z, et al. Hydroxyurea is associated with lower costs of care of young children with sickle cell anemia. Pediatrics 2013;132(4): 677–83.

95. Locatelli F, Pagliara D. Allogeneic hematopoietic stem cell transplantation in children with sickle cell disease. Pediatr Blood Cancer 2012;59(2):372–6.

96. Chakravorty S, Williams TN. Sickle cell disease: a neglected chronic disease of increasing global health importance. Arch Dis Child 2015;100(1):48–53.

97. Dallas MH, Triplett B, Shook DR, et al. Long-term outcome and evaluation of organ function in pediatric patients undergoing haploidentical and matched related hematopoietic cell transplantation for sickle cell disease. Biol Blood Marrow Transplant 2013;19(5):820–30.

98. Pule G, Wonkam A. Treatment for sickle cell disease in Africa: should we invest in haematopoietic stem cell transplantation? Pan Afr Med J 2014;18:46.

Progress Toward the Control and Management of the Thalassemias

Suthat Fucharoen, MD[a,*], David J. Weatherall, MD, FRCP, FRS[b]

KEYWORDS

- Different forms of thalassemia • Screening • Prevention • Management
- National partnerships • Role of non-governmental organizations

KEY POINTS

- The prevention and management of the thalassemias is reasonably advanced in several countries in Asia.
- Partnerships are being developed between these countries and those in which facilities for the control and development of thalassemia are not yet established.
- There is urgent need for support on behalf of international health agencies for the further development of these programs.

PROGRESS OF THALASSEMIA CONTROL IN THAILAND

Thalassemia in Thailand

Both α-thalassemia and β-thalassemia and some abnormal hemoglobins (Hb), such as Hb E and Hb Constant Spring (CS), are prevalent in Thailand. The frequencies are 20% to 30% for α-thalassemia, 3% to 9% for β-thalassemia, 10% to 50% for Hb E, and 1% to 8% for Hb CS (**Table 1**).[1,2] Different combinations of these abnormal genes lead to more than 60 thalassemia syndromes. The 2 major alpha thalassemic diseases are Hb Bart's hydrops fetalis or homozygous α^0-thalassemia and Hb H disease that results from the interaction between α^0-thalassemia and α^+-thalassemia or between α^0-thalassemia and Hb CS. Almost all fetuses with Hb Bart's hydrops die intrautero or a few

Disclosure Statement: The authors have nothing to disclose.

This work was supported by a Research Chair Grant from the National Science and Technology Development Agency (P-11-00435) and Mahidol University, Thailand, The Wellcome Trust and Medical Research Council, United Kingdom, and the Anthony Cerami and Ann Dunne Foundation for World Health.

[a] Thalassemia Research Center, Institute of Molecular Biosciences, Mahidol University, Nakhon Pathom 73170, Thailand; [b] Weatherall Institute of Molecular Medicine, John Radcliffe Hospital, University of Oxford, Oxford OX3 9DS, UK

* Corresponding author.

E-mail address: suthat.fuc@mahidol.ac.th

Table 1	
Thalassemia in Thailand	
Major Types of Thalassemia	**Frequencies, %**
α-Thalassemia (α⁰-thalassemia and α⁺-thalassemia)	20–30
Hemoglobin Constant Spring (α⁺-thalassemialike effect)	1–8
β-thalassemia	3–9
Hemoglobin E	10–53

minutes after birth and their mothers often suffer from obstetric complications, such as toxemia of pregnancy (preeclampsia and eclampsia), postpartum hemorrhage due to an enlarged placenta, and the psychological burden of carrying a nonviable fetus to term. Interaction between β-thalassemia genes or β-thalassemia and Hb E genes leads to homozygous β-thalassemia or β-thalassemia/Hb E disease, which are major beta thalassemic syndromes in this region. In β-thalassemia/Hb E disease, although the patients have identical genotypes, the degree of anemia varies greatly, with hemoglobin levels ranging from 3 to 13 g/dL.[3–5] The birth rates of major thalassemic diseases are shown in **Table 2**.

Since 2002, Thailand has implemented the Universal Health Care policy that resulted in a 99% universal coverage among Thai nationals using a mix of health protection schemes. Under this policy, all Thais will receive free treatment, either at the nearby district hospital or by referral for treatment in a medical center for cases that need special care. Almost all patients with thalassemia can have access to free blood transfusion and iron chelation, such as desferrioxamine and deferiprone. To reduce the cost of the iron chelators, the Government Pharmaceutical Organization has synthesized deferiprone for local use. The product is effective in the treatment of iron overload in all thalassemia syndromes, except major thalassemia cases that need regular blood transfusion that still need desferrioxamine treatment as a combination therapy.[6,7] The estimated direct cost for the management of a patient with major thalassemia who receives regular blood transfusion and desferrioxamine treatment who lives to be 10 to 30 years old is approximately 1.3 to 6.6 million Baht (US\$ 39,393–200,000).[8] Even though thalassemia may be cured by stem cell transplantation, it is still expensive and it is difficult to find appropriate HLA-matched donors. Thus, the best approach to cope with thalassemia in

Table 2			
Total number of patients with thalassemia and the number of births per year (total births = 800,000/year)			
Diseases	**Couples at Risk (per year)**	**Births (per year)**	**Living Patients**
Homozygous β-thalassemia	828	207	2070
β-Thalassemia/Hb E	12,852	3213	96,390
Hb Bart hydrops fetalis	3332	833	0
Hb H disease	22,400	5600	336,000
Total	39,412	9853	434,460

Abbreviation: Hb, hemoglobin.

Modified from Fucharoen S, Winichagoon P. Problems of thalassemia in Thailand. ICMR Ann 1988;8:30; with permission.

developing countries, including Thailand, is to prevent the birth of new cases with major thalassemic diseases.

PREVENTION AND CONTROL PROGRAM FOR THALASSEMIA IN THAILAND

A nationwide program has commenced to prevent and control homozygous β-thalassemia, compound heterozygote β-thalassemia/Hb E, and Hb Bart's hydrops fetalis. The program started in 1997, after some preparation in technology transfer to the Minister of Public Health. Three major departments are involved in this program, namely Department of Medical Services, Department of Health, and Department of Medical Sciences. The 3 departments are involved in the prevention and control of thalassemia as follows:

1. The Department of Medical Services is involved in the improvement of treatment to improve the quality of life of patients with thalassemia. The department has worked in collaboration with the Thalassemia Foundation of Thailand and Thai Hematology Society to develop a clinical practice guideline as a reference for how to manage thalassemia in Thailand.
2. The Department of Health is involved more in the screening, counseling, and prenatal diagnosis under the policy "Select partner, Select pregnancy, Select birth," which will lead to thalassemia-free infants born in the kingdom.
3. The Department of Medical Science is involved in the training of laboratory technicians at various levels to learn how to screen for thalassemia carriers and high-risk couples by using both simple screening tests and standard procedures for the accurate diagnosis of thalassemia.

During 1997 through 2010 we had conducted many workshops and trained medical staff, including pediatricians, physicians, nurses, medical technologists, and technicians, in basic knowledge about thalassemia, laboratory diagnosis, and management. Declaration of the nationwide policy by the Permanent Secretary of the Ministry of Public Health for thalassemia control was announced on February 9, 2005 (**Box 1**). We are still conducting refresher courses and have held a National Annual Meeting on Thalassemia for the past 20 years.

Box 1
National policy for the prevention of severe thalassemia delivered by the Permanent Secretary of the Ministry of Public Health, Bangkok, Thailand on February 9, 2005

1. Every pregnant woman should receive genetic counseling for thalassemia.
2. Every pregnant woman should receive thalassemia screening by consent. If the result is found to be positive for thalassemia/hemoglobinopathies trait, the husband should be screened as well.
3. Every pregnant woman and husband with thalassemia/hemoglobinopathies trait should receive a confirmation test to be a COUPLE AT RISK of having severe thalassemia offspring.
4. Pregnant women who are diagnosed to be a COUPLE AT RISK should receive prenatal diagnosis.
5. Every health care unit should organize a thalassemia promote/prevent/control service system that is high standard. If any service exceeds the unit capability, the case should be transferred to the service network.
6. Students, reproductive women, and married couples will extensively receive the information about thalassemia.

The target group for thalassemia screening is pregnant women. This is done by a simple 1-tube osmotic fragility test for β and α^0-thalassemia carriers and Hb E by dichlorophenol-indolphenol dye test (DCIP dye test).[9] The husband of those pregnant women who have a positive screening test will be called up for further screening. The couples that have positive screening of both husband and wife will be further referred for a confirmation test by standard methods of blood counts and hemoglobin analysis by automatic high-performance liquid chromatography (HPLC) (Variant System, Bio-Rad Laboratories, Hercules, CA) or by capillary zone electrophoresis in some centers.[10,11] **Fig. 1** demonstrates the schematic outline of thalassemia screening in Thailand. The result of nationwide screening for high-risk couples shows that it varies from the north to south related to the abnormal gene frequencies in each region (**Fig. 2**). Wanapirak,[12] Chiangmai University, has shown that the total cost of screening for high-risk couples plus the cost of prenatal diagnosis in 21,975 pregnant women and prevention of the birth of 80 severe thalassemic diseases (both α-thalassemia and β-thalassemia) is much less than the costs of treatment of these patients if they were born (**Box 2**).

The overall result of thalassemia control program at Chiangmai Medical School is summarized in **Table 3** and the result of national screening cases is summarized in **Table 4**. After 20 years of launching a nationwide control program for severe thalassemia, we still achieve only approximately 50% screening of pregnant women because many of them attend the antenatal care clinic late. Moreover, we still have the problem of investigating the husband because some of them work in other places, and even abroad. At the moment, we are planning to move further to perform premarital screening and screening of nonpregnant women as well.

THALASSEMIA IN OTHER REGIONS OF ASIA

Thalassemia is common in almost all Asian countries; α-thalassemia, β-thalassemia, and Hb E are commonly noted as the hallmark of Southeast Asia, Sri Lanka, Bangladesh, Maldives, and the eastern region of India and south China. Hemoglobin CS is also prevalent in the Southeast Asia region. The most serious form of thalassemia, Hemoglobin Bart's hydrops fetalis, is almost exclusively found in Southeast Asia and south China.[1,2] The frequency of these abnormal genes in Asian countries is summarized in **Tables 5** and **6**; however, the capability to cope with this magnitude of a public health problem varies widely (**Tables 7** and **8**). Because of this, the Asian Network for Thalassemia Control (ANTC) was established during a conference on Genetics and Population Health held in Fremantle, Australia, in 2004. Representatives

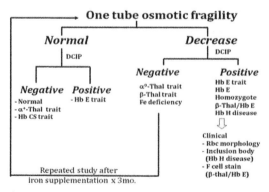

Fig. 1. Schematic of thalassemia screening in Thailand.

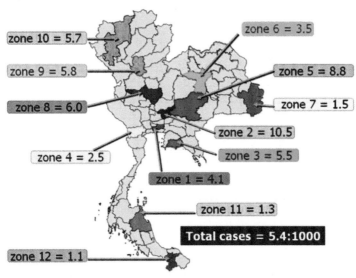

Fig. 2. Infants with thalassemia born per 1000 live births in different parts of Thailand. (*From* the summary of the Department of Health, Ministry of Public Health, Thailand, during the National Annual Thalassemia meeting in Chiangmai, Thailand, October 30-November 1, 2013; with permission.)

from a number of Asian countries together with workers in the thalassemia field from the United Kingdom, Canada, and Australia agreed to work together with Asian people toward the prevention and control of thalassemia in Asia. It was agreed that the ANTC should focus on fact-finding regarding the extent of the problem in individual countries together with an account of the facilities that exist for the diagnosis and management of the different forms of thalassemia in each country. The health burden of the thalassemias in Asia should be translated into disability-adjusted life years (DALYs). Using this approach. it is possible to compare the health burden of the thalassemias with other health problems in Asia (see Kassebaum NJ: The Global Burden of Anemia, in

---

Box 2
The cost-benefit analyses of thalassemia screening versus cost of treatment at Chiangmai University

- Period of screening test: 8 years
- 21,975 pregnant women have been screened
- The program prevented birth of 80 severe thalassemia cases
- Total cost of screening (husband and wife) and PND = 3091,000 Thai Baht (US$ 93,667)
- The cost of treatment of thalassemia patients = 222,961,250 Thai Baht (US$ 6,756,401)

  Benefit:Cost = 72:1

From Wanapirak C. Cost-benefit analysis between screening for high risk couples to prevention of birth of severe thalassemia at Chiangmai University Medical School. Proceeding, National Annual Thalassemia Meeting. Kosa Hotel, Khon Kaen, 2002; with permission.

Table 3
Accumulative data of the prevention and control among pregnant women for severe thalassemia at Chiangmai Medical School between 2003 and 2013

Year	2003	2004	2005	2006	2007	2008	2009	2010	2011	2012	2013	Total
Total screened	2152	1765	1737	1504	1563	1580	1400	1269	1202	1100	1215	16,487
Positive cases	634	697	697	487	598	633	403	383	312	322	373	5539
Couple at risk	41	43	47	31	31	32	25	23	25	23	27	348
Hb Bart hydrops	13	12	12	10	12	12[a]	10	8	5	5	8	107[a]
Homo. β thal	7	8	6	3	5	4	2	3	3	2	4	47
β thal/Hb E	21	23	29	18	14	17[a]	13	12	17	16	15	195[a]
Affected	5	7	10	10	7	8	5	6	5	5	7	75

The overall affected severe thalassemic fetus (Hb Bart hydrops fetus, homozygous β-thalassemia, and β-thalassemia/Hb E disease) detected and prevented birth was 75 cases.
Abbreviations: Hb, hemoglobin; Homo, homozygous; thal, thalassemia.
[a] Double risk.

this issue). Although the preliminary data indicate that thalassemia will pose a health burden comparable to some of the major communicable diseases, far more data are required, particularly gene frequency and accurate costing of both prevention and treatment regimens. During the past 10 years, many Asian countries have made progress in thalassemia.

Guangxi, south China, where thalassemia and Hb E are very common, launched a prevention program in 2010. They have set a "1-stop service unit" for thalassemia screening at marriage registration centers (in China, all couples must be registered at these centers). This is where they educate newly married couples about birth control, human immunodeficiency virus, and other issues including thalassemia, after which blood is drawn and sent to the hospital for a test. Those couples who show a

Table 4
Results of national screening for couples at risk in different parts of Thailand in 2013

Zone	Screened	Screening Pos/Pos	%CAR	%CAR (Predicted)	Efficiency, %
Zone 1	52,046	394	0.76	2.28	33.3
Zone 2	32,700	263	0.80	2.32	34.5
Zone 3	28,633	306	1.07	2.4	44.6
Zone 4	37,263	228	0.61	4.2	14.5
Zone 5	44,326	205	0.46	1.0	46.0
Zone 6	47,767	194	0.46	2.2	20.9
Zone 7	48,534	994	2.05	1.4	100.0
Zone 8	54,112	775	1.43	1.4	100.0
Zone 9	61,063	1019	1.67	3.52	47.4
Zone 10	45,626	—	No data	—	—
Zone 11	41,915	182	0.43	0.52	82.7
Zone 12	48,730	147	0.30	0.52	57.7
Total	536,948	4707	0.88	2.16	40.7

Abbreviations: CAR, couple at risk; Pos, positive.

Table 5
Carriers of α-thalassemia and expected number of new affected births with Hb Bart hydrops fetus in Asian countries

Country	Total Population, Millions	%Carriers of α⁰-thal	%Carriers of α⁺-thal	Estimated Number of Carriers α-thal (α⁰-thal + α⁺-thal)	Estimated Number of Carriers α⁰-thal	Estimated Number of Carriers α⁺-thal	Expected New Affected Births Hb Bart Hydrops
Australia	23.62	0.1	0	23,624	23,624	0	0
Bangladesh	163.09	0	41	66,870,680	0	66,870,680	0
Brunei Darussalam	0.44	0	4.3	18,780	0	18,780	0
Cambodia	15.74	4	33.4	5,887,423	629,671	5,257,752	566
China Guangxi	49.2	0	3.54	1,741,680	0	1,741,680	0
China Hong Kong	7.28	5	14.5	1,419,989	364,100	1,055,889	5.7
India	1293.93	0	41	530,511,824	0	530,511,824	0
Indonesia	256.09	3.2	7.7	27,914,880	8,195,194	19,719,686	1942
Laos	7.03	2	34	2,532,410	140,689	2,391,720	29
Malaysia	30.84	1.8	3.1	1511096	555,096	955,999	85
Maldives	0.4	0	32	128,000	0	128,000	0
Myanmar	54.77	0.4	32	17,746,907	219,098	17,527,810	7
Philippines	103.11	2	18.4	21,034,408	2,062,197	18,972,211	416
Singapore	5.46	3.5	12.1	852,098	191,176	660,922	23
Sri Lanka	21.5	0	6.5	1,397,500	0	1,397,500	0
Thailand	68.08	5	21	17,702,076	3,404,245	14,297,830	918
Vietnam	92.07	2.6	9.1	10,772,471	2,393,882	8,378,588	435
Total	2192.65	—	—	708.1 million (32.3%)	18.2 million (0.83%)	689.9 million (31.5%)	4478

Abbreviations: Hb, hemoglobin; thal, thalassemia.

Table 6
Carriers and expected number of β-thalassemia and new affected births with β-thalassemic diseases in Asian countries

Country	Total Population, Millions	% Carriers of β-thal	% Carriers of Hb E	Estimated Number of Carriers β-thal and Hb E	Estimated Number of Carriers β-thal	Estimated Number of Carriers Hb E	Expected New Affected Births β-thal/Hb E	Expected New Affected Births Homozygous β-thal
Australia	23.62	0.4	0.4	188,988	94,494	94,494	8	2
Bangladesh	163.09	4.1	6.1	16,636,120	6,687,068	9,949,052	15,694	2536
Brunei Darussalam	0.44	2	0	8735	8735	0	1	1
Cambodia	15.74	3	30	519,475	472,253	4,722,532	38,555	319
China Guangxi	49.2	6.78	0.42	3,542,400	3,335,760	206,640	306	271
China Hong Kong	7.28	3.5	0.3	276,716	254870	21,846	33	28
India	1293.93	3.9	1	63,402,633	50,463,320	12,939,313	26,422	16,738
Indonesia	256.09	5	6	28,170,979	12,804,991	15,365,989	22,942	4740
Laos	7.03	6	18	1,688,273	422,068	1,266,205	4244	265
Malaysia	30.84	4.5	5.5	3,083,869	1,387,741	1,696,128	2616	530
Maldives	0.4	18	0.9	75,600	72,000	3600	76	69
Myanmar	54.77	2.2	25	14,898,638	1,205,037	13,693,601	32,008	209
Philippines	103.11	1.2	0.4	1,649,758	1,237,318	412,439	266	150
Singapore	5.46	3	0.64	198,823	163,865	34,958	25	17
Sri Lanka	21.5	2.5	2.5	105,000	537,500	537,500	376	94
Thailand	68.08	5.3	33	26,076,519	3,608,500	22,468,019	53,837	1031
Vietnam	92.07	2.6	1	3,314,606	2,393,882	920,724	833	435
Total	2192.65	—	—	169.5 million (7.7%)	85.2 million (3.9%)	84.4 million (3.8%)	198,241	27,434

Abbreviations: Hb, hemoglobin; thal, thalassemia.

Table 7
Thalassemia diagnosis in different Asian countries

Country	Blood Cell Analyzer	OF	Hb Analysis Electrophoresis	Hb Analysis HPLC/LPLC/CE	DNA Analysis α	DNA Analysis β
Australia	+	−	+	+	+	+
Bangladesh	(+)	−	(+)	(+)	(+)	(+)
Cambodia	(+)	(+)	(+)	(+)	−	−
China: Guangxi	+	−	+	+	+	+
China: Hong Kong	+	−	+	+	+	+
India	(+)	+	+	(+)	+	+
Indonesia	(+)	−	+	(+)	(+)	(+)
Laos	(+)	−	(+)	−	−	−
Malaysia	+	−	+	+	+	+
Maldives	+	−	−	+	(+)	−
Myanmar	+	(+)	+	(+)	(+)	(+)
Singapore	+	−	+	+	+	+
Sri Lanka	+	−	+	(+)	(+)	(+)
Thailand	+	(+)	+	+	+	+
Vietnam	+	−	+	(+)	(+)	(+)

(+) indicates that such diagnostic test is available only in a larger hospital or medical center. Patients who live in rural areas may have to travel hundreds of kilometers for definite diagnosis of thalassemia or blood samples may need to be transported to a nearby medical center for diagnosis.

Abbreviations: CE, capillary electrophoresis; Hb, hemoglobin; HPLC, high-performance liquid chromatography; LPLC, low-pressure liquid chromatography.

positive blood test will be called back for further counseling. In general, this is preconception counseling followed by prenatal diagnosis when they become pregnant. **Table 9** shows some preliminary data of the prevention and control program in Guangxi. Approximately 50% of pregnant women were screened for thalassemia and they can prevent births of severe and intermedia thalassemia in 6940 cases within 5 years.

Malaysia started a National Thalassemia Program in 2004 and a year later the Malaysian government provided a 40 million Ringgit (US$ 10.6 million) grant to support the program. This budget is for public awareness and health education, population screening and laboratory diagnosis, comprehensive management of patients, and a thalassemia registry. Up to 2014, the number of patients with thalassemia was as follows: β-thalassemia major 2415 cases, β-thalassemia/Hb E 1961 cases, β-thalassemia intermedia 590, and 359 cases of Hb H disease. The method of screening for couples at risk is through cascade screening and is voluntary (Hishamshah B, Mohd Ibrahim, Personal communication, 2015).

Sri Lanka launched a National Prevention Program in 2006 (see Allen A, Allen S, Olivieri N: Improving laboratory and clinical hematology services in resource limited settings, in this issue). The aim of the program is as follows:

1. Draft guidelines and protocols on prevention and management,
2. Support for transferring affordable resources and technologies, and
3. Promotion of community empowerment and mobilization.

Table 8
Treatment available in different Asian countries

Country	Blood Transfusion	Iron Chelation DFO	L1	Exjade	BM Transplant	PND	National Program
Australia	+	+	+	+	+	+	(+)
Bangladesh	(+)	(+)	(+)	(+)	−	−	−
Cambodia	(+)	(+)	−	−	−	−	−
Guangxi	+	(+)	(+)	(+)	+	+	+
Hong Kong	+	+	+	+	+	+	+
India	(+)	(+)	+	+	(+)	(+)	(+)
Indonesia	(+)	(+)	+	+	−	(+)	(+)
Laos	(+)	(+)	(+)	−	−	−	−
Malaysia	+	+	+	+	+	+	+
Maldives	+	+	+	+	−	+	+
Myanmar	(+)	(+)	+	(+)	−	−	−
Singapore	+	+	+	+	+	+	+
Sri Lanka	+	+	+	+	−	−	+
Thailand	+	+	+	(+)	+	+	+
Vietnam	(+)	(+)	(+)	(+)	(+)	(+)	−

(+) indicates that such treatment is available only in a larger hospital or medical center. Patients who live in rural areas may have to travel hundreds of kilometers for a blood transfusion and other treatment.

The government provided 40 million Rs (US\$ 298,982) for equipment to the regional thalassemia screening centers in 2008. Under this program, they have screened more than 100,000 individuals; 16.3% have received a "pink card," which means thalassemia carrier, and those who are healthy received a "green card."[13]

Indonesia is preparing for a nationwide thalassemia prevention program. Epidemiologic studies and genotyping to determine the distribution of abnormal hemoglobin genes, including α-thalassemia, β-thalassemia, and Hb E in different islands/ethnic groups has been conducted. This will help to plan an appropriate strategy for a future prevention program in the country. Currently, the government provides a budget to buy deferasirox (Exjade) for patients with thalassemia with iron overload. A clinical practice guideline has been developed. Some pilot models of thalassemia screening have been conducted in several medical centers.[13]

Table 9
Some results of the thalassemia control program in Guangxi between 2010 and 2014

Year	Number Screening (Hb Typing)	Genotyping	Prenatal Diagnosis	Severe and Intermedia Thalassemia Fetus Detected
2010	907,217	27,000	2712	768
2011	1,494,201	50,199	4373	815
2012	1,885954	92,907	5717	1264
2013	1,860,416	96,241	7955	1596
2014	1,892,267	106,489	8279	2013
Total	8,567,608	395,015	30,878	6940

India has also conducted an epidemiologic study for abnormal hemoglobin genes in different parts of the country (see Das R, Ahluwalia J, Sachdeva MUS: Hematological Practice in India, in this issue). A pilot model for mass screening, genetic counseling has been developed in 6 centers: Maharashtra, Gujarat, West Bengal, Assam, Karnataka, and Punjab. The results show that among the 21,645 cases screened, including 10,673 college students and 10,972 antenatal cases, the prevalence of β-thalassemia trait varies from 2% to 4%. The major problem in India is that 50% of pregnant women first attended hospital in the third trimester.[13]

Even in other Asian countries that do not have a nationwide program for the prevention of thalassemia some progress has been made. Almost all Asian countries have established a nongovernment society/foundation for parents and patients. This is partly supported by the Thalassemia International Federation (TIF). TIF has also arranged to donate an automatic HPLC system to Cambodia and is planning for the second Pan-Asian Conference on Haemoglobinopathies in Hanoi, Vietnam, from September 26 to 27, 2015 (the first Pan-Asian Conference on Haemoglobinopathies was held in Bangkok, February 2012). Although without support from international agencies, collaboration between Asian countries is developing. At the moment, Thailand is working with their colleagues in Bangladesh, Cambodia, Myanmar, Laos, and Vietnam to identify molecular defects of both α-thalassemias and β-thalassemias and is also helping to train technicians and scientists from these countries. It also supports each country to conduct education meetings and workshops on laboratory diagnosis of thalassemia by helping them to organize the program and send speakers to give lectures. August 7 to 8, 2014, was the first time that the Southeast Asian Regional Office of the World Health Organization called for a meeting on management and prevention of thalassemia in the region in New Delhi. The objective of the meeting was to review and learn from the experiences of the countries and to review their draft regional guidelines on management and prevention of thalassemia.

GLOBAL ISSUES

It has been recognized for some time that the thalassemias, like the sickle cell disorders, are producing an increasingly serious global health problem.[1,14] As well as the remarkable diversity of these conditions in Asian countries, particularly the severe forms of α-thalassemia as well as β-thalassemia, the latter occur at variable rates throughout the Middle East, the Mediterranean region, and localized parts of Africa. Like some of the Asian countries, slow progress has been made in many of these regions toward the prevention and better management of the different forms of thalassemia, but, given the remarkable diversity of acquired communicable and other diseases, it has been very difficult for the governments of some of these countries to either recognize or develop programs for the control of the thalassemias.

In 2002, the World Health Organization published a report entitled *Genomics and World Health* that recommended both North/South and South/South partnerships as an approach to the control and management of common genetic diseases such as the hemoglobin disorders. These recommendations were later confirmed by the World Health Organization Executive Board, and at the 59th World Health Assembly, resolutions were passed to urge member states to develop programs for the prevention and management of the hemoglobin disorders. Later, a meeting was held under the auspices of the World Health Organization and TIF that published further recommendations for the development of international partnerships of this kind for the control of the hemoglobin disorders.[15] Recently, and for the first time, the inherited hemoglobin disorders have been included in the latest edition of the Global Burden of Disease Program and they have been clearly defined as major factors in the global burden of anemia[16,17] (see Kassebaum NJ: The Global Burden of Anemia, in this issue).

Although there is evidence that the governments of developing countries are slowly becoming aware of the importance of the inherited disorders of hemoglobin, progress is still very slow. The World Health Organization and related international bodies have done very little to support the concept of North/South and South/South partnerships and with a few notable exceptions the major international medical funding charities have shown little interest in inherited diseases. It seems likely that this situation will continue unless these bodies can be persuaded to produce more balanced support between inherited and acquired diseases in the future.

An important factor for the future will be work directed at determining the true global burden of the inherited hemoglobin disorders. It is becoming clear that our knowledge of the true frequency of these conditions is still rather limited. There is growing evidence that these conditions vary in their frequency in many countries over short geographic distances and much of the published data are based on measurements of gene frequency in 1 or 2 centers that is then extrapolated to the whole country. Hence, the true burden of these conditions will only become apparent by detailed micro mapping of their frequency throughout high-frequency countries.[18–20]

SUMMARY

Thalassemia is one of the major global public health problems. The strategy for control programs consists of treatment and prevention, that is, treatment of existing patients in the most cost-benefit way and reducing the birth of new cases. The specific target is to set up the core of effective treatment, prevention, and training services in each country. This should define the methods of treatment and prevention appropriate to individual countries. To achieve success in the prevention and control of thalassemia, it needs continuity and a holistic approach. It is expected that with optimal collaboration between countries in high-frequency regions and north-south collaboration, effective prevention and control can be achieved.

REFERENCES

1. Weatherall DJ, Clegg JB. The thalassaemia syndromes. 4th edition. Oxford: Blackwell Science; 2001.
2. Fucharoen S, Winichagoon P. Thalassemia in Southeast Asia: problems and strategy for prevention and control. Southeast Asian J Trop Med Public Health 1992; 23:647–55.
3. Winichagoon P, Thonglairoam V, Fucharoen S, et al. Severity differences in β-thalassaemia haemoglobin E syndromes: implication of genetic factors. Br J Haematol 1993;83:633–9.
4. Sripichai O, Makarasara W, Munkongdee T, et al. A scoring system for the classification of beta-thalassemia/Hb E disease severity. Am J Hematol 2008;83: 482–4.
5. Premawardhena A, Fisher CA, Olivieri NF, et al. Haemoglobin E β thalassaemia in Sri Lanka. Lancet 2005;366:1467–70.
6. Viprakasit V, Nuchprayoon I, Chuansumrit A, et al. Deferiprone (GPO-L-ONE((R))) monotherapy reduces iron overload in transfusion-dependent thalassemias: 1-year results from a multicenter prospective, single arm, open label,

dose escalating phase III pediatric study (GPO-L-ONE; A001) from Thailand. Am J Hematol 2013;88:251–60.

7. Songdej D, Sirachainan N, Wongwerawattanakoon P, et al. Combined chelation therapy with daily oral deferiprone and twice-weekly subcutaneous infusion of desferrioxamine in children with beta-thalassemia: 3-year experience. Acta Haematol 2015;133:226–36.

8. Leelahavarong P, Chaikledkaew U, Hongeng S, et al. A cost-utility and budget impact analysis of allogeneic hematopoietic stem cell transplantation for severe thalassemic patients in Thailand. BMC Health Serv Res 2010;10:209.

9. Fucharoen G, Sanchaisuriya K, Sae-ung N, et al. A simplified screening strategy for thalassaemia and haemoglobin E in rural communities in south-east Asia. Bull World Health Organ 2004;82:364–72.

10. Fucharoen S, Winichagoon P, Wisedpanichkij R, et al. Prenatal and postnatal diagnoses of thalassemias and hemoglobinopathies by HPLC. Clin Chem 1998;44:740–8.

11. Winichagoon P, Svasti S, Munkongdee T, et al. Rapid diagnosis of thalassemias and other hemoglobinopathies by capillary electrophoresis system. Transl Res 2008;152:178–84.

12. Wanapirak C. Cost-benefit analysis between screening for high risk couples to prevention of birth of severe thalassemia at Chiangmai University Medical School. Proceeding, National Annual Thalassemia Meeting. Kosa Hotel, Khon Kaen, Thailand, 8–9 August, 2002.

13. SEARO/WHO. Thematic group meeting on management and prevention of thalassaemia. New Delhi: Lalit Hotel; 2014.

14. Weatherall DJ. The inherited diseases of hemoglobin are an emerging global health burden. Blood 2010;115:4331–6.

15. WHO. Management of haemoglobin disorders. Report of a joint WHO-TIF meeting. Nicosia, Cyprus, November 16–18, 2007. World Health Org. 2008.

16. Kassebaum NJ, Jasrasaria R, Naghavi M, et al. A systematic analysis of global anemia burden from 1990 to 2010. Blood 2014;123:615–24.

17. Murray CJ, Vos T, Lozano R, et al. Disability-adjusted life years (DALYs) for 291 diseases and injuries in 21 regions, 1990-2010: a systematic analysis for the Global Burden of Disease Study 2010. Lancet 2012;380:2197–223.

18. Colah R, Gorakshakar A, Phanasgaonkar S, et al. Epidemiology of beta-thalassaemia in Western India: mapping the frequencies and mutations in sub-regions of Maharashtra and Gujarat. Br J Haematol 2010;149:739–47.

19. Weatherall DJ. The importance of micromapping the gene frequencies for the common inherited disorders of haemoglobin. Br J Haematol 2010;149:635–7.

20. Weatherall DJ. The challenge of haemoglobinopathies in resource-poor countries. Br J Haematol 2011;154:736–44.

Glucose-6-Phosphate Dehydrogenase Deficiency

Lucio Luzzatto, MD, FRCP, FRCPath[a,b,*], Caterina Nannelli, MSc[c], Rosario Notaro, MD[c]

KEYWORDS

- Glucose-6-phosphate dehydrogenase • Hemolytic anemia • Favism
- X-linked genetic polymorphism • Malaria selection

KEY POINTS

- Glucose-6-phosphate dehydrogenase (G6PD) deficiency, expressed in red cells, is mostly asymptomatic; however, G6PD-deficient persons develop acute hemolytic anemia (AHA) when exposed to fava beans, to infection, or to certain drugs, including primaquine.
- The gene encoding G6PD maps to the X chromosome. Therefore, full-blown G6PD deficiency is more common in males, but female heterozygotes are also at risk of hemolysis.
- G6PD deficiency is widespread in the entire world and its epidemiology correlates with that of malaria; different mutant alleles underlie G6PD deficiency in different populations.
- Primaquine is still the only drug that can eradicate *Plasmodium vivax* hypnozoites; to promptly prevent or to treat hemolytic anemia, it is important to test for G6PD before administering primaquine.

INTRODUCTION

G6PD was discovered and biochemically characterized in 1932 by Otto Warburg and Walter Christian[1] in yeast and in red cells as an enzyme with a redox function. It was one of the first enzymes of glucose metabolism to be identified, but, although Warburg did not know that, the clinical manifestations of what later became known as G6PD deficiency had been already described. In the nineteenth century, pediatricians in Greece, Portugal, and Italy observed severe anemia and hemoglobinuria in children who had eaten fava beans – hence, the term *favism*[2]; it was noticed that favism tended to recur in the same persons and also that it ran in families. Subsequently, since the 1920s, it was observed[3] that an adverse side effect of 8-aminoquinolines (primaquine and plasmoquine), used for the treatment and the prophylaxis of malaria, was AHA. No connection to favism was suspected at the time, but again it was reported that it was

[a] Scientific Direction, Istituto Toscano Tumori, Viale Pieraccini 6, Florence 50139, Italy; [b] University of Florence, Florence, Italy; [c] Core Research Laboratory-Istituto Toscano Tumori, Azienda Universitaria-Ospedaliera Careggi, Viale Pieraccini 6, Florence 50139, Italy
* Corresponding author. Department of Haematology and Blood Transfusion, Muhimbili University College of Health Sciences (MUHAS), P. O. Box 65001, Dar-es-Salaam, Tanzania.
E-mail address: lluzzatto@blood.ac.tz

Hematol Oncol Clin N Am 30 (2016) 373–393
http://dx.doi.org/10.1016/j.hoc.2015.11.006
0889-8588/16/$ – see front matter © 2016 Elsevier Inc. All rights reserved.

only in certain people that this side effect occurred, and in those people it could happen again on rechallenge with the same drug; this became known as the *primaquine sensitivity syndrome.*

In 1956, Paul Carson's group in Chicago[4] reported that red cells from primaquine-sensitive persons were deficient in G6PD (enzyme activity <15% of normal), and in 1958 Gennaro Sansone's group in Genoa, Italy,[5] found the same deficiency in children with a previous history of favism. It was promptly proved that G6PD deficiency was genetically determined and that its inheritance was X-linked.[6] Almost as soon as Mary Lyon[7] discovered the X-chromosome inactivation phenomenon in mice, Ernie Beutler's group[8] found independently, using G6PD as a marker, that the same applied to humans. At the time this was the first example of a hemolytic anemia due to an inherited abnormality expressed in red cells; hence, the term *enzymopathy* was coined, in analogy to hemoglobinopathy. Reassuringly, however, it was clear that in the absence of an exogenous trigger, G6PD-deficient persons had no pathology; hence, primaquine-induced or fava bean–induced AHA became a prototype of a disease arising from a specific interaction between a gene and an environmental factor, just at the time when the term *pharmacogenetics* was coined.[9]

At approximately the same time, Tony Allison[10] and Arno Motulsky[11] hypothesized that genetically determined G6PD deficiency might have been favored by malaria selection; this spurred a flurry of studies aiming to determine the frequency of this trait in many countries. It quickly emerged that G6PD deficiency was widespread in human populations in all continents; a wealth of epidemiologic data were tabulated by David Livingstone as early as 1967.[12] In the meantime, the World Health Organization (WHO) Human Genetics, then headed by Italo Barrai, was prompt in taking on board the public health implications of such a widespread genetic abnormality; in 1966, a study group was arranged with the remit to review available data and to agree on a measure of standardization for the study of G6PD deficiency.[13]

This article focuses on the essentials of G6PD deficiency as a global health problem and on the essentials of its clinical manifestations, which are a paradigmatic example of a highly specific interaction between an inherited abnormality and exogenous agents that trigger hemolysis. Space does not permit a comprehensive coverage, particularly with respect to management, for which existing literature is referred to.[14,15]

BIOCHEMISTRY OF GLUCOSE-6-PHOSPHATE DEHYDROGENASE AND GLUCOSE-6-PHOSPHATE DEHYDROGENASE DEFICIENCY

G6PD is a housekeeping enzyme, expressed in all cells of the body, that catalyzes the oxidation of glucose 6-phosphate (G6P) to 6-phosphoglucono-δ-lactone (**Fig. 1**), which is then hydrolyzed to 6-phosphoglucono-∂-lactone this, in turn, through the action of the enzyme phosphogluconate dehydrogenase (6PGD), is further oxidized and decarboxylated to the pentose sugar ribulose 5-phosphate.[16] Both G6PD and 6PGD have NADP as coenzyme, and therefore 2 molecules of NADPH are formed per molecule of G6P oxidized by G6PD (see **Fig. 1**). Because the product of these reactions is pentose, G6PD is commonly referred to as the first enzyme of the pentose phosphate pathway. On the other hand, from targeted inactivation of G6PD in embryonic stem cells[17] and from other lines of evidence it became clear that the prime physiologic role of G6PD is the production of NADPH.

In most cells of the human body NADPH is the key electron donor required for many biosynthetic processes, including several reactions in the pathways of fatty acid synthesis, cholesterol, and steroid hormone synthesis, as well as in the formation

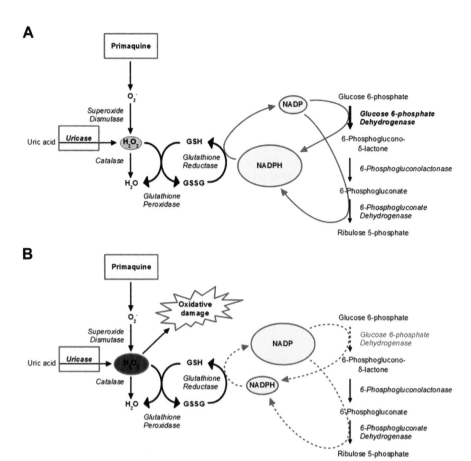

Fig. 1. Role of G6PD in protection against oxidative damage. (*A*) In G6PD-normal red cells, G6PD and 6-phosphogluconate dehydrogenase—2 of the first enzymes of the pentose phosphate pathway—provide ample supply of NADPH, which in turn regenerates GSH when this is oxidized by reactive oxygen species (eg, O_2^- and H_2O_2). O_2^- is one of the most reactive oxygen species that can be generated from the metabolism of pro-oxidant compounds, such as primaquine; uricase, on the other hand, directly produces hydrogen peroxide in equimolar amount to uric acid degraded. (*B*) In G6PD-deficient red cells, where the enzyme activity is reduced, NADPH production is limited and it may not be sufficient to cope with the excess of reactive oxygen species generated in the presence of pro-oxidant compounds.

from ribose of deoxyribose required for DNA synthesis.[16] In most cells there are several enzymes catalyzing dehydrogenase reactions – other than G6PD – that produce NADPH, and therefore even when G6PD is deficient there may be no shortage of NADPH. The situation is radically different in red blood cells, because the other NADPH-producing enzymes have been sacrificed in the course of erythroid cell differentiation; at the same time, these cells do not need NADPH for the biosynthetic pathways (discussed previously) because they do not exist, having been sacrificed as well.[18] On the other hand, red cells have a great need for the other major function of NADPH: defense against oxidative stress or oxidative attack.[19] This defense is largely mediated through the glutathione cycle, whereby a steady regeneration of reduced glutathione (GSH) depends on a steady supply of NADPH (see **Fig. 1**). Because the red cell is a professional loader, carrier, and unloader of hemoglobin-bound oxygen, and because free radicals can be formed in the process,[20] it is crucially important that it can defend itself against endogenous oxidative stress, even when there is no exogenous attack in sight.

G6PD deficiency is due to inherited mutations in the *G6PD* gene (discussed later) that are expressed in all cells; and it is already clear from the above that erythrocytes, more than other cells, are vulnerable to the consequences of this defect. But there is an additional important reason for this. As red cells age in circulation, there tends to be a gradual decrease in many of their functions, because individual proteins underlying those functions decay exponentially in these ribosome-less cells that cannot make new protein[21]; as a result, G6PD activity is approximately 50 times less in a normal red cell that is ready to be removed on day 120 compared with when it itself was a reticulocyte.[22] This process is further magnified with those mutations—the large majority—that compromise the in vivo stability of the G6PD protein.[23]

G6PD deficiency is never complete; if it were complete, it would be lethal.[24] Therefore, in most cases, in the steady state, the consequences of G6PD deficiency are not noticeable (see **Fig. 1**); the NADPH produced by the residual G6PD activity and by 6PGD activity is just enough to keep the red cell going, with marginal reduction of its life span. If an exogenous oxidative stress is applied, however, G6PD-deficient red cells are unable to step up NADPH production (which normal red cells do); as a consequence, GSH is rapidly depleted (see **Fig. 1**), hemoglobin and other proteins are damaged, and eventually the red cell becomes prey to macrophages or hemolyzes altogether.[25]

MOLECULAR-GENETIC BASIS OF GLUCOSE-6-PHOSPHATE DEHYDROGENASE DEFICIENCY

The *G6PD* gene consists of 13 exons (the first of which is noncoding) and it encodes a 515–amino acids (AAs) protein subunit,[26] the homodimer of which is enzymatically active; the dimer can further dimerize to give an enzymatically active homotetramer.[27] Each subunit has 1 molecule of tightly bound NADP[28] in addition to binding sites for the NADP substrate and the G6P substrate.

As discussed previously, G6PD deficiency was known from formal genetics to be inherited as an X-linked trait,[6] and the *G6PD* gene maps to the long arm of the X chromosome (band Xq28).[29] X-linkage has important implications with respect to G6PD deficiency. First, in males there are only 2 genotypes: hemizygous normal and hemizygous G6PD deficient. In females there are 3 genotypes: homozygous normal, homozygous deficient, and heterozygous. Second, although it is often stated that G6PD deficiency is more common in males, this is not correct; according to the fundamental principle of population genetics (the Hardy-Weinberg equilibrium), homozygous females are much more rare than hemizygous males, but heterozygous females are much more numerous (**Table 1**). A bonus of X-linkage is that male frequencies indicate directly allele frequencies (see **Table 1**). Third, as a result of X-chromosome inactivation, heterozygous females are genetic mosaics[8,30]; on average, one-half of their red cells are G6PD normal and one-half are G6PD deficient. There is a wide distribution around this average, whereby in some females the enzyme activity phenotype overlaps with normal, whereas in others it overlaps with the G6PD deficiency as seen in homozygotes[31]; this has obvious clinical implications.

All *G6PD* mutations known (**Table 2**), except *G6PD* A, are associated with more or less severe enzyme deficiency but never with complete loss of activity; there are no frameshift mutations in the database (such mutations presumably are lethal; discussed previously and later), and the only nonsense mutation has been found in a heterozygous woman.[32] The mutations that underlie G6PD deficiency are spread

Table 1
The frequency of glucose-6-phosphate dehydrogenase deficiency is markedly different in males and in females (Hardy-Weinberg rule)

Glucose-6-Phosphate Dehydrogenase Deficiency Allele Frequency, q	Glucose-6-Phosphate Dehydrogenase– Deficient Hemizygous Males, %	Glucose-6-Phosphate Dehydrogenase– Deficient Homozygous Females, %	Glucose-6-Phosphate Dehydrogenase– Deficient Heterozygous Females, %
0.01	1	0.01	2
0.05	5	0.25	9.5
0.25	25	6.25	37.5

In the first column, q is the conventional symbol for the rarer allele in a 2-allele polymorphism. The frequency of G6PD-deficient males in column 2 is simply the value of q expressed in %. The frequency of G6PD-deficient homozygous females (column 3) is q^2, and the frequency of G6PD-deficient heterozygous (column 4) is $2(1-q)q$, as from the Hardy-Weinberg rule. It is seen that at low allele frequency heterozygous females are approximately double the hemizygous males, whereas homozygous females are rare.

throughout the coding region (**Fig. 2**). The most recent compilation[33] lists 186 *G6PD* alleles in addition to the normal or wild-type gene, referred to traditionally as *G6PD B*.

A large majority of mutations (159) are missense mutations due to single nucleotide substitutions causing single AA replacements; however, there are also multiple missense mutations within the same allele as well as in frame deletions and rare mutations that affect splicing. The frequency of single and multiple nucleotide substitutions is approximately the same among variants that are or may be polymorphic and those that are not. In contrast, deletions are only found within the nonpolymorphic variants (see **Table 2**).

Not surprisingly, different mutations cause both quantitative and qualitative changes in the enzyme. This has led to a classification of G6PD variants based on the degree of deficiency and on clinical manifestations (**Table 3**). A cluster of mutations, most of them in exon 10, encode AAs that are in the dimerization domain[34]; they affect markedly the stability of the dimer and they produce class I variants (see **Table 3**), causing chronic nonspherocytic hemolytic anemia (CNSHA).

A remarkable feature at the genomic level is that the *G6PD* gene overlaps with the *IKBKG/NEMO* gene, which is transcribed in the opposite direction and mutations of

Table 2
Molecular basis of allelic variants of glucose-6-phosphate dehydrogenase[a]

	Class	Single Nucleotide Substitutions	Multiple Nucleotide Substitutions	Deletions	Intronic Mutations	Total Number
Polymorphic	II, III, and IV	27	4	0	0	31
Perhaps polymorphic[b]	II and III	55	6	0	0	61
Nonpolymorphic	I	69	5	10	1	85
Undefined	—	8	0	0	1	9
Total number	—	159	15	10	2	*186*

[a] *G6PD* B is regarded as the human wild type and, therefore, is not included in the count.
[b] Not every G6PD variant in class II or III has been proved polymorphic, but this is probable.

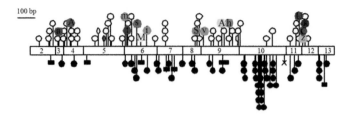

○ Union ; ● Canton ; M Mediterranean ; ▲ A–(202A); ● Kaiping ; ● Taipei;

● Viangchan ; m Mahidol ; ● Chatham ; i Coimbra ; S Seattle ; S Santamaria ;

● Aures ; z Cosenza ; A A–(968C).

Fig. 2. Many structural mutations are found within the coding region of the human *G6PD* gene. All variants shown, except *G6PD* A, are associated with enzyme deficiency. Below the diagram with numbered exons are mutations associated with the most severe clinical phenotype (class I: see **Table 3**), all of which are sporadic and rare. Above the exon diagram are mutations associated with a milder phenotype (class II or III), many of which are polymorphic; and some of those that have been more extensively investigated are shown by initialed lollipop symbols. A– is heterogeneous because it can result from a combination of the N126D replacement with any of three additional mutations, the most common of which is V68M. (*From* Luzzatto L, Poggi, VE. Glucose 6-phosphate dehydrogenase deficiency. In: Orkin SH, Nathan DG, Ginsburg D, et al, editor. Hematology of infancy and childhood. Philadelphia: Saunders; 2009. p. 887; with permission.)

Table 3
Classification of glucose-6-phosphate dehydrogenase variants

	Current Classification			Proposed Revision	
Class	Residual Glucose-6-Phosphate Dehydrogenase Activity (% of Normal)[a]	Clinical Manifestations	Examples of Genetic Variants	Class	Residual Glucose-6-Phosphate Dehydrogenase Activity (% of Normal)[a]
I[b]	<10[c]	CNSHA[d] (NNJ, acute exacerbations)	Guadalajara, Nara, Sunderland	I	<10
II	<10[c]	None in the steady state	Mediterranean, Canton, Union	II + III	<30[e]
III	10–60	None in the steady state	A–, Mahidol, Seattle		
IV	100	None	A, B	IV	>85
V	>100	None	—	—	—

[a] Levels of residual G6PD activity in hemizygous males.
[b] The definition of class I variants is not biochemical but clinical (ie, class I variants cause CNSHD).
[c] The range of G6PD activity is similar in class I and class II variants, which may seem strange because the clinical phenotype is significantly different. It must be considered, however, that (1) in CNSHD, there is always reticulocytosis, which increases G6PD levels, and (2) in some class I variants, the residual G6PD activity may be similar to a class II or even a class III variant, but the enzyme kinetics may be unfavorable.
[d] When hemolysis is not compensated, chronic anemia is present and blood transfusions may be necessary at times or even at regular intervals.
[e] Cutoff is indicated as 30%, because all G6PD variants in class II and III described so far have a residual activity of less than 30%.

which are responsible for the serious disease *incontinentia pigmenti*.[35] Some of these mutations are lethal in males, but in females they include large deletions of *G6PD*, which are compatible with life thanks to selection for cells in which the active X chromosome has an intact *G6PD* allele.

EVOLUTION

From full genome databases, it is inferred that G6PD is not present in *Archaebacteria*, which, because they live in environments with low or no oxygen, hardly need defense against oxidative stress.[36] In all other living organisms, G6PD is highly conserved; the AA sequence similarity from microorganisms to mammals ranges from 43% to 98%. This high degree of conservation must mean that the G6PD protein has been shaped by evolution early and robustly to perform its enzymatic function well. In many plants, there are 2 *G6PD* genes—1 encodes cytosolic G6PD and the other G6PD present in plastids[37]—and a human pseudogene is known.[38]

In the alignment of *G6PD* coding sequences from all organisms, those of *Plasmodia* stand out because they have a long 5′ extension,[39] which encodes the metabolically related enzyme 6-phosphoglucono-δ-lactonase.[40] It has been suggested that the protein product of the parasite's bifunctional gene[41] might be a new target for antimalarials.[42,43]

It is often thought that in an enzyme protein, functionally critical AA residues are less likely to change over evolutionary times; as a result, mutations that cause disease in general are more likely to affect the most evolutionarily conserved residues.[44,45] This simple correlation, however, is not always seen,[46] and it seems that it does not exactly hold for G6PD. An analysis of 103 *G6PD* mutants causing G6PD deficiency in humans, as against 52 *G6PD* sequences from 45 different organisms, has shown that most mutations (74%) are in highly and moderately conserved (50%–99% of similarity) AAs, whereas few mutations are in fully conserved or in poorly conserved AAs (**Fig. 3**).[36] This distinct relationship suggests that mutations in poorly conserved AAs may remain inconspicuous because they do not cause significant G6PD deficiency, whereas mutations in fully conserved AAs might be lethal, which is not

Amino Acid Conservation

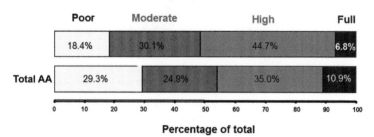

Fig. 3. Conservation and human G6PD mutants. The upper bar reports the distribution of G6PD mutants among evolutionary AA conservation categories: full, 100% of similarity; high, 76%–99% of similarity; moderate, 50%–75% of similarity; and poor, less than 50% of similarity. The lower bar reports the distribution of the 515 AAs of the human G6PD among the conservation categories. The distribution among evolutionary conservation categories of the mutants is statistically different from the distribution of AAs: $\chi^2 = 9.36$; *P*<.03. (*Adapted from* Notaro R, Afolayan A, Luzzatto L. Human mutations in glucose 6-phosphate dehydrogenase reflect evolutionary history. FASEB J 2000;14:491; with permission.)

surprising in the case of a gene, such as G6PD, present in a single functioning copy and indispensable for life.

EPIDEMIOLOGY AND MALARIA SELECTION

The geographic distribution of G6PD deficiency is spectacular, because it spares no continent[47] (**Fig. 4**), yet population frequencies are highly variable, because they reflect 2 major factors in the epidemiology of a genetic abnormality: environmental selection and migration. The correlation with the epidemiology of malaria, discussed previously, is obvious, for instance, in areas as distant as tropical Africa, Southeast Asia, and the Vanuatu archipelago in the Pacific; and parts of Southern Europe can be included, where malaria was endemic until 2 to 3 generations ago.[48] G6PD deficiency is also common in the Americas, however, including areas that have never had malaria; this is largely accounted for by migrations, voluntary or otherwise, from Africa, Asia, and Europe. G6PD deficiency has no significant frequency in native American populations.

The wealth of data on the frequency of G6PD deficiency (reflected in **Fig. 4**) originates from many population surveys, carried out by a variety of methods; therefore, a margin of error must be allowed in the classification of individual samples. Also, in collecting data there may have been several sources of inadvertent sampling bias (blood donors, school children, and so forth). The most common type of confusion relates, however, to some cases of a single figure reported as the overall frequency of G6PD deficiency, observed in a mixed group of males and females, despite that the *G6PD* gene is X-linked. Most tests for G6PD deficiency classify as deficient all G6PD-deficient hemizygous males, all G6PD-deficient homozygous females, and some (variable and difficult to estimate) portion of heterozygous females. It is

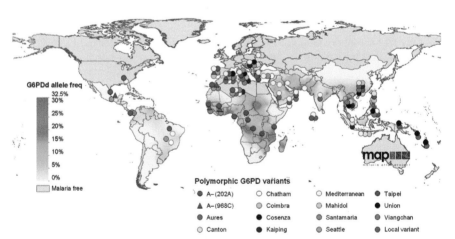

Fig. 4. Global distribution of G6PD deficiency. This map is a combination of 3 previous maps.[47,49,59] Color shades on the map indicate the median predicted allele frequency of G6PD deficiency in malaria-endemic and malaria-eliminating countries, according to the geostatistical model designed by Howes and coworkers.[49] Each colored circle illustrates the geographic distribution of 1 polymorphic *G6PD* allele present in more than 1 population. (triangles used for G6PD A− [968C, L323P] to distinguish it from *G6PD* A− [202A, V68M]; note that both of these mutations are always found associated with 376G, N126D). Dark gray circles indicate local polymorphic variants that have been detected only in 1 population. (*Data from* Refs.[47,49,59])

preferable to carry out a population survey by testing males only; from the G6PD frequency value obtained, the frequencies of the female genotypes can be calculated by using the Hardy-Weinberg rule (see **Table 1**).

The striking geographic similarity between the distribution of G6PD deficiency and that of malaria[49] does not itself constitute proof that the latter has selected for genes that cause the former, but more pieces of evidence exist.[50] Natural selection has to do with prereproductive mortality, and in malaria-endemic countries, malaria mortality is mostly in children. Numerous field studies in Africa have tested this evolutionary hypothesis by comparing, in G6PD-normal children and G6PD-deficient children, the rate of malaria incidence, the levels of parasitemia, or the severity of malaria[51–54]; an additional large multicentric study has been published recently.[55] All studies have been concordant in finding that G6PD deficiency is malaria protective (especially against severe malaria); however, again it is highly relevant that the *G6PD* gene is X-linked. The dynamics of natural selection for an X-linked gene are such that if both males and females with the protective gene have increased fitness, the gene tends to fixation: however, there is no instance where, despite high levels of malaria, the entire population has become G6PD deficient. This is a strong argument identifying females who are heterozygous for G6PD deficiency as the genotype that is most protected.[56]

Until recently it was thought that among malaria parasites, *P falciparum* was the selective agent for G6PD deficiency; however, recent data suggest that *P vivax*, where present, may have played a role as well.[57,58] Finally, a strong argument in favor of malaria as the main force that has selected for G6PD deficiency is that many different G6PD deficiency alleles have reached polymorphic frequencies in populations in disparate parts of the world, a glaring example of convergent evolution.[59]

CLINICAL MANIFESTATIONS OF GLUCOSE-6-PHOSPHATE DEHYDROGENASE DEFICIENCY

Perhaps the most important point to consider about the clinical implications of G6PD deficiency is that this genetic abnormality remains largely or totally asymptomatic throughout life; thus, what is outlined previously is the epidemiology of a genetic abnormality, not of a disease. G6PD-deficient persons do develop a disease only under specific circumstances.

- In newborns, G6PD deficiency entails an increased risk of neonatal jaundice (NNJ), including severe NNJ.[60] The reason for this has not been fully elucidated, but in countries where G6PD deficiency is prevalent this is probably the most frequent cause of NNJ, which, if not appropriately treated, can lead to invalidating neurologic consequences. Thus, serious complications can take place not only in G6PD-deficient hemizygous baby boys but also in G6PD-deficient heterozygous baby girls.[15] Also, in this type of NNJ, the peak bilirubin is usually on day 3; this implies that if the onset of NNJ is not taken seriously enough, it may get worse after the baby is discharged.
- Ingestion of fava beans (*Vicia faba*), also known as broad beans, can trigger AHA (ie, *favism*) in G6PD-deficient persons.[61,62] It was thought that favism was an allergic reaction, which could be triggered not only by ingestion of the beans but also even just by inhalation of pollen; this is not correct, as it is now known that the offending chemicals, present at a high concentrations in fava beans, are nonvolatile glucosides (vicine and convicine), the aglycones of which produce free radicals.[63] These glucosides are not present in other beans, which, contrary to mistaken if well-meaning counseling, are safe for G6PD-deficient

persons. Favism can happen at any age, but it is more common and more commonly severe in children. The AHA can be brisk; a fall in hemogloblin from normal levels to 4 g/dL can take place over 48 hours or less, and it is associated with macroscopic hemoglobinuria, indicating that much of the hemolysis is intravascular.

- Since the time when G6PD deficiency was discovered through the use of primaquine (discussed previously), several other drugs have been found to entail the risk of hemolysis in G6PD-deficient persons[64] (**Table 4**). Once the list of risky drugs is well known, any drug on the list should be avoided in G6PD-deficient persons; the literature on drug-induced AHA consists almost entirely of individual case reports, most of them with favorable outcome, because, fortunately, after AHA is over, there is full recovery. Drug-triggered AHA is markedly dose dependent; therefore, in rare cases when there is no alternative, a reduced dose may be given deliberately under appropriate surveillance. Two recent mishaps, however, deserve mention.
  - In 2004, a combination of dapsone and chlorproguanil (Lapdap, GlaxoSmithKline, London) was launched as an effective antimalarial and was marketed in 17 African countries where G6PD deficiency is prevalent (male frequency of 10%–23%), in spite of AHA recorded as a serious adverse event in clinical trials.[65–68] There was no mortality in the trials, because the children who developed AHA

Table 4
Drugs that may trigger acute hemolytic anemia in glucose-6-phosphate dehydrogenase–deficient patients

Type of Drug	Evidence Based (Youngster et al,[74] 2010)	Definite Risk of Acute Hemolytic Anemia (British National Formulary, March 2015)	Possible Risk of Acute Hemolytic Anemia (British National Formulary[100])	Additional Possible Association (Other Sources)
Antimalarials	Dapsone-containing combinations Primaquine	Dapsone-containing combinations Pamaquine Primaquine	Chloroquine Quinidine Quinine	—
Other drugs	Methylthioninium chloride[a] Nitrofurantoin Phenazopyridine[b] Rasburicase Tolonium chloride[c]	Ciprofloxacin Methylthioninium chloride[a] Moxifloxacin Nalidixic acid Niridazole Nitrofurantoin[d] Norfloxacin Ofloxacin Rasburicase Sulfamethoxazole/cotrimoxazole	Aspirin[e] Menadiol sodium phosphate Sulfadiazine Sulfasalazine Sulfonylureas	Chloramphenicol[94] Dimercaptosuccinic acid[95,96] Glibenclamide[f,95] mepacrine[94] Vitamin K analogs[94]

[a] Methylene blue.
[b] Pyridium.
[c] Toluidine blue.
[d] Furadantin.
[e] Acetylsalicylic acid.
[f] Glyburide.
Data from Refs.[74,94–96]

were appropriately treated; it is not known whether there was mortality in the field until 2008, when Lapdap was withdrawn by the manufacturers because of these complications.[69] A thorough post-trial analysis found that AHA developed in all the G6PD-deficient children (**Fig. 5**), including many of the heterozygous girls.[70] It took this epidemic of serious adverse events to persuade the national and international regulatory bodies that G6PD testing is mandatory when a potentially hemolytic drug is administered (discussed later).

  ○ In 2007, rasburicase (the enzyme uricase) was introduced as a potent uricolytic agent, indicated to prevent severe hyperuricemia, particularly as part of the tumor lysis syndrome.[71] Subsequently rasburicase was also used in neonates who had evidence of kidney injury.[72] Unlike with other drugs, for which the biochemical mechanism whereby they produce oxidative damage is incompletely understood, rasburicase is known to produce 1 mol of H_2O_2 for each mole of uric acid catabolized; this produces oxidative damage directly (see **Fig. 1**). A G6PD-deficient newborn may die from rasburicase,[64,73] and it is imperative that a G6PD test is carried out before this drug is administered, especially to a child.

- Infections make it extremely important to be aware of which drugs are potentially capable of causing hemolytic anemia before administration to patients. In the literature, however, there is considerable confusion concerning this topic. One of the main reasons is that infection itself can be a triggering factor for hemolysis; therefore, it is highly probable that many compounds have been considered dangerous because they were administered to patients in whom hemolytic anemia had been triggered by preexisting infection.[74] It has been also observed that after severe trauma, G6PD-deficient persons are at higher risk of sepsis.[75]

- The epidemiology of favism must correspond to the intersection of the prevalence of G6PD deficiency and of the use of fava beans as a foodstuff (**Box 1**). Fava beans are not grown in tropical Africa, but they are popular in the

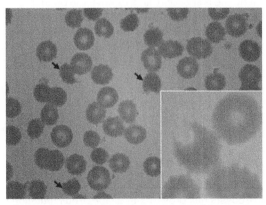

Fig. 5. Blood smear from a 3-year-old boy who was treated for acute malaria with a combination of dapsone and chlorproguanil (Lapdap) and who was G6PD deficient. Three days after starting treatment is the picture of AHA due to severe oxidative damage: (Giemsa staining, original magnification ×63) contracted erythrocytes, spherocytes, and hemighosts (also called bite cells [*arrows*]). (*Inset*) A hemighost at a higher magnification (original magnification ×100). The missing part of the erythrocyte is the negative image of a Heinz body. (*From* Pamba A, Richardson ND, Carter N, et al. Clinical spectrum and severity of hemolytic anemia in glucose 6-phosphate dehydrogenase-deficient children receiving dapsone. Blood 2012;120(20):4129; with permission.)

Box 1
Countries with documented cases of favism

Algeria, Australia, Bulgaria, Chile, China, Croatia, Cyprus, Egypt, France, Germany, Greece, India, Iran, Iraq, Israel, Italy, Japan, Jordan, Lebanon, Morocco, Poland, Portugal, Republic of Macedonia, Romania, Russia, Saudi Arabia, Spain, Taiwan, Thailand, The Netherlands, Tunisia, Turkey, UK, USA.

Mediterranean, in the Middle East as far as Iran, and in Southeast Asia.[76] In a recent report from Gaza, of 80 G6PD-deficient children admitted with AHA, 65 had consumed fava beans.[77] Although no quantitative data are available, on a global basis favism is almost certainly still today the most common form of AHA associated with G6PD deficiency.

MANAGEMENT OF GLUCOSE-6-PHOSPHATE DEHYDROGENASE DEFICIENCY

In someone who is known to be G6PD deficient, hemolytic anemia from fava beans or from drugs should not take place, because exposure can be avoided; however, acute infection can trigger an attack. In any known G6PD-deficient person with an acute illness and a fall in hemoglobin, it is not difficult to recognize AHA, and the telltale sign of intravascular hemolysis, namely hemoglobinuria, should be sought not only by asking the patient but also by inspecting the urine. If the G6PD status is not previously known, but a patient spontaneously reports eating fava beans and comes from an area or from a population where G6PD deficiency is common, the index of suspicion for favism ought to be high. Whenever such circumstances do not occur, a diagnosis can be made in most cases with near certainty by an inexpensive approach rarely carried out nowadays—examination of a blood film (see **Fig. 5**)—that often reveals evidence, ranging from suspicious to spectacular, of oxidative hemolysis. A test helpful by virtue of being negative is the direct antiglobulin (Coombs) test.

In terms of treatment, the first priority is to remove the offending agent, if any, and to control infection, if any. Next, in adults, the most important measure is to provide fluids to prevent hemodynamic shock that entails the threat of acute renal failure. In children, more often than in adults, blood transfusion may be indicated; in a child with favism, it may be life-saving.[15] Fortunately, once AHA is overcome, full recovery without sequelae is the rule rather than the exception.

For the rare cases of CNSHA that are associated with G6PD deficiency, the management is different from that discussed previously; it is more similar to that of CNSHA related to other causes (eg, hereditary spherocytosis and pyruvate kinase deficiency). This specialized topic is discussed in other reviews.[15,78]

ANIMAL MODELS AND DRUG SCREENING

Knocking out *G6PD* in mouse embryonic stem cells revealed that the cells were viable, but transfer into blastocysts has proved that a *G6PD*-null mutation is lethal in embryonic life[24]; this explains why *G6PD*-null mutations are never found in humans and also proves conclusively that the irreplaceable function of G6PD is not pentose synthesis but defense against oxidative stress.[79,80] Recently, it has been found in *Caenorhabditis elegans* (**Table 5**) that G6PD RNA interference knockdown was associated with enhanced germ cell apoptosis and oxidative damage to DNA.[81]

Apart from helping to understand physiology, a good animal model would be useful if it predicts whether a new drug will cause AHA in G6PD-deficient persons. In the past, studies performed in vitro on red blood cells from G6PD-deficient donors were

Table 5
Animal models of glucose-6-phosphate dehydrogenase deficiency

Model Type	Methodology	Residual Glucose-6-Phosphate Dehydrogenase Activity (%)	Chemicals Tested	Effects
C elegans[81]	Knockdown of G6PD by RNA interference	11	H_2O_2	Enhanced germ-cell death; decreased egg production
Mouse[84]	Genetic cross of Gpdx[a-m1Neu] mice with C57L/J mice	5–10	Naphthalene[a]	AHA[b]
Mouse[85]	G6PD-deficient mice (y/-) on a C3H background	10–20	Primaquine, pamaquine Chloroquine[c]	AHA[b] No AHA
Mouse[86]	NOD/SCID mice, intraperitoneal injection daily for 14 d with human G6PD-deficient red blood cells	5–20[d]	Primaquine, pamaquine[e] Chloroquine[c]	AHA[b] No AHA
Zebrafish[87]	Morpholino targeting of G6PD	Visibly reduced	α-Naphthol, primaquine	Significant hemolysis and cardiac edema

[a] The metabolite of naphthalene, α-naphtol, was shown in vitro to cause reduction of GSH in G6PD-deficient mouse red cells.
[b] In general, the doses of drugs causing significant effects have been much higher than those that cause hemolysis in G6PD-deficient humans.
[c] Similar results were obtained with mefloquine, doxycycline, and pyrimethamine.
[d] G6PD activity of human red cells; the G6PD activity of coexisting mouse red cells is normal.
[e] Similar results were obtained with sitamaquine, tafenoquine and dapsone.
  Data from Refs.[81,84–87]

disappointing in this respect, partly because such studies poorly mimic hemolysis in vivo and partly because oxidative damage may be caused by metabolites rather than by the drug itself.[82,83]

Recently, Ko and colleagues[84] produced a mouse model (see **Table 5**) with residual G6PD activity comparable to that found in human class II G6PD-deficient subjects. Oxidized glutathione increased and GSH decreased in mouse red cells treated with the pro-oxidative agent α-naphthol, whereas its precursor naphthalene produced dose-dependent AHA in vivo. In a similar model, with characteristics comparable to those of class III G6PD-deficient subjects, Zhang and colleagues[85] obtained dose-dependent AHA through oral administration of primaquine and pamaquine, known to be hemolytic in G6PD-deficient humans, but not with the nonhemolytic drugs chloroquine and mefloquine.

Also, recently, a humanized mouse model of G6PD deficiency has been produced by Rochford and colleagues[86] by injecting human red blood cells from G6PD-deficient donors (G6PD A− or G6PD Med) into nonobese diabetic (NOD)/severe combined immunodeficiency (SCID) mice. When treated with primaquine and pamaquine, these mice hemolyzed their human red cells and developed dose-dependent AHA with (endogenous) reticulocytosis. Moreover, the spleen size increased significantly. On the contrary, nonhemolytic drugs produced no hemolysis.

Recently, Patrinostro and colleagues[87] developed a model of G6PD deficiency in the zebrafish (*Danio rerio*). G6PD expression was knocked down with morpholinos. When exposed to different pro-oxidant compounds, *g6pd* morphants had significant hemolysis and cardiac edema.

It seems reasonable to expect that 1 or more of these models will become validated for preclinical testing of new drugs before they are administered to G6PD-deficient humans.

TESTING FOR GLUCOSE-6-PHOSPHATE DEHYDROGENASE DEFICIENCY AND MALARIA CONTROL

Even though the term, primaquine sensitivity syndrome (discussed previously), has been appropriately supplanted by the term, G6PD deficiency, the fact remains that primaquine is probably the drug that has caused the largest number of cases of AHA in persons who were G6PD deficient.[88] The well-established indications for primaquine in malaria control are 2 (**Table 6**).[1] With *P vivax*, any of several drugs can successfully terminate an acute attack, but primaquine is the only drug that eradicates the *P vivax* hypnozoites hiding in the liver and thus prevents endogenous recurrence. For this purpose, the recommended dose of primaquine (for an adult) has been 45 mg/d for 14 days.[2] With *P falciparum*, after an acute attack is successfully treated with appropriate medication (currently an artemisinin-containing combination), the only drug that eliminates gametocytes is primaquine; the recommended (adult) dose was 45 mg just once, but recently this has been reduced to 15 mg.[89]

These recommendations have been widely ignored for different reasons. With respect to *P falciparum* malaria, every episode is a threat to life, and the urgency to terminate a clinical attack has understandably obfuscated the public health concern about gametocytes, which are clinically irrelevant for a patient but, through a mosquito, become a threat to the next person bitten by the same mosquito. In addition, in hyperendemic areas there is a huge amount of malaria transmission by people

Table 6
The resurgence of primaquine and the advent of tafenoquine

Drug	Parasite Type	Recommended Use	Standard Adult Dose	G6PD Testing
Primaquine	*P falciparum*	After treatment of the acute disease, to eliminate gametocytes responsible for malaria transmission	Single dose of 15 mg[a]	Not necessary
	P vivax	After treatment of the acute disease or to eliminate liver hypnozoites responsible for relapse	30 mg/d for 14 d	Necessary
Tafenoquine[b]	*P vivax*	Alternative to the use of primaquine (see above)	300–600 mg once only[c]	Necessary

[a] In the past, the recommended dose was 45 mg, but recently this has been lowered to 15 mg.[89]
[b] Not a licensed drug.
[c] Doses tested in 3 clinical trials conducted in G6PD-normal subjects.[90,97,98] In a recent trial in women heterozygous for the G6PD Mahidol variant who had 40% to 60% G6PD-deficient red cells, 100 to 200 mg of tafenoquine caused clinically significant but not severe hemolytic anemia.[99]
Data from Refs.[89,90,97–99]

with asymptomatic malaria; hence, elimination of gametocytes from the minority of patients with clinical malaria has little impact on transmission. With respect to *P vivax*, this infection is endemic in areas where G6PD deficiency is common; with the G6PD status of individual patients unknown, and with the need of a prolonged course of administration, there has been justified concern about causing AHA in those who are G6PD deficient.[88] It might also have been regarded as reasonable to hope that, over decades, an alternative to primaquine would turn up. The only alternative today is tafenoquine[90] (not yet an approved drug) (see **Table 6**), but this too is an 8-aminoquinoline and, although its pharmacokinetics is different from primaquine (it last for weeks in circulation), it causes AHA in G6PD-deficient persons just as primaquine does.

In recent years there have been 2 positive developments. First, more countries are moving toward malaria elimination[91]; therefore, the public health importance of reducing relapse (*P vivax*) and reducing transmission (*P falciparum*) has increased. Second, in spite of screening tests for G6PD deficiency available for half a century, it has been thought by many malariologists and public health professionals that they were too cumbersome or not sufficiently reliable and that, therefore, it was not realistic to adopt their use in endemic areas before giving primaquine. Recently it has become accepted that testing is necessary, and, therefore, there has been a revival of interest by WHO, by public health authorities, and by the diagnostics industry in point- of-care tests for G6PD deficiency. At least 2 kits are on the market[92,93]; they are being extensively validated in the field and, although more expensive than older screening tests, they may come down to less than $1 per test. Having a strip not unlike a pregnancy test that comes in a kit with primaquine tablets can be looked forward to in a not too distant future.

The WHO has worked out recommendations, whereby, for preventing relapse of *P vivax*, primaquine is given whenever indicated to those who have tested G6PD normal, whereas it is not given, or given only under medical/health worker surveillance, to those who have tested G6PD deficient (see http:www.who.int/malaria/mpac/mpac_sep13_erg_g6pd_testing.pdf). For the clearance of *P falciparum* gametocytes, a single adult dose of 25 mg[89] is probably safe for all. The authors expect that implementation of these measures will be straightforward with respect to males; in females, again, the fact that most heterozygotes have intermediate enzyme levels cannot be circumvented. Those who test deficient or doubtful will have to be managed like those who test G6PD deficient; those who test normal may still be heterozygotes, but in their blood the proportion of G6PD-deficient red cells is sufficiently small to make it unlikely that they will develop clinically significant AHA.

CONCLUSION

G6PD is at the crossroads of haematology, pharmacogenetics and malariology. Indeed, one can perceive a remarkable triangular relationship: (1) malarial *Plasmodia* select for (2) G6PD deficient human mutants, (3) primaquine is a potent anti-malarial, but it is dangerous for those G6PD deficient mutants that malaria has selected for. From this triangle we have learnt several of lessons in evolutionary biology and in medicine, but not yet enough: for instance, if we understood fully how G6PD deficiency protects from malaria we might be able to mimic the mechanism in order to protect other people as well. In the meantime, we now do have the means to protect G6PD deficient persons from exposure to fava beans or to iatrogenic risks, and in the interest of global health we have a duty to do so.

REFERENCES

1. Warburg O, Christian W. Uber ein neues oxydationsferment und sein absorptionsspektrum. Biochem Z 1932;254:438–58.
2. Fermi C, Martinetti P. Studio sul favismo. Annali di Igiene Sperimentale 1905;15: 75–112.
3. Cordes W. Zwischenfälle bei der plasmochinbehandlung. Arch. Schiffs- u. Tropenhyg 1928;32:143–8.
4. Carson PE, Flanagan CL, Ickes CE, et al. Enzymatic deficiency in primaquine-sensitive erythrocytes. Science 1956;124:484–5.
5. Sansone G, Segni G. Nuovi aspetti dell'alterato biochimismo degli eritrociti dei favici: assenza pressoche' completa della glucoso-6-P deidrogenasi. Bollettino della Società Italiana di Biologia Sperimentale 1958;34:327–9.
6. Adam A. Linkage between deficiency of glucose 6-phosphate dehydrogenase and colour-blindness. Nature 1961;189:686–8.
7. Lyon MF. Gene action in the X chromosome in the mouse (Mus musculus L.). Nature 1961;190:372–3.
8. Beutler E, Yeh M, Fairbanks VF. The normal human female as a mosaic of X-chromosome activity: studies using the gene for G6PD deficiency as a marker. Proc Natl Acad Sci U S A 1962;48:9–16.
9. Vogel F. Moderne problem der humangenetik. Ergeb Inn Med U Kinderheilk 1959;12:52–125.
10. Allison AC. Glucose 6-phosphate dehydrogenase deficiency in red blood cells of East Africans. Nature 1960;186:531–2.
11. Motulsky AG. Metabolic polymorphisms and the role of infectious diseases in human evolution. Hum Biol 1960;32:28–62.
12. Livingstone FB. Abnormal hemoglobins in human populations. Chicago: Aldine; 1967.
13. Betke K, Brewer GJ, Kirkman HN, et al. Standardization of procedures for the study of glucose-6-phosphate dehydrogenase. World Health Organ Tech Rep Ser 1967;366:53.
14. Cappellini MD, Fiorelli G. Glucose-6-phosphate dehydrogenase deficiency. Lancet 2008;371(9606):64–74.
15. Luzzatto L, Poggi VE. Glucose 6-phosphate dehydrogenase deficiency. In: Orkin SH, Nathan DG, Ginsburg D, et al, editors. Hematology of infancy and childhood. Philadelphia: Saunders; 2009. p. 883–907.
16. Berg JM, Tymoczko JL, Stryer L. Biochemistry. 5th edition. New York: W. H. Freeman and Co; 2002.
17. Pandolfi PP, Sonati F, Rivi R, et al. Targeted disruption of the housekeeping gene encodinbg glucose 6-phosphate dehydrogenase (G6PD): G6PD is dispensable for pentose synthesis but essential for defense against oxidative stress. EMBO J 1995;14:5209–15.
18. Prankerd TAJ. The red cell. Oxford (United Kingdom): Blackwell; 1961.
19. Beutler E. Haemolytic anaemia in disorders of red cell metabolism (topics in haematology). New York; London: Plenum Medical; 1978.
20. Bunn HF, Forget BG. Hemoglobin: molecular, genetic, and clinical aspects. Philadelphia: Saunders; 1986.
21. Luzzatto L, Karadimitris A. The molecular basis of anemia. In: Provan D, Gribben J, editors. Molecular haematology. 3rd edition. Oxford (United Kingdom): Wiley-Blackwell; 2010. p. 140–64.

22. Marks PA, Johnson AB. Relationship between the age of human erythrocytes and their osmotic resistance: a basis for separating young and old erythrocytes. J Clin Invest 1958;37:1542–8.
23. Morelli A, Benatti U, Gaetani GF, et al. Biochemical mechanisms of glucose-6-phosphate dehydrogenase deficiency. Proc Natl Acad Sci U S A 1978;75:1979–83.
24. Longo L, Vanegas OC, Patel M, et al. Maternally transmitted severe glucose 6-phosphate dehydrogenase deficiency is an embryonic lethal. EMBO J 2002;21(16):4229–39.
25. Arese P, De Flora A. Pathophysiology of hemolysis in glucose 6-phosphate dehydrogenase deficiency. Semin Hematol 1990;27:1–40.
26. Persico MG, Viglietto G, Martini G, et al. Isolation of human glucose-6-phosphate dehydrogenase (G6PD) cDNA clones: primary structure of the protein and unusual 5' non-coding region. Nucleic Acids Res 1986;14:2511–22, 7822.
27. Cohen P, Rosemeyer MA. Subunit interactions of human glucose 6-phosphate dehydrogenase from human erythrocytes. Eur J Biochem 1969;8:8–15.
28. Au SW, Gover S, Lam VM, et al. Human glucose-6-phosphate dehydrogenase: the crystal structure reveals a structural NADP(+) molecule and provides insights into enzyme deficiency [In Process Citation]. Structure 2000;8(3):293–303.
29. Chen EY, Zollo M, Mazzarella R, et al. Long-range sequence analysis in Xq28: thirteen known and six candidate genes in 219.4 kb of high GC between RCP/GCP and G6PD loci. Hum Mol Genet 1996;5:659–68.
30. Migeon BR. Glucose 6-phosphate dehydrogenase as a probe for the study of X-chromosome inactivation in human females. In: Rattazzi MC, Scandalios JC, Whitt GS, editors. Isozymes: current topics in biological and medical research, vol. 9. New York: Alan Liss; 1983. p. 189–200.
31. Rinaldi A, Filippi G, Siniscalco M. Variability of red cell phenotypes between and within individuals in an unbiased sample of 77 certain heterozygotes for G6PD deficiency in Sardinians. Am J Hum Genet 1976;28:496–505.
32. Xu W, Westwood B, Bartsocas CS, et al. Glucose 6-phosphate dehydrogenase mutations and haplotypes in various ethnic groups. Blood 1995;85:257–63.
33. Minucci A, Moradkhani K, Hwang MJ, et al. Glucose-6-phosphate dehydrogenase (G6PD) mutations database: review of the "old" and update of the new mutations. Blood Cells Mol Dis 2012;48(3):154–65.
34. Mason PJ, Bautista JM, Gilsanz F. G6PD deficiency: the genotype-phenotype association. Blood Rev 2007;21(5):267–83.
35. Fusco F, Paciolla M, Conte MI, et al. Incontinentia pigmenti: report on data from 2000 to 2013. Orphanet J Rare Dis 2014;9:93.
36. Notaro R, Afolayan A, Luzzatto L. Human mutations in glucose 6-phosphate dehydrogenase reflect evolutionary history. FASEB J 2000;14:485–94.
37. Wendt UK, Wenderoth I, Tegeler A, et al. Molecular characterization of a novel glucose-6-phosphate dehydrogenase from potato (Solanum tuberosum L.). Plant J 2000;23(6):723–33.
38. Yoshida A, Lebo RV. Existence of glucose-6-phosphate dehydrogenase-like locus on chromosome 17. Am J Hum Genet 1986;39:203–6.
39. Kurdi-Haidar B, Luzzatto L. Expression and characterization of glucose-6-phosphate dehydrogenase of Plasmodium falciparum. Mol Biochem Parasitol 1990;41(1):83–91.

40. Clarke JL, Sodeinde O, Mason PJ. A unique insertion in Plasmodium berghei glucose-6-phosphate dehydrogenase-6-phosphogluconolactonase: evolutionary and functional studies. Mol Biochem Parasitol 2003;127(1):1–8.

41. Jortzik E, Mailu BM, Preuss J, et al. Glucose-6-phosphate dehydrogenase-6-phosphogluconolactonase: a unique bifunctional enzyme from Plasmodium falciparum. Biochem J 2011;436(3):641–50.

42. Maloney P, Hedrick M, Peddibhotla S, et al. A selective inhibitor of plasmodium falciparum Glucose-6-phosphate dehydrogenase (PfG6PDH). Probe Reports from the NIH Molecular Libraries Program [Internet]. Bethesda (MD): National Center for Biotechnology Information (US); 2010. 2011 Dec 16 [updated 2013 Mar 7]. PMID: 23762930.

43. Guiguemde WA, Shelat AA, Bouck D, et al. Chemical genetics of plasmodium falciparum. Nature 2010;465(7296):311–5.

44. Kimura M, Ohta T. On some principles governing molecular evolution. Proc Natl Acad Sci U S A 1974;71(7):2848–52.

45. Miller MP, Kumar S. Understanding human disease mutations through the use of interspecific genetic variation. Hum Mol Genet 2001;10(21):2319–28.

46. Miller MP, Parker JD, Rissing SW, et al. Quantifying the intragenic distribution of human disease mutations. Ann Hum Genet 2003;67(Pt 6):567–79.

47. WHO Working Group. Glucose-6-phosphate dehydrogenase deficiency. Bull World Health Organ 1989;67:601–11.

48. Nkhoma ET, Poole C, Vannappagari V, et al. The global prevalence of glucose-6-phosphate dehydrogenase deficiency: a systematic review and meta-analysis. Blood Cells Mol Dis 2009;42(3):267–78.

49. Howes RE, Piel FB, Patil AP, et al. G6PD deficiency prevalence and estimates of affected populations in malaria endemic countries: a geostatistical model-based map. PLoS Med 2012;9(11):e1001339.

50. Luzzatto L. Genetics of red cells and susceptibility to malaria. Blood 1979;54:961–76.

51. Bienzle U, Ayeni O, Lucas AO, et al. Glucose-6-phosphate dehydrogenase deficiency and malaria. Greater resistance of females heterozygous for enzyme deficiency and of males with non-deficient variant. Lancet 1972;1:107–10.

52. Ruwende C, Khoo SC, Snow RW, et al. Natural selection of hemi- and heterozygotes for G6PD deficiency in Africa by resistance to severe malaria. Nature 1995;376:246–9.

53. Guindo A, Fairhurst RM, Doumbo OK, et al. X-linked G6PD deficiency protects hemizygous males but not heterozygous females against severe malaria. PLoS Med 2007;4(3):e66.

54. Clark TG, Fry AE, Auburn S, et al. Allelic heterogeneity of G6PD deficiency in West Africa and severe malaria susceptibility. Eur J Hum Genet 2009;17(8):1080–5.

55. Reappraisal of known malaria resistance loci in a large multicenter study. Nat Genet 2014;46(11):1197–204.

56. Luzzatto L. G6PD deficiency and malaria selection. Heredity (Edinb) 2012;108(4):456.

57. Bouma MJ, Goris M, Akhtar T, et al. Prevalence and clinical presentation of glucose-6-phosphate dehydrogenase deficiency in Pakistani Pathan and Afghan refugee communities in Pakistan; implications for the use of primaquine in regional malaria control programmes. Trans R Soc Trop Med Hyg 1995;89:62–4.

58. Louicharoen C, Patin E, Paul R, et al. Positively selected G6PD-mahidol mutation reduces plasmodium vivax density in Southeast Asians. Science 2009; 326(5959):1546–9.
59. Luzzatto L, Notaro R. Malaria. Protecting against bad air. Science 2001; 293(5529):442–3.
60. Doxiadis SA, Valaes T, Karaklis A, et al. Risk of severe jaundice in glucose 6-phosphate dehydrogenase deficiency of the newborn. Differences in population groups. Lancet 1964;2:1210.
61. Luisada L. Favism: a singular disease affecting chiefly red blood cells. Medicine 1941;20:229–50.
62. Meloni T, Forteleoni G, Dore A, et al. Favism and hemolytic anemia in glucose-6-phosphate dehydrogeanse deficiency subjects in North Sardinia. Acta Haematol 1983;70:83–90.
63. Chevion M, Navok T, Glaser G, et al. The chemistry of favism-inducing compounds. The properties of isouramil and divicine and their reaction with glutathione. Eur J Biochem 1982;127:405–9.
64. Luzzatto L, Seneca E. G6PD deficiency: a classic example of pharmacogenetics with on-going clinical implications. Br J Haematol 2014;164(4):469–80.
65. Alloueche A, Bailey W, Barton S, et al. Comparison of chlorproguanil-dapsone with sulfadoxine-pyrimethamine for the treatment of uncomplicated falciparum malaria in young African children: double-blind randomised controlled trial. Lancet 2004;363(9424):1843–8.
66. Fanello CI, Karema C, Avellino P, et al. High risk of severe anaemia after chlorproguanil-dapsone+artesunate antimalarial treatment in patients with G6PD (A-) deficiency. PLoS One 2008;3(12):e4031.
67. Tiono AB, Dicko A, Ndububa DA, et al. Chlorproguanil-dapsone-artesunate versus chlorproguanil-dapsone: a randomized, double-blind, phase III trial in African children, adolescents, and adults with uncomplicated Plasmodium falciparum malaria. Am J Trop Med Hyg 2009;81(6):969–78.
68. Premji Z, Umeh RE, Owusu-Agyei S, et al. Chlorproguanil-dapsone-artesunate versus artemether-lumefantrine: a randomized, double-blind phase III trial in African children and adolescents with uncomplicated Plasmodium falciparum malaria. PLoS One 2009;4(8):e6682.
69. Luzzatto L. The rise and fall of the antimalarial Lapdap: a lesson in pharmacogenetics. Lancet 2010;376(9742):739–41.
70. Pamba A, Richardson ND, Carter N, et al. Clinical spectrum and severity of hemolytic anemia in glucose 6-phosphate dehydrogenase-deficient children receiving dapsone. Blood 2012;120(20):4123–33.
71. Tosi P, Barosi G, Lazzaro C, et al. Consensus conference on the management of tumor lysis syndrome. Haematologica 2008;93(12):1877–85.
72. Hobbs DJ, Steinke JM, Chung JY, et al. Rasburicase improves hyperuricemia in infants with acute kidney injury. Pediatr Nephrol 2010;25(2):305–9.
73. Zaramella P, De Salvia A, Zaninotto M, et al. Lethal effect of a single dose of rasburicase in a preterm newborn infant. Pediatrics 2013;131(1): e309–12.
74. Youngster I, Arcavi L, Schechmaster R, et al. Medications and glucose-6-phosphate dehydrogenase deficiency: an evidence-based review. Drug Saf 2010;33(9):713–26.
75. Spolarics Z, Siddiqi M, Siegel JH, et al. Increased incidence of sepsis and altered monocyte functions in severely injured type A- glucose-6-phosphate

dehydrogenase-deficient African American trauma patients. Crit Care Med 2001; 29(4):728–36.

76. Belsey MA. The epidemiology of favism. Bull World Health Organ 1973;48:1–13.

77. Sirdah M, Reading NS, Vankayalapati H, et al. Molecular heterogeneity of glucose-6-phosphate dehydrogenase deficiency in gaza strip palestinians. Blood Cells Mol Dis 2012;49(3–4):152–8.

78. Fiorelli G, Martinez di Montemuros F, Cappellini MD. Chronic non-spherocytic haemolytic disorders associated with glucose-6-phosphate dehydrogenase variants. Baillieres Best Pract Res Clin Haematol 2000;13(1):39–55.

79. Filosa S, Fico A, Paglialunga F, et al. Failure to increase glucose consumption through the pentose-phosphate pathway results in the death of glucose-6-phosphate dehydrogenase gene-deleted mouse embryonic stem cells subjected to oxidative stress. Biochem J 2003;370(Pt 3):935–43.

80. Paglialunga F, Fico A, Iaccarino I, et al. G6PD is indispensable for erythropoiesis after the embryonic-adult hemoglobin switch. Blood 2004;104(10):3148–52.

81. Yang HC, Chen TL, Wu YH, et al. Glucose 6-phosphate dehydrogenase deficiency enhances germ cell apoptosis and causes defective embryogenesis in Caenorhabditis elegans. Cell Death Dis 2013;4:e616.

82. Beutler E. G6PD deficiency. Blood 1994;84(11):3613–36.

83. Bashan N, Makover O, Livne A, et al. Effect of oxidant agents on normal and G6PD-deficient erythrocytes. Isr J Med Sci 1980;16:531–6.

84. Ko CH, Li K, Li CL, et al. Development of a novel mouse model of severe glucose-6-phosphate dehydrogenase (G6PD)-deficiency for in vitro and in vivo assessment of hemolytic toxicity to red blood cells. Blood Cells Mol Dis 2011;47(3):176–81.

85. Zhang P, Gao X, Ishida H, et al. An In vivo drug screening model using glucose-6-phosphate dehydrogenase deficient mice to predict the hemolytic toxicity of 8-aminoquinolines. Am J Trop Med Hyg 2013;88(6):1138–45.

86. Rochford R, Ohrt C, Baresel PC, et al. Humanized mouse model of glucose 6-phosphate dehydrogenase deficiency for in vivo assessment of hemolytic toxicity. Proc Natl Acad Sci U S A 2013;110(43):17486–91.

87. Patrinostro X, Carter ML, Kramer AC, et al. A model of glucose-6-phosphate dehydrogenase deficiency in the zebrafish. Exp Hematol 2013;41(8):697–710.e2.

88. Baird KJ, Maguire JD, Price RN. Diagnosis and treatment of Plasmodium vivax malaria. Adv Parasitol 2012;80:203–70.

89. White NJ, Qiao LG, Qi G, et al. Rationale for recommending a lower dose of primaquine as a Plasmodium falciparum gametocytocide in populations where G6PD deficiency is common. Malar J 2012;11:418.

90. Llanos-Cuentas A, Lacerda MV, Rueangweerayut R, et al. Tafenoquine plus chloroquine for the treatment and relapse prevention of Plasmodium vivax malaria (DETECTIVE): a multicentre, double-blind, randomised, phase 2b dose-selection study. Lancet 2014;383(9922):1049–58.

91. WHO. World malaria report. Geneva (Switzerland): World Health Organization; 2014.

92. Bancone G, Chu CS, Chowwiwat N, et al. Suitability of capillary blood for quantitative assessment of G6PD activity and performances of G6PD point-of-care tests. Am J Trop Med Hyg 2015;92(4):818–24.

93. Adu-Gyasi D, Asante KP, Newton S, et al. Evaluation of the diagnostic accuracy of carestart G6PD deficiency Rapid Diagnostic Test (RDT) in a malaria endemic area in Ghana, Africa. PLoS One 2015;10(4):e0125796.

94. Kliegman RM, Behrman RE, Jenson HB, et al. Nelson textbook of pediatrics. 18th edition. Philadelphia: WB Saunders Co; 2007.
95. Lichtman M, Beutler E, Kaushansky K, et al. Williams hematology. 7th edition. New York: McGraw-Hill, Medical Pub. Division; 2006.
96. Manganelli G, Masullo U, Passarelli S, et al. Glucose-6-phosphate dehydrogenase deficiency: disadvantages and possible benefits. Cardiovasc Hematol Disord Drug Targets 2013;13(1):73–82.
97. Walsh DS, Looareesuwan S, Wilairatana P, et al. Randomized dose-ranging study of the safety and efficacy of WR 238605 (Tafenoquine) in the prevention of relapse of Plasmodium vivax malaria in Thailand. J Infect Dis 1999;180(4): 1282–7.
98. Walsh DS, Wilairatana P, Tang DB, et al. Randomized trial of 3-dose regimens of tafenoquine (WR238605) versus low-dose primaquine for preventing Plasmodium vivax malaria relapse. Clin Infect Dis 2004;39(8):1095–103.
99. Bancone G, Beelen AP, Carter N, et al. A phase I study to investigate the haemolytic potential of tafenoquine in healthy subjects with Glucose-6-phosphate dehydrogenase deficiency. The American Society of Tropical Medicine and Hygiene 61st Annual Meeting; Atlanta, USA. Am J Trop Med Hyg 2012;87(Suppl. 5):130.
100. British Medical Association and the Royal Pharmaceutical Society of Great Britain. British National Formulary. 69th edition. BMJ Publishing Group: United Kingdom; 2015.

Hematologic Changes Associated with Specific Infections in the Tropics

David J. Roberts, DPhil, MRCP, FRCPath

KEYWORDS

- Anemia • Malaria • Leishmaniasis • Schistosomiasis • Trypanosomiasis
- Hookworm • Bartonellosis

KEY POINTS

- Malaria is responsible for approximately 600,000 deaths each year, although the epidemiologic picture over the last decade has been one of a substantial reduction in the burden of malaria.
- Malaria causes severe and life-threatening anemia by reducing erythropoiesis and increasing red cell destruction.
- Blood transfusion is beneficial in the group of children with malaria who have both anemia and respiratory distress, but bolus fluid supplementation of severely ill children on admission may result in higher mortality.
- Ill children should be carefully assessed clinically, and appropriate fluid or blood transfusion should be given to correct hypovolemia or severe anemia.
- Visceral leishmaniasis can cause considerable diagnostic difficulty and may be mislabeled as leukemia or myelodysplasia when the diagnosis of leishmaniasis was not considered.

Anemia frequently accompanies and plays a minor role in the presentation and course of parasitic, bacterial, or viral infection. However, a variety of infections, many of which are common in Africa and Asia, cause specific hematologic syndromes. The pathophysiology of these syndromes is complex and, to some extent, reduced red cell production may form part of an innate protective host response to infection. Across the world and in endemic areas, malaria, the most important among this group of infections, forms a major part of everyday practice across all clinical specialities and laboratory work. Several other parasitic diseases and bacterial infections, including visceral leishmaniasis, schistosomiasis, trypanosomiasis, hookworm, and bartonellosis, may present with major hematologic syndromes. These diseases may have restricted geographic distribution, but through travel, may present anywhere and must be recognized, diagnosed, and treated.

Disclosure Statement: The author has nothing to disclose.
National Health Service Blood and Transplant, John Radcliffe Hospital, University of Oxford, Level 2, Headington, Oxford OX3 9BQ, UK
E-mail address: david.roberts@ndcls.ox.ac.uk

Hematol Oncol Clin N Am 30 (2016) 395–415
http://dx.doi.org/10.1016/j.hoc.2015.11.007
0889-8588/16/$ – see front matter © 2016 Elsevier Inc. All rights reserved.

MALARIA

Malaria is the most important parasitic illness of humans.[1-3] The total burden of disease in 2013 was estimated to be 200 million episodes annually, and malaria is responsible for approximately 600,000 deaths each year.[4,5] Despite the huge number of cases and deaths, the epidemiologic picture over the last decade has been one of a substantial reduction in the burden of malaria. The prevalence of infection and malaria-related mortality decreased dramatically in sub-Saharan Africa during the period 2000 to 2013. Across Africa, the average infection prevalence in children aged 2 to 10 years decreased from 26% in 2000 to 14% in 2013, a relative decline of 46%.[2,5] Nevertheless, substantial problems remain for successful malaria control. There remains the perennial problem of increasing drug resistance of the malarial parasite and of resistance of the mosquito vector to insecticides used to impregnate bed nets, and malaria still remains one of the major global problems of public health.

The Life Cycle of Malaria Infection and Human Infection

Because of its peculiar life cycle (**Fig. 1**), the malarial parasite is particularly prone to cause hematologic manifestations. Female anopheline mosquitoes inject sporozoites that enter liver parenchymal cells, where they proliferate into thousands of merozoites. Merozoites rupture from liver cells, pour into the bloodstream, and invade erythrocytes. Further development of the intraerythrocytic parasite follows 1 of 2 pathways: asexual differentiation or differentiation into sexual parasites called gametocytes. Asexual parasites develop from young ring forms through trophozoites to dividing forms called schizonts. On rupture of infected erythrocytes, forms called merozoites are released, invade other erythrocytes, and thus continue the erythrocyte cycle. When billions of schizonts rupture simultaneously and release cytokine-inducing toxins, they cause paroxysms of malarial fever.

When a child is infected with malaria for the first time, the result is usually an intermittent febrile illness lasting a few weeks, although a significant proportion of children and a high proportion of nonimmune adults experience severe disease (see later discussion). In the phase between cessation of the fever and final resolution of the infection, the child may appear well, but the destruction of red cells continues. From a hematologic viewpoint, the major question is how soon will the child be reinfected, for in some communities reinfection occurs almost every day, and immunity to malaria is slowly acquired and never complete. In regions of high transmission, children eventually acquire the ability to maintain a parasite density below the level that causes fever, but chronic or repeated infections cause a state of chronic anemia.

Four species of Plasmodium infect humans—*Plasmodium falciparum*, *Plasmodium vivax*, *Plasmodium ovale*, and *Plasmodium malariae*—and a fifth species, *Plasmodium knowlesi*, normally restricted to macaque monkeys, has recently been discovered in the human population in Borneo.[6] *P falciparum* is the predominant cause of clinical malaria in Africa and much of Southeast Asia, whereas *P vivax* tends to predominate in Central America and the Indian subcontinent. *P vivax* is essentially absent in populations of Central and West Africa because their erythrocytes fail to express the Duffy antigen or interleukin-8 (IL-8) receptor, to which the merozoites of this species attach during invasion.[7]

Another peculiarity of *P vivax*, shared also with *P ovale*, is the ability to form hypnozoites, which can remain dormant in cells for months or years. This ability results in relapsing infections that are often associated with mild chronic anemia. However, profound anemia and other grave complications are almost always seen with *P falciparum* malaria, and the following sections apply mainly to this particular species.

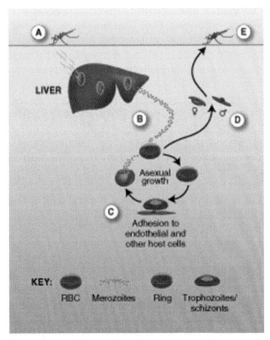

Fig. 1. Plasmodia life cycle. (*A*) The asexual life cycle begins when sporozoites from a female mosquito taking a blood meal enter the circulation and invade hepatocytes. (*B*) Up to 10,000 merozoites are formed. Following rupture of the hepatocyte, infective merozoites are released and invade erythrocytes (red blood cells [RBC]). (*C*) Within RBC, the parasite develops through the stages of rings, trophozoites, and schizonts. Mature schizonts burst to release erythrocytic merozoites that invade new RBC. (*D*) A small proportion of merozoites in RBC transform into male and female gametocytes that are ingested by the mosquito. (*E*) The male and female gametes fuse and transform into an oocyst, which divides asexually into many sporozoites that migrate to the salivary gland from where they are released during the next blood meal. (*From* Roberts DJ. Hematological manifestations of parasitic disease. In: Hoffman, Benz, Shattil, et al, editors. Hematology: basic principles and practice. 5th edition. Churchill Livingstone; 2009. p. 2342; with permission.)

SEVERE MALARIA

Life-threatening complications are estimated to occur in about 1% of episodes of *P falciparum* infection in African children, and it has been estimated that a child in rural Africa has a 15% lifetime risk of a malaria infection requiring hospital admission as a result of complications.[8] Such complications include profound anemia, cerebral malaria (a syndrome of unarousable coma, often accompanied by severe convulsions), hypoglycemia, jaundice, renal failure, pulmonary edema, and coagulation abnormalities.[9] In Southeast Asia, all the aforementioned complications are commonly seen, whereas in Africa, cerebral malaria, severe malarial anemia, and hypoglycemia are common, but the other complications of *P falciparum* malaria are surprisingly rare. Malarial illness affects mostly children in Africa, where transmission rates are high, whereas adults are more commonly affected in some other parts of the world. It appears that higher rates of malarial transmission lead to a greater prevalence of anemia but, paradoxically, a low incidence of cerebral malaria.[10]

The lethality of P falciparum as compared with other species of Plasmodium probably stems from 2 biologic properties. First, the parasite density that it achieves is typically a hundred times higher than that of other species before its growth is curtailed by host defense mechanisms. Second, mature intraerythrocytic forms of P falciparum adhere to the endothelium of postcapillary venules and thus sequester in tissues.[11,12] Parasite sequestration is mediated by a parasite-derived molecule known as PfEMP1 that is expressed on the surface of a mature infected erythrocyte and binds to a variety of endothelial adhesion molecules, including CD36, intracellular adhesion molecule-1, E-selectin, and vascular cell adhesion molecule-1.[13]

Another potentially important pathophysiologic mechanism is vascular sludging, which results from the clumping of parasitized erythrocytes, with either unparasitized erythrocytes ("rosettes") or platelets ("autoagglutination" or "clumps").[14,15]

There is an association between salmonellosis and malarial infection. This association goes beyond the growing recognition that a significant proportion of cases of severe malaria in the tropics is bacteremic[16] in that salmonellosis in Africa seems to be specifically associated with malarial anemia.[17]

Malarial Anemia

The pattern of hematologic changes in malaria varies considerably, depending on the type of patient. During an acute attack of P falciparum malaria in a nonimmune person, the hematocrit starts to decrease after 1 or 2 days and continues to decrease for about 1 week after antimalarial treatment.[18] Subsequently, there is usually a steady increase in the hematocrit, although it may take several weeks before the hematologic picture is back to normal. The anemia, which is not usually life-threatening, is characterized by both hemolysis and an ineffective marrow response,[18] features that have also been documented in acute P vivax infection.[19] When profound anemia occurs with acute P falciparum malaria, it is often associated with multi-organ failure, although it can occur as an isolated complication, particularly in African children.

From the perspective of tropical child health, the most important hematologic problem is seen in a child chronically infected with P falciparum, whose anemia is debilitating and sometimes fatal. The most striking pathophysiologic findings are hemolysis, hypersplenism, and a suboptimal bone marrow response (**Fig. 2**).[18] In the sections that follow, some of the mechanisms for these components of the acute and chronic anemia of malaria are discussed in more detail.

Role of Hemolysis

Normal children living in rural Africa typically have extremely low levels of haptoglobin that increase significantly after reduced transmission,[20] thus providing some indication of the burden of chronic hemolysis that malaria causes in many tropical communities. The mechanisms of red cell destruction in P falciparum malaria are complex and not fully understood.[21] Clearly, erythrocytes are destroyed when schizonts rupture and release their progeny, and a proportion of the parasitized erythrocytes are destroyed by the host before schizont rupture can take place. In most infections, less than 1% of erythrocytes are infected, a loss that is important in the context of chronic infection but would not account for the severity of anemia that is commonly observed. Both mathematical modeling and clinical observation suggest that 10 times as many uninfected erythrocytes are removed from the circulation for each infected erythrocyte.[22] Indeed, cross-transfusion experiments clearly indicate that erythrocyte survival is shortened both in the acute phase of malaria and during convalescence.[23,24]

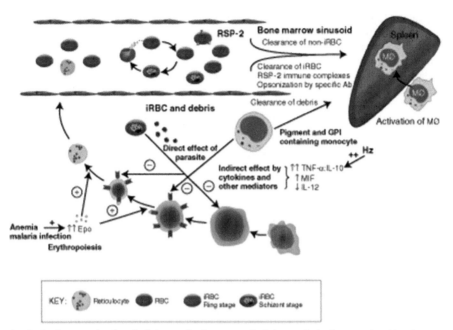

Fig. 2. Pathogenesis of malarial anemia. Severe malarial anemia is characterized by destruction of infected red blood cells (iRBC) following schizogony and clearance of both iRBC and uninfected RBC. During malarial infection, changes in membrane protein composition occur and the resultant immune complexes of RBC, Ag, and immunoglobulin (eg, RBC-RSP2-Ig) are cleared by macrophages to the spleen where they become activated. Pigment-containing macrophages may release inflammatory cytokines and other biologically-active mediators, such as 4-hydroxy-nonenal. Macrophage inhibitory factor (MIF) may be released by macrophages or a Plasmodial homolog may suppress erythropoiesis. Malarial pigment or other parasite products may have a direct inhibitory effect on erythropoiesis. Inhibition of erythropoiesis may be at one or more sites in the growth and differentiation of hematopoietic progenitors. Both indirect and direct effects may cause suppression of the bone marrow and spleen, resulting in inadequate reticulocyte counts for the degree of anemia. Ab, antibody; Epo, erythropoietin; GPI, glycophosphatidylinositol anchors of merozoite proteins; Hz, hemozoin; M, macrophage; RSP-2, ring surface protein-2. (*From* Roberts DJ. Hematological manifestations of parasitic disease. In: Hoffman, Benz, Shattil, et al, editors. Hematology: basic principles and practice. 5th edition. Churchill Livingstone; 2009. p. 2343; with permission.)

Role of the Spleen

Some degree of splenomegaly is a normal feature of malarial infection, and the prevalence of splenomegaly in regions of malarial transmission is used as a major indicator of the level of malarial endemicity. The phenomenon of parasitic sequestration, discussed earlier, is thought to have evolved primarily as an immune evasion strategy whereby the mature parasite can avoid passing through the spleen.

Several studies have attempted to define the pathophysiologic changes in the spleen during acute malaria. In studies of human malaria, it has been found that increased splenic clearance of heated red cells occurs during acute attacks.[25] Reduced deformability of uninfected red cells is observed in *P falciparum* malaria and is a significant predictor of the severity of anemia, consistent with the notion that these cells are being removed by the spleen.[26] It has also been found that immunoglobulin G (IgG) -sensitized red cells are rapidly removed from the circulation by the spleen and that unusually rapid clearance persists well into the convalescent phase.[27] Undoubtedly, the activity and number of macrophages are increased during human malarial infection, and this may therefore also contribute to the increased removal of uninfected cells.[28,29]

Clinical studies have also uncovered a curious phenomenon whereby some erythrocytes appear to be returned to the circulation after having had their parasites removed,[30] but killing parasites usually means destroying erythrocytes, and it appears that the survival of uninfected red cells is reduced in the process.

Experimental evidence supports the notion that with relatively nonspecific effector mechanisms such as erythrophagocytosis within the spleen, anemia is part of the price that the host has to pay for protection against overwhelming parasitemia.

Massive Intravascular Hemolysis

A peculiar and striking example of malaria-associated hemolysis is blackwater fever. The classic form of this syndrome, often reported in colonial times among Europeans living in Africa, was characterized by fever and massive intravascular hemolysis associated with low or no parasitemia. It was suspected that intermittent quinine ingestion might have led to a drug-induced immune hemolysis, although this mechanism was never proved and recent reports have implicated newer antimalarial drugs, such as halofantrine and mefloquine/artemisinin combinations.[31,32] Classic blackwater fever is now much less common, but massive intravascular hemolysis remains an important complication of P falciparum malaria in Southeast Asia in both children and adults. A survey of cases in Vietnam found considerable overlap of quinine ingestion, glucose-6-phosphate dehydrogenase deficiency, and concurrent malaria, thus suggesting that these different factors may interact but certainly do not all have to be present for blackwater fever to occur.[33]

Decreased Erythrocyte Deformability

The increased clearance of uninfected erythrocytes is due, not only to the activation of splenic macrophages, but also to extrinsic and intrinsic factors that enhance their recognition and phagocytosis. Uninfected erythrocytes have reduced deformability, although the mechanism responsible for the loss of deformability is not completely understood. However, increased oxidation of membranes in uninfected erythrocytes has been demonstrated in children with severe P falciparum malaria, and the ongoing inflammatory insults associated with acute malaria (proinflammatory cytokines) or the direct effects of parasite products have been shown to cause loss of red cell deformability.[34,35] Intriguingly, a severe reduction in red cell deformability measured on admission is also a strong predictor, not just for anemia, but also for mortality in both adults and children with severe malaria.[36,37]

Immune Complex–Mediated Hemolysis

It is also possible that at least part of the hemolysis in P falciparum malaria might have an immune basis. A positive direct Coombs antiglobulin test (DAT) is seen in some patients with malaria.[38,39] However, in Thai children or adults during their first attack or with subsequent attacks in those who live in areas where a degree of immunity has not developed, DAT results are invariably negative.[40]

The position is different in African children who have suffered repeated attacks of malaria. Positive DAT results have been found in up to 50% of these children, and the incidence is significantly higher in children with active malarial infection than in those who are not infected.[38,39] DAT results may remain positive for several weeks after an acute infection. The most common type of red cell sensitization occurs with C3. The IgG that can be eluted from these cells has specific activity against *P falciparum* schizont antigen,[40] which suggests that the erythrocyte coating results from passive attachment of circulating complement-fixing malarial antigen-antibody complexes. It is therefore likely that the development of positive DAT results is part of the immune response to *P falciparum*.

Other studies have suggested that the *P falciparum* ring surface protein 2 (RSP-2) may be one component of the immunoglobulin-antigen complexes deposited on un-infected erythrocytes. This protein is expressed on infected erythrocytes shortly after merozoite invasion. RSP-2 is also deposited on uninfected erythrocytes and forms im-mune complexes that contribute to the phagocytosis of uninfected erythrocytes. Limited clinical studies have shown that high levels of anti-RSP-2 antibodies are found in the sera of immune adults and children with severe anemia.[41]

However, it is far from clear whether the presence of positive DAT results indicates that immune destruction of red cells occurs in African children with malaria. Several studies have shown that there is no correlation between the degree of anemia and positive DAT results, and other measured parameters of hemolysis have not corre-lated with coating of red cells.

In short, there is little evidence for immune destruction of red cells in *P falciparum* malarial infections in nonimmune adults. Although a varying proportion of children with chronic malaria in Africa has positive DAT results, only occasionally is evidence of genuine immune destruction of red cells seen. However, the persistence of short-ened red cell survival of nonparasitized cells in the absence of any consistent sero-logic abnormalities suggests that there must be another factor involved in the shortened red cell survival in malaria. This factor appears to be nonspecific over-activity of the monocyte/macrophage populations of the spleen and liver, as dis-cussed earlier.

Defective Marrow Response

In addition to the hemolytic components of the anemia of *P falciparum* malaria, there is undoubtedly an inappropriate marrow response.[18,42–44] The reticulocytosis in response to the decrease in hematocrit is often inappropriately low and delayed (see **Fig. 2**). It remains unclear whether defective erythropoietin production is a signif-icant cause, with some studies suggesting an appropriate increase[45] or even enhanced response[46] and others observing a blunted response,[47] but there is no question that significant dysfunction of marrow takes place and appears to have a complex, multifactorial basis.

Some of the features of iron metabolism and bone marrow morphology and function in acute malaria resemble those of other acute infections. Thus, the serum iron level rapidly decreases and iron appears to be sequestrated into the storage compartments of the marrow.[18,42] It is now clear that disturbances in iron metabolism are mediated by hepcidin. Hepcidin is regulated by pro-inflammatory mediators, such as tumor necrosis factor (TNF) and IL-6, which are elevated in both murine infections and in patients presenting with severe falciparum malaria, although other parasite-derived and host factors may be involved in stimulating hepcidin production. High hepcidin levels stimulated by blood stage malaria infection are associated with inhibition of liver stage malaria infection in mice[48] and reduced incorporation of iron into red cells in humans.[49] Hepcidin levels decrease in the most severely ill children as hypoxia inhibits hepcidin production.[50] Evidence from murine malaria suggests that low serum iron caused by elevated hepcidin reduced parasite growth and progression to severe dis-ease.[51] These experimental and clinical findings are consistent with a role for iron as a growth factor for malaria parasites and a role for raised hepcidin and reduction in available iron as a protective innate response to malaria infection.

During acute malarial infections, there are marked dyserythropoietic changes in the bone marrow.[18,42–44] These morphologic abnormalities, which have been studied by both light and electron microscopy, consist of erythroblast multinuclearity, karyorrhexis, incomplete and unequal amitotic nuclear divisions, and cytoplasmic bridging (**Fig. 3**).[42]

There is a significant abnormality of red cell proliferation in the bone marrow that occurs in acute malaria. Changes include an increased proportion of red cell precursors in the G2 phase and arrest in progress of cells in the S phase.[43] Gene expression is profoundly altered in erythroid precursors exposed to malarial products, and this pattern of dyserythropoiesis is distinct from dyserythropoiesis induced by inflammatory cytokines.[52,53]

In addition to these dyserythropoietic changes, erythrophagocytosis is particularly common in the bone marrow in *P falciparum* malaria.[42] This phenomenon is not restricted to the marrow and may be seen in the spleen and other organs and, as mentioned earlier, may play a role in the hemolytic component of the disease.

Although the mechanism of dyserythropoietic changes is unknown, it was thought possible that they are an exaggerated example of the bone marrow suppression that occurs in other situations of chronic infection. An important factor may be the high levels of TNF production that occur during malarial infection because this cytokine has been strongly implicated in the anemia of chronic infection, and severe malarial anemia has been associated with certain TNF promoter polymorphisms.[54] TNF suppresses the proliferation of erythroid progenitor cells in human marrow culture, although the effect declines as the cells differentiate.[55] On the other hand, TNF stimulates fibroblasts to secrete growth factors for colony-forming-unit–granulocyte-erythrocyte-monocyte-macrophage and burst-forming-unit–erythrocyte.[56] Furthermore, experimental findings in mice are consistent with a role for TNF in the dyserythropoietic changes of malaria.[57]

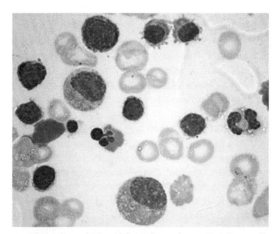

Fig. 3. Bone marrow aspirate in malaria. Although erythropoiesis is usually normoblastic in individuals with acute or chronic malaria, the examination of bone marrow frequently shows changes reflecting dyserythropoiesis, such as the irregular nuclei and cytoplasmic bridges in erythroblasts seen in this figure. Two young rings of P falciparum can be seen in an erythrocyte (Giemsa stain, ×900). (*From* Roberts DJ. Hematological manifestations of parasitic disease. In: Hoffman, Benz, Shattil, et al, editors. Hematology: basic principles and practice. 5th edition. Churchill Livingstone; 2009. p. 2344; with permission.)

IL-10 is an anti-inflammatory cytokine, and 2 clinical studies in African children with severe malarial anemia have found a low ratio of IL-10 to TNF in plasma, thus leading the investigators to propose that defective IL-10 production may pave the way to marrow suppression by TNF.[58,59] Anti-inflammatory cytokines may be associated with a more favorable outcome. IL-12 protects against severe anemia in experimental murine malaria, which might reflect both its antiparasitic actions and its effects on erythropoiesis.[60]

Several studies have suggested that a parasite byproduct of hemoglobin digestion, hemozoin, may have an indirect or direct role in impaired erythroid development.[44,52] Hemozoin stimulates the secretion of biologically active endoperoxides from monocytes, such as 15(S)-hydroxyeicosatetraenoic acid and hydroxynonenal, via oxidation of membrane lipids, which may affect erythroid growth.[61]

Hemozoin and TNF-α also have additive effects on erythropoiesis *in vitro*, and in a clinical study, hemozoin-containing macrophages and plasma hemozoin were associated with anemia and reticulocyte suppression.[44] Moreover, bone marrow sections from children who died with severe malaria show a significant association between the quantity of hemozoin (located in erythroid precursors and macrophages) and the proportion of erythroid cells that were abnormal. These findings are consistent with a direct inhibitory effect of hemozoin on erythropoiesis.

Coagulation Abnormalities

Modest thrombocytopenia is not uncommon during acute *P falciparum* attacks, and occasionally, the platelet count decreases to as low as 10,000 to 20,000/mL.[18] The mechanisms have not been determined but probably involve platelet activation and adhesion of infected erythrocytes to platelets, and experimental studies in mice suggest that platelets sequester in venules during malarial infection.[62]

In some patients with severe *P falciparum* malaria, a severe bleeding diathesis may develop during the acute phase of the illness. Although it has been suggested that the diathesis results from disseminated intravascular coagulation, studies in Thailand have not substantiated this supposition.[18] Rather, the bleeding appears to reflect gross thrombocytopenia together with liver damage. However, it is becoming apparent that approximately 10% of African children with severe malaria also have bacteremia,[16,17] so when disseminated intravascular coagulation occurs, the cause may be complex.

MALARIA IN PREGNANCY

In endemic regions, malaria in pregnancy is extremely common and may present with severe disease in the mother. The placenta also provides a favorable environment for parasite replication, and specific pathways of adhesion of infected erythrocytes to the surface of syncytiotrophoblasts have now been unraveled. A specific variant antigen, PfEMP1, expressed on the surface of infected erythrocytes (varCSA-2), mediates adhesion of infected erythrocytes to chondroitin sulfate. Apart from effects on the mother, it is an important cause of low birth weight and increased perinatal mortality. Studies of cord hemoglobin levels indicate that it is also a significant cause of fetal anemia. Because the severity of the fetal anemia is out of proportion to the degree of maternal anemia, it has been suggested that intrauterine hemolysis may be involved.[63] Malaria in pregnancy is a preventable illness, although it has become more difficult to control with the increase of resistance to antimalarial drugs. Studies in different parts of Africa have found placental malaria to be an important risk factor for anemia in the first 6 months of life.[64]

Given the high prevalence of malaria in pregnancy and the strong association of placental malaria with infantile anemia, it is surprising how few infants have overt symptoms of congenital malaria in the tropics. On the rare occasions when it does occur, it can result in a perplexing hematologic disorder. The manifestations of malaria may not be seen until several months after birth, presumably because of passive immunization from the mother and possibly the fact that *P falciparum* tends to grow less effectively in cells containing relatively large amounts of fetal hemoglobin. The disease is characterized by a febrile illness associated with anemia that may often be profound.[63] As in conventionally-acquired malaria, the pathophysiologic course of the anemia is a complex combination of hemolysis and marrow suppression. Thus, it is important to obtain a careful travel history from the parents of any infant with unexplained hemolysis. This condition is commonly misdiagnosed because it is not considered.

MALARIA IN SPLENECTOMIZED PATIENTS

It is generally thought that malaria may be associated with particularly severe infections in individuals who have been splenectomized. It is wise to advise visitors to the tropics who have had their spleens removed and splenectomized patients who live in regions where malaria is endemic to be particularly careful about continuing to maintain malaria prophylaxis.

HYPERREACTIVE MALARIAL SPLENOMEGALY SYNDROME

Although splenomegaly is a feature of many tropical disorders, there is increasing evidence, particularly from work in East and West Africa and Papua New Guinea, that a specific entity, formerly known as tropical splenomegaly syndrome, occurs widely throughout Africa, India, and Southeast Asia.[65] This condition is characterized by gross splenomegaly, high malarial antibody titer, and serum IgM levels at least 2 SD greater than the local mean. The classic syndrome regresses after prolonged antimalarial prophylaxis with proguanil, a dihydrofolate reductase inhibitor marketed outside the United States as Paludrine.

Epidemiologic studies indicate that its prevalence is related to patterns of malarial transmission and that affected individuals have higher malarial antibody titer than do those who live in the same environment and are unaffected; this seems to involve IgM rather than IgG. There is usually a good clinical response to prolonged antimalarial treatment. These observations suggest that the condition probably results from an unusual form of immune response to chronic malarial infection. For this reason, it is now commonly referred to as hyperreactive malarial splenomegaly (HMS).

With progressive splenomegaly, there is pooling of the formed elements of blood. Such sequestration produces a dilutional anemia, and there is also pooling of neutrophils and platelets, so the hematologic picture is characterized by pancytopenia. No characteristic changes in the bone marrow morphology are seen.

Some evidence of a genetic predisposition to HMS exists. A recent study in Ghana found that splenomegaly, high IgM levels, and anemia were more common in relatives of HMS patients than in the general population, but there was no clear pattern of mendelian segregation, thus suggesting that the cause in this population is likely to be complex and involve multiple genetic and environmental factors. For some years, researchers have debated whether HMS is premalignant because it sometimes becomes refractory to antimalarial treatment, and it can also be associated with a lymphocytosis resembling chronic lymphocytic leukemia (CLL). Clonal rearrangements of the joining (JH) region of the immunoglobulin gene have been noted in some patients whose clinical syndrome appears to be intermediate between HMS and CLL, thus suggesting that HMS has premalignant potential.[66]

The clinical picture of HMS is typical and consists of massive splenomegaly, weight loss, and a variable degree of anemia.[65] Serum IgM levels are high, and a relative increase in T lymphocytes in peripheral blood may be seen. Serum may also show increased cold agglutinin titers and an increase in rheumatoid factor, antibodies to thyroglobulin and antinuclear factor, and circulating immune complexes.

The prognosis for patients with this condition is remarkably poor in parts of Africa, with up to 50% mortality in some populations. It is managed by long-term antimalarial prophylaxis, most commonly with proguanil.

ASPECTS OF THE CLINICAL MANAGEMENT OF MALARIAL ANEMIA

There is no scope for a full exposition of the clinical management of severe anemia in the many different medical arenas across the world. However, some considerations are relevant to the management of severe anemia in malaria. The definition of severe anemia depends on the clinical context, and the normal level of hemoglobin in the community has to be considered. In an African child with malaria, a hemoglobin level of approximately 5 g/dL is commonly used as the criterion for transfusion, although a transfusion would normally be given sooner if the parasitemia were extremely high. The fatality rate for severe malarial anemia varies widely between clinics, but a typical figure is approximately 7%.[67]

An urgent need exists to define the clinical criteria that make transfusion absolutely essential. Decision trees have been devised,[68] but the underlying risk-benefit equation may vary from place-to-place, and a meta-analysis found no clear evidence of benefit for transfusion in anemic children whose conditions are clinically stable.[69] One issue that has become clear is the prognostic importance of respiratory distress. For example, in Kenyan children, malarial anemia rarely causes death unless respiratory distress is present,[69] and the only clear evidence that blood transfusion is beneficial is seen in the group of children who have both anemia and respiratory distress.[70]

Investigations into the clinical physiologic course of severe malarial anemia in African children have yielded important insights into the management of this condition. Lactic acidosis appears to be the main cause of the relationship between anemia and respiratory distress, and there is a substantial oxygen debt. However, it is now clear that bolus fluid supplementation of severely ill children on admission may result in higher mortality.[71–73] Ill children should therefore be carefully assessed clinically, and appropriate fluid or blood transfusion should be given to correct hypovolemia or severe anemia.

As the criteria for transfusion become stricter, there is a need for more data on optimal hematinic therapy for children with malarial anemia. The practices of pediatricians vary, but many prescribe both iron and folic acid in addition to antimalarial therapy. One concern has been that iron deficiency may help suppress parasite growth, and these observations have been supported by experimental studies that have shown *P falciparum* infects iron-deficient erythrocytes less efficiently than iron-replete erythrocytes.[74]

Another concern has been that folic acid supplements might reduce the efficacy of the antifolate drugs that are increasingly being used to treat chloroquine-resistant malaria in the community. These issues were addressed in a study of moderately anemic Gambian children with *P falciparum* infection.[75] Supplementary iron therapy was found to result in a small, but significant improvement in hemoglobin levels after 1 month and did not increase the risk for reinfection within this period. Folic acid supplements failed to improve hemoglobin levels and increased the risk for parasite recrudescence if sulfadoxine-pyrimethamine was used to treat the infection. However, it cannot be assumed that these findings would necessarily apply to regions with different rates of malarial transmission and different nutritional problems, and the need for locally based research into this type of problem and indeed many other aspects of clinical malaria cannot be overemphasized.

VISCERAL LEISHMANIASIS (KALA-AZAR)

Leishmaniasis is an infection caused by intracellular protozoan parasites transmitted by various species of sandflies.[76] Human infections can result in 3 main forms of disease: cutaneous, mucocutaneous, and visceral (kala-azar). The important hematologic manifestations of leishmanial infection are found in the visceral forms.

The generalized form of leishmanial disease involves the liver, spleen, bone marrow, and lymph nodes and is caused by organisms belonging to the *Leishmania donovani* complex. The parent species, *L donovani*, is found throughout Asia and Africa and can affect individuals of all ages. However, the parasite that causes kala-azar in countries bordering the Mediterranean, in southern Europe, and in North Africa primarily affects young children and infants. It differs from *L donovani* to such an extent that it warrants the designation of a special species and is called *Leishmania infantum*. Similarly, in the Western Hemisphere, kala-azar is also a disease of very young children; the causative organism is *Leishmania chagasi*.

Although visceral leishmaniasis is primarily a disease of indigenous populations, it may be contracted on short-term visits. For example, in the United Kingdom, it is being recognized increasingly after return from Mediterranean holidays, and particularly in young children, it can cause considerable diagnostic difficulty; occurrences have been mislabeled as leukemia when the diagnosis of leishmaniasis was not considered. The risk for leishmaniasis is greatly increased in individuals infected with HIV.[77]

Although the incubation period is usually 1 to 3 months, it can be as short as a few weeks. The onset is usually insidious and consists of fever, sweating, malaise, and anorexia, although a much more acute onset may be seen. As the disease progresses, the acute symptoms abate, but there is gradual enlargement of the spleen and liver for several months. By this time, there may be marked splenomegaly, cachexia, and anorexia. Generalized lymphadenopathy is also present.

Hematologic findings in later stages of the illness include anemia, neutropenia, and thrombocytopenia, manifestations characteristic of hypersplenism. The bone marrow is hyperplastic with dyserythropoietic changes, and the diagnosis can usually be made by finding Leishman-Donovan bodies—macrophages containing intracellular organisms with characteristic staining properties. The diagnosis can also be made by splenic or lymph node puncture.

Red cell survival studies and ferrokinetic analyses have suggested that hemolysis is the major cause of anemia in leishmaniasis,[18] but that there may also be plasma volume expansion associated with the massively enlarged spleen. Surprisingly, ferrokinetic studies have shown very little evidence of ineffective erythropoiesis, but a reduced plasma iron level in the presence of greatly increased iron stores suggests that the reticuloendothelial hyperplasia is accompanied by abnormal iron retention by macrophages, typical of the anemia of chronic disorders[78]; this may limit the marrow response to hemolysis.

In babies or young children with acute visceral leishmaniasis, the clinical and hematologic findings may differ from those described earlier. For example, in Mediterranean populations, a very rapid onset of anemia with severe hemolysis is commonly observed.[79] Occasionally, both IgG and complement components are found on the red cells, but this finding is not consistent and its significance remains to be determined. In most instances, there is no evidence of immune hemolysis, and it appears that nonsensitized red cells are destroyed by macrophages recruited to the spleen and liver as part of the inflammatory response to the parasite. Severe neutropenia may also occur in young children, and this, together with dyserythropoietic changes in the marrow, marked erythrophagocytosis, and bizarre mononuclear infiltrates, may cause confusion with leukemia.

SCHISTOSOMIASIS

The schistosomes are a group of trematodes that cause major health problems in many parts of the developing world.[79] The major human parasites include *Schistosoma haematobium*, *Schistosoma mansoni*, and *Schistosoma japonicum*. Schistosomiasis affects mainly children and young adults. Two hundred million people worldwide are estimated to have schistosomiasis, 80% in sub-Saharan Africa.[80,81]

The location of adult worms in the human host varies with the parasite species: *S haematobium* in the veins of the bladder, *S mansoni* in the superior mesenteric veins, and *S japonicum* in the inferior mesenteric veins. Sexual maturity of female schistosomes depends on their interaction with living male worms. Egg deposition occurs in the small venules of the bladder or portal venous system. When freshly deposited, the ova are partially developed. Hatching of the eggs leads to the liberation of miracidia. Further development occurs when miracidia penetrate a snail intermediate host. After 2 generations, cercariae are released that are capable of penetrating intact skin and migrating through tissues to reach their final home.

S haematobium infections occur in Africa and the Middle East, whereas *S mansoni* is found in Africa, the Middle East, and parts of South America. *S japonicum* occurs in Japan, the Philippines, and together with the related species *Schistosoma mekongi*, in mainland Indochina.

The most consistent hematologic changes are found in association with *S mansoni* infection. The acute phase is characterized by fever, myalgia, and progressive hepatosplenomegaly. At this time, the most common finding in peripheral blood is eosinophilia. As the disease progresses, there may be massive hepatosplenomegaly associated with anemia, neutropenia, and thrombocytopenia.[82] Good descriptions of the appearance of bone marrow in this condition are few, and the data available suggest that the anemia is predominantly due to hypersplenism and hemodilution from the massive splenomegaly.

S haematobium infection leads to urinary tract symptoms, in particular, hematuria and dysuria. The hematuria may be gross and persistent and lead to iron deficiency anemia. In addition, affected children have typical features of the anemia of chronic disorders.

A major advance in control of schistosomiasis is the availability of a highly effective drug, praziquantel, which is safe in both children and pregnant women. The cost of control programs may be reduced by combination therapy for schistosomiasis, gastrointestinal helminths, and filariasis; in 2001, the World Health Assembly resolved that at least 75% of school-aged children in high-burden areas should be treated for schistosomiasis and soil-transmitted helminth infections by 2010 to reduce morbidity.[80]

TRYPANOSOMIASIS

Trypanosomal infections are a major cause of ill health throughout the world. The disease syndromes produced by these infections vary widely but, in general, are divided into the American and African forms.[83,84]

American Trypanosomiasis (Chagas Disease)

American trypanosomiasis is a zoonosis caused by *Trypanosoma cruzi*, which is transmitted to humans by blood-sucking insects. It was first described by Carlos Chagas in 1909.

In its invertebrate host, *T cruzi*, grows extracellularly. Epimastigotes divide in the insect gut and differentiate into metacyclic trypomastigotes, which are the infective form for mammalian hosts. They are released close to the site of a bite and enter the host via the skin or mucous membranes. After invasion, they enter cells, where they replicate as rounded amastigote forms that differentiate into trypomastigotes, which are released into the circulation and tissues. A variety of organs are involved, but the most important pathophysiologic result is a chronic cardiomyopathy.

There are characteristic clinical findings at each of these different stages of infection. After penetration of the skin, a local cutaneous lesion called an inoculation chagoma develops and is accompanied by swelling of the local lymph glands. Occasionally, the route of inoculation is through the eye, where the initial lesion is characterized by unilateral conjunctivitis with edema of the eyelids. Invasion may or may not be followed by an acute phase consisting of fever, generalized lymphadenopathy, hepatosplenomegaly, and acute myocarditis.

The chronic phase of Chagas disease takes several forms. If cardiac involvement is predominant, a slowly progressive cardiomyopathy with heart failure, arrhythmias, and embolic complications is seen. In other patients, gastrointestinal symptoms predominate as a result of denervation and destruction of the myenteric plexus, which may give rise to megaesophagus or megacolon.

A congenital form of Chagas disease may occur. The organism can traverse the placental villi and from there be released into the fetal circulation. The most common findings include growth retardation, hepatosplenomegaly, acute myocarditis, neurologic lesions, including a meningoencephalitic picture with tremors and convulsions, and occasionally, a generalized hemorrhagic tendency with purpura or more widespread bleeding. The prognosis for patients with congenital Chagas disease is poor, and most infants die during the first week of life.

The hematologic changes in Chagas disease are nonspecific. In the acute phase, mild anemia and lymphocytosis may occur. At this stage, the parasite can be found in the blood or in leukocyte concentrates. Parasites may be concentrated by sedimentation of heparinized blood cells with the addition of phytohemagglutinin. Similarly, it is possible to find amastigote forms of *T cruzi* in muscle or lymph node biopsy samples. The results of serologic tests for anti–*T cruzi* IgM antibodies typically become positive about 20 to 40 days after the onset of symptoms.

African Trypanosomiasis

In Africa, these conditions are caused by subspecies of the hemoflagellate *Trypanosoma brucei* known as *T brucei gambiense*, which causes a chronic illness called sleeping sickness, and *T brucei rhodesiense*, which is associated with a more acute illness. *T brucei* is transmitted by the tsetse fly Glossina, in which it undergoes a variety of developmental changes.

At the site of the tsetse bite, a small nodule called a trypanosomal chancre forms from which organisms may be isolated. After this self-limited lesion subsides, the parasite invades and multiplies extracellularly in the blood, which leads to the systemic phase of the illness characterized by fever, lymphadenopathy, and splenomegaly. In the later phase of African trypanosomiasis, invasion of the central nervous system takes place and results in meningoencephalitis.

During the acute phase, normochromic normocytic anemia associated with hypoalbuminemia may be present. Occasionally, patients have hemorrhagic manifestations and evidence of disseminated intravascular coagulation. The total white blood cell count is either normal or elevated with relative lymphocytosis. The sedimentation rate is markedly elevated, and circulating immune complexes may be present together with rheumatoid factor.

The parasite can often be demonstrated in thin or thick blood films stained with Giemsa or Field stain. Several concentration techniques have been developed to increase the likelihood of finding the parasite. A variety of immunodiagnostic tests are available, notably indirect immunofluorescence and enzyme-linked immunosorbent assay, but visualization of the parasite is necessary for a confident diagnosis. In the more chronic stage, it is important to examine cerebrospinal fluid, which often shows lymphocytosis, an elevated protein level, and the presence of morular cells of Mott or motile trypanosomes. High levels of IgM in cerebrospinal fluid may suggest the diagnosis in advanced disease if trypanosomes have not been found.

A novel test for African trypanosomiasis involves analysis of serum samples by mass spectrometry to detect distinct proteomic signatures; this test appears to provide more sensitive and specific detection than other diagnostic tests.[85]

HOOKWORM

It has been estimated that more than 900 million people are infected with hookworms.[86] There are 2 main species, *Ancylostoma duodenale* and *Necator americanus*, sometimes called the Old World and the New World hookworms, respectively. Both species are widely distributed in tropical and subtropical Asia and Africa. The prevalence of infection ranges from 80% to 90% in rural areas in the moist parts of the tropics, such as West Bengal, to 10% to 20% in relatively dry countries, such as those of the Middle East and Pakistan.

Both species of hookworm produce enormous numbers of eggs—approximately 20,000 per day per female hookworm. The eggs are discharged into the intestinal lumen, where they undergo several cell divisions before being passed in stool. Given appropriate conditions, the eggs develop further and hatch, with liberation of larvae. These free-living stages go through a series of developments designated L1 to L3, after which they penetrate the skin and the infective filarial larval forms migrate to the intestinal tract via the circulation, lungs, and respiratory tract. The final larval stage, L4, and the adult worms are found in the small intestine.

Hookworms attach to the mucosa of the upper intestine by their buccal capsules. Although they are found mainly in the jejunum, in very heavy infections they may be distributed as low as the ileum. Attachment of the worm results in bleeding into the gastrointestinal tract.

The worms change their attachment site every few hours. Continuous or intermittent suction causes tissue and blood to be drawn into the worm's intestinal tract. Only about 50% of the iron lost as hemoglobin into the gut may be reabsorbed. Therefore, there is a marked increase in fecal iron concentration that is related directly to the worm load, which can be assessed by the fecal egg count. Direct recordings of blood loss have given values of the order of 0.03 mL/d per worm for *N americanus* and up to 0.26 mL/d per worm for *A duodenale*, and the latter species tends to cause more profound levels of iron deficiency in the community.[87]

The hematologic findings in children or adults with heavy hookworm infections are characteristic. Because the condition is usually chronic, anemia is the major clinical feature. In severe cases, hemoglobin values of 2 to 5 g/dL are common.[88] The blood film shows the typical changes of iron deficiency anemia, such as microcytosis, hypochromia, and a normal reticulocyte count. The serum iron level is low, and iron is absent from bone marrow stores. Because of associated protein loss, these children often have hypoalbuminemia.[89] Mild eosinophilia may be present in patients with established illness, although very high eosinophil counts may occur during the phase of the illness in which the worms are migrating from the skin to the gastrointestinal tract.

The diagnosis is made by analysis of stool for eggs. In heavy infections, a fecal film can be examined directly after the sample is mounted in saline or iodine solution. In lighter infections, concentration by zinc sulfate flotation is required.

Affected children require oral iron treatment to restore the iron stores, as well as treatment with anthelmintic drugs. Although many of these children are severely anemic, they have had chronic anemia for many years, and rapid restoration of the hemoglobin level is not usually required. However, in profoundly anemic children with high-output failure and associated hypoalbuminemia, it may be necessary to administer red cells slowly, together with appropriate diuretics.

In recent years, a growing number of tropical countries have made concerted efforts to reduce the effects of hookworm infection by anthelmintic strategies in the community. For example, mass administration of mebendazole to 30,000 schoolchildren in Zanzibar was estimated to prevent 1260 cases of moderate to severe anemia and 276 cases of severe anemia in 1 year, although it appeared that at least 2 doses per year would be necessary to maintain this level of protection, thus raising the issue of long-term sustainability.[90]

BARTONELLOSIS

Bartonellosis (Carrión disease, Oroya fever) is an infectious disease that is endemic in the western Andes of Peru and is seen occasionally in Colombia and Ecuador.[91] It results from infection by an aerobic, gram-negative bacillus, *Bartonella bacilliformis*. It is usually transmitted through a sandfly bite. After inoculation, the organism multiplies in endothelial and red blood cells. In severe disease, almost 100% of red cells are infected with numerous bacteria. Hence, the major feature of the disease is profound anemia resulting from the infection and subsequent phagocytosis of red cells. Although the precise mechanisms of the anemia are not fully understood, it seems to have many of the features of anemia of acute malarial infection. Survival of infected and noninfected red cells is shortened, and a limited response to the hemolysis associated with dyserythropoietic changes in the bone marrow is seen.

The disease has 2 stages, anemic and eruptive, with an asymptomatic period between the stages. After an incubation period of approximately 60 days, the onset of the condition is acute and consists of malaise, chills, fever, and headache. The clinical picture is then dominated by severe hemolytic anemia associated with hepatosplenomegaly, lymphadenopathy, and occasionally, a fine petechial rash. In the later eruptive stage, nodule lesions of varying size appear on the face, trunk, and limbs. Arthralgia and fever may also be present. The lesions, which are widespread on the arms and legs, may be confused with leprosy, yaws, or even Kaposi sarcoma. Although the infection is often present for a prolonged period, the eruptive phase tends to regress spontaneously.

During the anemic stage, moderate to severe hemolytic anemia is seen with reticulocyte counts in the 5% to 10% range. The organisms can be seen on thick and thin blood films stained with Giemsa, Wright, or related stains. The bone marrow is hyperactive with dyserythropoietic changes. The white blood cell count is not usually elevated, but thrombocytopenia is common.

The principal complication of this disease, apart from profound anemia, is superinfection with other organisms, particularly *Salmonella typhi* and *Mycobacterium tuberculosis*. Fortunately, *B bacilliformis* is extremely sensitive to chloramphenicol, penicillin, and tetracyclines. Supportive treatment includes regular transfusion through the anemic phase of the illness.

SUMMARY

Malaria, visceral leishmaniasis, schistosomiasis, trypanosomiasis, hookworm, and bartonellosis cause hematologic syndromes that can dominate the clinical presentation of infected cases. The pathophysiology of anemia and cytopenias is complex, often involving reduced production and increased destruction of cells accompanied by restricted availability of iron. These features may prevent untrammeled multiplication of the respective microbe. Many public health initiatives have begun to reduce the incidence of these infections, but patients with these diseases will continue to present with hematologic problems and require careful diagnosis and management for some time to come.

REFERENCES

1. Fleming AF, Menendez C. Blood. In: Parry E, Godfrey R, Mabey D, et al, editors. Principles of medicine in Africa. Cambridge (UK): Cambridge University Press; 2005. p. 924–70.
2. World Health Organization. World malaria report 2014. Available at: http://www.who.int/malaria/publications/world_malaria_report_2014/wmr-2014-no-profiles.pdf. Accessed July 13, 2015.
3. Lamikanra AA, Brown D, Potocnik A, et al. Malarial anemia: of mice and men. Blood 2007;110(1):18–28.
4. Snow RW, Guerra CA, Noor AM, et al. The global distribution of clinical episodes of Plasmodium falciparum malaria. Nature 2005;434:214–7.
5. Gething PW, Battle KE, Bhatt S, et al. Declining malaria in Africa: improving the measurement of progress. Malar J 2014;13:39.
6. Singh B, Kim Sung L, Matusop A, et al. A large focus of naturally acquired Plasmodium knowlesi infections in human beings. Lancet 2004;363:1017–24.
7. Horuk R, Chitnis CE, Darbonne WC, et al. A receptor for the malarial parasite Plasmodium vivax: the erythrocyte chemokine receptor. Science 1993;61:1182–4.
8. Greenwood BM, Bradley AK, Greenwood AM, et al. Mortality and morbidity from malaria among children in a rural area of The Gambia, West Africa. Trans R Soc Trop Med Hyg 1987;81:478–86.
9. Warrell DA, Molyneux ME, Beales P. Severe and complicated malaria. Trans R Soc Trop Med Hyg 1990;84(Suppl 2):1–65.
10. Slutsker L, Taylor TE, Wirima JJ, et al. In-hospital morbidity and mortality due to malaria-associated severe anaemia in two areas of Malawi with different patterns of malaria infection. Trans R Soc Trop Med Hyg 1994;88:548–51.

11. Berendt AR, Ferguson DJP, Newbold CI. Sequestration in Plasmodium falciparum malaria: sticky cells and sticky problems. Parasitol Today 1990;6:247–54.
12. McCormick CJ, Craig AC, Roberts DJ, et al. Intracellular adhesion molecule-1 and CD36 synergize to mediate adherence of Plasmodium falciparum-infected erythrocytes to cultured human microvascular endothelial cells. J Clin Invest 1997;100:2521–9.
13. Roberts DJ, Craig AG, Berendt AR, et al. Rapid switching to multiple antigenic and adhesive phenotypes in malaria. Nature 1992;357:689–92.
14. Rowe JA, Moulds JM, Newbold CI, et al. P. falciparum rosetting mediated by a parasite-variant erythrocyte membrane protein and complement-receptor 1. Nature 1997;388:292–5.
15. Pain A, Ferguson DJ, Kai O, et al. Platelet-mediated clumping of Plasmodium falciparum–infected erythrocytes is a common adhesive phenotype and is associated with severe malaria. Proc Natl Acad Sci U S A 2001;98:1805–10.
16. Berkley J, Mwarumba S, Bramham K, et al. Bacteraemia complicating severe malaria in children. Trans R Soc Trop Med Hyg 1999;93:283–6.
17. Graham SM, Walsh AL, Molyneux EM, et al. Clinical presentation of non-typhoidal Salmonella bacteraemia in Malawian children. Trans R Soc Trop Med Hyg 2000; 94:310–4.
18. Phillips RE, Looareesuwan S, Warrell DA, et al. The importance of anaemia in cerebral and uncomplicated falciparum malaria: role of complications, dyserythropoiesis and iron sequestration. Q J Med 1986;58:305–23.
19. Wickramasinghe SN, Looareesuwan S, Nagachinta B, et al. Dyserythropoiesis and ineffective erythropoiesis in Plasmodium vivax malaria. Br J Haematol 1989;72:91–9.
20. McGuire W, D'Alessandro U, Olaleye BO, et al. C-reactive protein and haptoglobin in the evaluation of a community-based malaria control programme. Trans R Soc Trop Med Hyg 1996;90:10–4.
21. Roberts DJ, Casals-Pascual C, Weatherall DJ. Malaria anemia-host resistance to parasite virulence. In: Sullivan D, Krishna S, editors. Malaria: drugs, disease and post-genomic biology. Current topics in microbiology and immunology volume on antimalarial chemotherapy. Heidelburg (Germany): Springer Heidelburg; 2005. Current Topics in Microbiology and Immunology.
22. Jakeman GN, Saul A, Hogarth WL, et al. Anaemia of acute malaria infections in non-immune patients primarily results from destruction of uninfected erythrocytes. Parasitology 1999;119:127–33.
23. Looareesuwan S, Merry AH, Phillips RE, et al. Reduced erythrocyte survival following clearance of malarial parasitaemia in Thai patients. Br J Haematol 1987;67:473–8.
24. Allred D. Immune evasion by Babesia bovis and Plasmodium falciparum: cliff-dwellers of the parasite world. Parasitol Today 1995;11:100–5.
25. Looareesuwan S, Ho M, Wattanagoon Y, et al. Dynamic alterations in splenic function during acute falciparum malaria. N Engl J Med 1987;317:675–9.
26. Buffet PA, Safeukui I, Deplaine G, et al. The pathogenesis of Plasmodium falciparum malaria in humans: insights from splenic physiology. Blood 2011;117(2):381–92.
27. Lee SH, Looareesuwan S, Wattanagoon Y, et al. Antibody-dependent red cell removal during P. falciparum malaria: the clearance of red cells sensitised with an IgG anti-D. Br J Haematol 1989;73:396–402.
28. Mohan K, Dubey ML, Ganguly NK, et al. Plasmodium falciparum: role of activated blood monocytes in erythrocyte membrane damage and red cell loss during malaria. Exp Parasitol 1995;80:54–63.

29. Ladhani S, Lowe B, Cole AO, et al. Changes in white blood cells and platelets in children with falciparum malaria: relationship to disease outcome. Br J Haematol 2002;119:839–47.
30. Angus BJ, Chotivanich K, Udomsangpetch R, et al. In vivo removal of malaria parasites from red blood cells without their destruction in acute falciparum malaria. Blood 1997;90:2037–40.
31. Price R, van Vugt M, Phaipun L, et al. Adverse effects in patients with acute falciparum malaria treated with artemisinin derivatives. Am J Trop Med Hyg 1999;60:547–55.
32. Mojon M, Wallon M, Gravey A, et al. Intravascular haemolysis following halofantrine intake. Trans R Soc Trop Med Hyg 1994;88:91.
33. Tran TH, Day NP, Ly VC, et al. Blackwater fever in southern Vietnam: a prospective descriptive study of 50 cases. Clin Infect Dis 1996;23:1274–81.
34. Dondorp AM, Omodeo-Sale F, Chotivanich K, et al. Oxidative stress and rheology in severe malaria. Redox Rep 2003;8:292–4.
35. Omodeo-Sale F, Motti A, Dondorp A, et al. Destabilisation and subsequent lysis of human erythrocytes induced by Plasmodium falciparum haem products. Eur J Haematol 2005;74:324–32.
36. Dondorp AM, Angus BJ, Chotivanich K, et al. Red blood cell deformability as a predictor of anemia in severe falciparum malaria. Am J Trop Med Hyg 1999;60:733–7.
37. Dondorp AM, Nyanoti M, Kager PA, et al. The role of reduced red cell deformability in the pathogenesis of severe falciparum malaria and its restoration by blood transfusion. Trans R Soc Trop Med Hyg 2002;96:282–6.
38. Facer CA, Bray RS, Brown J. Direct Coombs' antiglobulin reactions in Gambian children with Plasmodium falciparum malaria. I. Incidence and class specificity. Clin Exp Immunol 1979;35:119–27.
39. Abdalla SH, Kasili FG, Weatherall DJ. The Coombs direct antiglobulin test in Kenyans. Trans R Soc Trop Med Hyg 1983;77:99–102.
40. Facer CA. Direct Coombs antiglobulin reactions in Gambian children with Plasmodium falciparum malaria. II: specificity of erythrocyte bound IgG. Clin Exp Immunol 1980;39:279–88.
41. Layez C, Nogueira P, Combes V, et al. Plasmodium falciparum rhoptry protein RSP2 triggers destruction of the erythroid lineage. Blood 2005;106:3632–8.
42. Abdalla S, Weatherall DJ, Wickramasinghe SN, et al. The anaemia of P. falciparum malaria. Br J Haematol 1980;46:171–83.
43. Wickramasinghe SN, Abdalla A, Weatherall DJ. Cell cycle distribution of erythroblasts in P. falciparum malaria. Scand J Haematol 1982;29:83–8.
44. Casals-Pascual C, Kai O, Cheung O, et al. Suppression of erythropoiesis in malarial anemia is associated with hemozoin in vitro and in vivo. Blood 2006;108:2569–77.
45. Burchard GD, Radloff P, Philipps J, et al. Increased erythropoietin production in children with severe malarial anemia. Am J Trop Med Hyg 1995;53:547–51.
46. Casals-Pascual C, Idro R, Gicheru N, et al. High plasma levels of erythropoietin are associated with protection against neurological sequelae in African children with cerebral malaria. Proc Natl Acad Sci U S A 2008;105(7):2634–9.
47. Burgmann H, Looareesuwan S, Kapiotis S, et al. Serum levels of erythropoietin in acute Plasmodium falciparum malaria. Am J Trop Med Hyg 1996;54:280–3.
48. Portugal S, Carret C, Recker M, et al. Host-mediated regulation of superinfection in malaria. Nat Med 2011;17:732–7.
49. Prentice AM, Doherty CP, Abrams SA, et al. Hepcidin is the major predictor of erythrocyte iron incorporation in anemic African children. Blood 2012;119:1922–8.

50. Casals-Pascual C, Huang H, Lakhal-Littleton S, et al. Hepcidin demonstrates a biphasic association with anemia in acute Plasmodium falciparum malaria. Haematologica 2012;97:1695–8.

51. Wang HZ, He YX, Yang CJ, et al. Hepcidin is regulated during blood-stage malaria and plays a protective role in malaria infection. J Immunol 2011;187:6410–6.

52. Lamikanra AA, Michel Theron M, Kooij TWA, et al. Malarial pigment directly promotes apoptosis of erythroid precursors. PLoS One 2009;4(12):e8446.

53. Lamikanra AA, Merryweather-Clarke AT, Tipping AJ. Distinct mechanisms of inadequate erythropoiesis induced by tumor necrosis factor alpha or malarial pigment. PLoS One 2015;10(3):e0119836.

54. McGuire W, Knight JC, Hill AV, et al. Severe malarial anemia and cerebral malaria are associated with different tumor necrosis factor promoter alleles. J Infect Dis 1999;179:287–90.

55. Roodman GD, Bird A, Hutzler D, et al. Tumor necrosis factor-alpha and hematopoietic progenitors: effects of tumor necrosis factor on the growth of erythroid progenitors CFU-E and BFU-E and the hematopoietic cell lines K562, HL60, HEL cells. Exp Hematol 1987;15:928–35.

56. Zucali JR, Broxmeyer HE, Gross MA, et al. Recombinant human tumor necrosis factors stimulates fibroblasts to produce hemopoietic growth factors in vitro. J Immunol 1988;140:840–4.

57. Johnson RA, Waddelow TA, Caro J, et al. Chronic exposure to tumor necrosis factor in vivo preferentially inhibits erythropoiesis in nude mice. Blood 1989;74:130–8.

58. Othoro C, Lal AA, Nahlen B, et al. A low interleukin-10 tumor necrosis factor-alpha ratio is associated with malaria anemia in children residing in a holoendemic malaria region in Western Kenya. J Infect Dis 1999;179:279–82.

59. Kurtzhals JA, Adabayeri V, Goka BQ, et al. Low plasma concentrations of interleukin 10 in severe malarial anaemia compared with cerebral and uncomplicated malaria. Lancet 1998;351:1768–72 [Erratum appears in Lancet 1998;352:242].

60. Mohan K, Stevenson MM. Dyserythropoiesis and severe anaemia associated with malaria correlate with deficient interleukin-12 production. Br J Haematol 1998; 103:942–9.

61. Giribaldi G, Ulliers D, Schwarzer E, et al. Hemozoin- and 4-hydroxynonenal-mediated inhibition of erythropoiesis. Possible role in malarial dyserythropoiesis and anemia. Haematologica 2004;89:492–3.

62. Grau GE, Tacchini-Cottier F, Vesin C, et al. TNF-induced microvascular pathology: active role for platelets and importance of the LFA-1/ICAM-1 interaction. Eur Cytokine Netw 1993;4:415–9.

63. Brabin B. Fetal anaemia in malarious areas: its causes and significance. Ann Trop Paediatr 1992;12:303.

64. Cornet M, Le Hesran JY, Fievet N, et al. Prevalence of and risk factors for anemia in young children in southern Cameroon. Am J Trop Med Hyg 1998;58:606–11.

65. Fakunle YM, Crane GG. Tropical splenomegaly. Part I: tropical Africa. Part 2: Oceania. Clin Haematol 1981;10:963–82.

66. Bates I, Bedu-Addo G, Bevan DH, et al. Use of immunoglobulin gene rearrangements to show clonal lymphoproliferation in hyper-reactive malarial splenomegaly. Lancet 1991;337:505–7.

67. Marsh K, Forster D, Waruiru C, et al. Indicators of life-threatening malaria in African children. N Engl J Med 1995;332:1399–404.

68. Obonyo CO, Steyerberg EW, Oloo AJ, et al. Blood transfusions for severe malaria-related anemia in Africa: a decision analysis. Am J Trop Med Hyg 1998;59:808–12.

69. Meremikwu M, Smith HJ. Blood transfusion for treating malarial anaemia. Cochrane Database Syst Rev 2000;(2):CD001475.
70. Lackritz EM, Campbell CC, Ruebush TKD, et al. Effect of blood transfusion on survival among children in a Kenyan hospital. Lancet 1992;340:524–8.
71. Maitland K, Kiguli S, Opoka RO, et al. Mortality after fluid bolus in African children with severe infection. N Engl J Med 2011;364:2483–95.
72. Murray MJ, Murray AB, Murray NJ, et al. The adverse effect of iron repletion on the course of certain infections. BMJ 1978;2:1113–5.
73. Oppenheimer SJ, Gibson FD, Macfarlane SB, et al. Iron supplementation increases prevalence and effects of malaria: report on clinical studies in Papua New Guinea. Trans R Soc Trop Med Hyg 1986;80:603–12.
74. Clark MA, Goheen MM, Fulford A, et al. Host iron status and iron supplementation mediate susceptibility to erythrocytic stage Plasmodium falciparum. Nat Commun 2014;5:4446.
75. van Hensbroek MB, Morris-Jones S, Meisner S, et al. Iron, but not folic acid, combined with effective antimalarial therapy promotes haematological recovery after acute falciparum malaria. Trans R Soc Trop Med Hyg 1995;89:672–6.
76. Herwaldt BL. Leishmaniasis. Lancet 1999;354:1191–9.
77. Alvar J, Canavate C, Gutierrez-Solar B, et al. Leishmania and human immunodeficiency virus coinfection: the first 10 years. Clin Microbiol Rev 1997;10:298–319.
78. Pippard MJ, Moir D, Weatherall DJ, et al. Mechanism of anaemia in resistant visceral leishmaniasis. Ann Trop Med Parasitol 1986;80:317–23.
79. Colley DG, Bustinduy AL, Secor WE, et al. Human schistosomiasis. Lancet 2014; 383(9936):2253–64.
80. Southgate VR, Rollinson D, Tchuem Tchuenté LA, et al. Towards control of schistosomiasis in sub-Saharan Africa. J Helminthol 2005;79:181–5.
81. Lai YS, Biedermann P, Ekpo UF, et al. Spatial distribution of schistosomiasis and treatment needs in sub-Saharan Africa: a systematic review and geostatistical analysis. Lancet Infect Dis 2015;15(8):927–40 [Erratum appears in Lancet Infect Dis 2015;15(7):761].
82. World Health Organization. Progress in assessment of morbidity due to schistosoma haematobium infection: a review of recent literature, WHO/Schisto/87.91. Geneva (Switzerland): World Health Organization; 1987.
83. Kennedy PG. Clinical features, diagnosis, and treatment of human African trypanosomiasis (sleeping sickness). Lancet Neurol 2013;12(2):186–94.
84. Bern C. Chagas' Disease. N Engl J Med 2015;373:456–66.
85. Papadopoulos MC, Abel PM, Agranoff D, et al. A novel and accurate diagnostic test for human African trypanosomiasis. Lancet 2004;363:1358–63.
86. Schad GA, Banwell JG. Hookworms. In: Warren KS, Mahmoud AAF, editors. Tropical and geographic medicine. New York: McGraw-Hill; 1989. p. 379–93.
87. Albonico M, Stoltzfus RJ, Savioli L, et al. Epidemiological evidence for a differential effect of hookworm species, Ancylostoma duodenale or Necator americanus, on iron status of children. Int J Epidemiol 1998;27:530–7.
88. Gilles HM, Watson-Williams EJ, Ball PA. Hookworm infection and anaemia. Q J Med 1964;33:1–24.
89. Variyam EP, Banwell JG. Nutrition implications of hookworm infection. Rev Infect Dis 1982;4:830–5.
90. Stoltzfus RJ, Albonico M, Chwaya HM, et al. Effects of the Zanzibar school–based deworming program on iron status of children. Am J Clin Nutr 1998;68:179–86.
91. Prutsky G, Domecq JP, Mori L, et al. Treatment outcomes of human bartonellosis: a systematic review and meta-analysis. Int J Infect Dis 2013;17(10):e811–9.

Global Approach to Hematologic Malignancies

Leslie Lehmann, MD[a],*, Alaa El-Haddad, MD[b], Ronald D. Barr, MB ChB, MD[c]

KEYWORDS

- Global • Low- and middle-income countries (LMIC) • Hematologic malignancies
- Leukemia • Lymphoma • Pediatric

KEY POINTS

- Pediatric hematologic malignancies are challenging to treat in low- and middle-resource settings owing to the complex, multidisciplinary, and longitudinal care required.
- Although outcomes are generally inferior to those reported by high-income countries, progress has been achieved particularly for acute lymphoblastic leukemia, Hodgkin lymphoma, and Burkitt lymphoma (BL).
- Capacity building to improve care includes pathology expertise, advances in supportive care and family support systems, and accessibility of palliative care.
- Developing an infrastructures that allows for collection of reliable data and supports clinical research is an essential component of strategies to improve outcomes for children globally.

GLOBAL APPROACH TO PEDIATRIC HEMATOLOGIC MALIGNANCIES

The treatment of childhood cancer requires complex, longitudinal, multidisciplinary care delivered by a dedicated team of providers in addition to reliable infrastructural support. There is marked variability in the intensity and duration of therapy as well as in the multidisciplinary expertise needed for the treatment of solid tumors in comparison with hematologic malignancies and also within different types of hematologic malignancies. As a result, creating a structure that can provide effective and safe therapy for this group of childhood diseases in resource-poor settings remains challenging. Therapy, ideally, would be tailored to the region, country, and specific medical center to ensure optimal matching of therapy intensity and resources. As an example, Hunger and colleagues[1] suggested a tiered hierarchy with treatments of increasing intensity for acute lymphoblastic leukemia (ALL); a program would move

[a] Pediatric Stem Cell Transplant, Dana-Farber Cancer Institute, Harvard Medical School, 450 Brookline Avenue, Boston, MA 02115, USA; [b] Department of Pediatric Oncology, 1 Fostat Street, Sayda Zainab, Cairo 11757, Egypt; [c] Department of Pediatric Oncology, McMaster University, 1200 Main Street West, Hamilton, Ontario L8S 4J9, Canada
* Corresponding author.
E-mail address: Leslie_Lehmann@DFCI.Harvard.edu

Hematol Oncol Clin N Am 30 (2016) 417–432
http://dx.doi.org/10.1016/j.hoc.2015.11.008
0889-8588/16/$ – see front matter © 2016 Elsevier Inc. All rights reserved.

hemonc.theclinics.com

to the next higher level of therapy once treatment-related mortality had been demonstrated to be acceptable at the current level. Another approach was taken in Asia, where a national summit meeting in 2013 was convened to generated guidelines for care delivery in both pediatric and adult ALL.[2] Recommendations concerning diagnosis, risk stratification, and supportive care measures were made and a model was proposed that intensified therapy based on both disease factors and the resource level of the treating facility. Guidelines for essential supportive care provisions have been generated by the International Society of Pediatric Oncology[3] and recommend hand washing hygiene, nutritional assessment and support, access to pain medications and antiemetics, as well as suggested therapy for febrile neutropenia.

Palliative care should be a component of all programs offering treatment to children with cancer and ideally programs would use a multifaceted approach of government-supported policy, education, and accessibility to pain medications and have a focus on home-based care.[4] Unfortunately, of the 192 member countries of the United Nations, almost two-thirds have no reported programs in pediatric palliative care[5]; in Africa, analysis of peer-reviewed and non–peer-reviewed literature found that fewer than 20% of 53 countries had any resources for pediatric palliative care identified.[5] It is crucial that initiatives in this arena are developed in parallel with advances in the scope and intensity of available oncologic therapies. There are sparse data on either the cost or cost effectiveness of treating childhood hematologic malignancies. In China it was estimated that it cost 11,000 USD per child treated for ALL.[6] The cost per patient treated was estimated to be 17,000 USD for ALL in Brazil and 50 USD for BL treated in Malawi; both met criteria for cost effectiveness according to the standard World Health Organization (WHO) definition of ratio of cost to disability-adjusted life-years prevented.[7] It would be enormously helpful to have similar data across the spectrum of low- and middle-income countries (LMICs).

Undertaking quality research is an essential exercise, not a luxury, in LMICs, in which resources by definition are limited. Understandably, priorities are in the areas of health services and outcomes,[8] with "scaling up" of research a necessary goal.[9] Particular challenges in conducting research in LMICs have been described.[10]

The importance of good data acquisition and management cannot be overemphasized; with proper training and a well-defined career trajectory as a priority.[11] Such investment has borne sound return, as exemplified by an audit of data quality in Honduras.[12] More recently, building on this foundation, regional pediatric cancer registries have been in operation in Central America since 2013.[9] It will be impossible to design appropriate treatment strategies for children from LMICs without robust data reporting on outcomes and toxicities.

THE ROLE OF ESSENTIAL MEDICINES

The high cost of drugs overall, and the marked disparities among LMICs and even within individual countries, is an enormous barrier to care.[13] Bulk purchasing provides some relief and it is worthy of note that the Pan-American Health Organization Strategic Fund includes important drugs for noncommunicable diseases, including cancers in children.[14] It has been estimated that the annual cost of all medicines for the treatment of incident cases of ALL in children in LMICs is less than US$150 million.[13] Arguably the biggest challenge to improving the care of children with cancer in LMICs is access to affordable, safe, and effective chemotherapy. At the World

Health Assembly in 2014, Resolution 67.22 requested that the WHO "support members states in sharing best practices in the selection of essential medicines and in developing processes for the selection of medicines for national essential medicines lists."[15] The WHO had established a Model List of Essential Medicines in 1977 and created a separate list (EMLc) for children in 2007. These lists are reviewed by an Expert Committee every 2 years and are used by national governments to guide drug procurement.[16]

In 2011, using a disease-based approach, the Expert Committee endorsed the inclusion in the List of Essential Medicines for children for the treatment of ALL, BL, and Wilms tumor; these diseases were selected as priorities based on incidence and curability.[17] This prompted the International Society of Pediatric Oncology's Working Group on Essential Medicines to propose a more comprehensive list of drugs[18] that served as a basis for recommendations to the Expert Committee for additions to the original list. The committee accepted all of these and 6 more cytotoxic agents were added in May 2015 to the List of Essential Medicines for children for the treatment of 6 more diseases, including Hodgkin lymphoma (**Table 1**). Further additions will be limited to steps 1 and 2 of the 5-level step ladder approach to the selection of essential medicines; that is, those used in common regimens for all children with a given disease and those used additionally for high-risk patients.[19] Decision makers continue to wrestle with the balance between magnitude of clinical benefit and cost effectiveness. Aiming to provide policymakers with evidence for deciding on interventions and programs that maximize health for the available resources, WHO has developed the WHO-CHOICE tool (*CHO*osing *I*nterventions that are *C*ost-*E*ffective).[20]

BUILDING CAPACITY

The vehicle most commonly associated with capacity building is twinning: establishing a sustainable program of cooperation between 1 or more institutions in an LMIC and partners in a high income country. The first example seems to have been an association that began almost 30 years ago between the Pediatric Clinic of the University of Milano-Bicocca in Monza, Italy, and Manuel de Jesus, 'La Mascota,' Hospital in Managua, Nicaragua. This experience led to the establishment at the Monza International School of Pediatric Hematology Oncology[21] that in turn spawned multiple twinning programs between children's hospitals in Italy and partner institutions in Central and South America. These endeavors contributed to the formation of regional groups that have sustained and expanded the building of capacity, namely, Asociación de Hemato-Oncología Pediátrica de Centro América in Central America[11] and GALOP (Latin American Pediatric Oncology Group) in South America,[9] the latter having a strong association with the US-based Children's Oncology Group. The sharing of resources within institutions in LMICs represents a different version of twinning, as in the use of flow cytometry serving several countries in Central America.[22] Recent initiatives have also developed North–South links and oncology facilities in Africa, for example, in Rwanda (**Fig. 1**). These developments are not only cost effective, but provide a basis and stimulus for mutual advancement and shared research opportunities.

Fundamental to the success of twinning is a strong focus on education. This was the primary purpose of Monza International School of Pediatric Hematology Oncology and is the basis of programs in Singapore,[9] Marrakesh,[23] and Guatemala City,[11] among others. Initially, such programs were limited to physicians, but important and measurable educational advances have also taken place for nurses,[24] clinical pharmacists,[25] and data managers.[11]

Table 1
Proposed list of cancers in children with nominated essential medicines for the EMLc, 2015

Disease	Medicine
Acute lymphoblastic leukemia	Asparaginase Cyclophosphamide Cytarabine Daunorubicin Dexamethasone Doxorubicin Etoposide Hydrocortisone Mercaptopurine Methotrexate Methylprednisolone Prednisolone Thioguanine Vincristine
Wilms tumor	Dactinomycin Doxorubicin Vincristine
Burkitt lymphoma	Cyclophosphamide Cytarabine Doxorubicin Etoposide Prednisolone Vincristine
Adjuvant medicines	Allopurinol Mesna
Ewing sarcoma	Cyclophosphamide Doxorubicin Etoposide Ifosfamide and mesna Vincristine
Hodgkin lymphoma	Cyclophosphamide Dacarbazine Doxorubicin Etoposide Prednisolone Vincristine

Abbreviation: EMLc, List of Essential Medicines for children.

Acute Lymphoblastic Leukemia

Incidence

ALL is the most common hematologic malignancy of childhood. The majority of incidence data are generated by high-income countries (HICs); in the United States, there are approximately 42 cases of ALL per 1 million children.[26] However, less than 15% of the population in Africa and Southeast Asia is captured by established cancer registries[27] and it is thus very difficult to know if these numbers are accurate on a global scale. Historically, the incidence has seemed to be lower in less-developed countries with a mean annual incidence of 16.5 cases per million population.[28] However, the incidence does seem to be steadily increasing at a greater rate than in HICs, likely owing to a combination of improved awareness, better reporting, and decreases in other contributors to childhood mortality.[26]

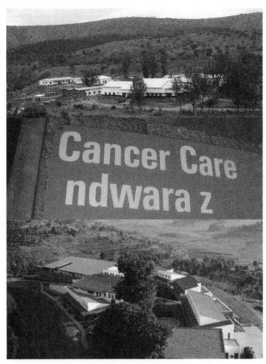

Fig. 1. Recent district general hospitals built in Rwinkwavu (*top*) and Butaro (*bottom*) in Rwanda with support from the Jeff Gordon Children's Foundation and Partners in Health incorporating up to date medical, pediatric and oncology facilities and a Cancer Centre of Excellence. (*Courtesy of* L. Lehmann, MD, Dana Farber Cancer Institute, Partners in Health, Boston, MA.)

Treatment and outcomes

ALL can be cured in almost 90% of children in HICs using multiagent systemic and intrathecal chemotherapy for a total duration of therapy of 2 to 3 years. Induction, the first phase of treatment, consists of more intensive therapy and patients often require prolonged hospitalization and systemic antimicrobials. Repeat examination of the marrow occurs at the end of induction to assess for early response and provide intensification of therapy in patients not in remission. High-risk patients receive a second induction course and a minority of children, primarily those with central nervous system involvement, will require cranial radiation therapy. Maintenance therapy is of much less intensity and occurs primarily in the outpatient setting. However, the care remains complex. Maintenance involves a rotating combination of oral, intravenous, and possibly intramuscular drugs, of which some are administered daily, some weekly, and some monthly. Repetitive visits to the cancer center are required.

Approaches to treatment and outcome have been quite variable in the LMIC setting; in general, as the intensity of therapy increases the number of relapses has decreased, but treatment-related mortality has increased. Thus, attempts have been made to match therapy intensity to the level of supportive care available,[1] as well as to use risk stratification to deliver the most intense therapy to the patients with the worst prognosis based on presenting features and early response to therapy. All approaches have used an induction phase and a maintenance phase with intermittent intrathecal chemotherapy administration.

Given that there are still reported differences in outcomes related to disparities in socioeconomic status in HICs,[29] the challenges of improving outcomes in the LMICs is enormous. There is, unsurprisingly, a wide range reported for disease-free survival (DFS), from as low as 15% to greater than 60%, depending on the patient population and resources available.[28,30–33] Standard factors used for risk stratification—namely, age, initial white blood count, and prednisone response—have been assumed to apply globally, although a large study from India found that age had no impact on outcome and that risk factors were center specific even with the use of one standardized protocol within 1 country.[34,35] There are many potential factors contributing to inferior survival with some more amenable to intervention than others:

1. Innate biological differences: TEL-AML1 is the most common acquired genetic abnormality in pediatric B precursor ALL, occurring in 20% to 30% of patients in the United States. Patients harboring this transcript are known to have an improved DFS. Although the impact on prognosis seems to be immutable, the proportion of TEL-AML1–positive patients may vary by region and occur less frequently in some areas of the world, such as south Asia.[35,36] Similarly, a higher percentage of patients are reported to have T-cell versus precursor B ALL in Egypt and rural India.[35] This biologic variability results in an increased incidence of high-risk features in some populations and thus would contribute to poorer outcomes for the group as a whole.

2. Delay in diagnosis: Delay between development of symptoms and initiation of therapy can impact survival from solid tumors at risk for metastasis. This may not be as problematic in hematologic malignancies, which are systemic at the time of presentation. In addition ALL may be recognized and therapy sought more quickly than in other childhood malignancies such as Hodgkin lymphoma (HL), even in resource-poor settings.[37] A separate issue is that some children with ALL may receive pretreatment with steroids for symptoms thought to reflect other diagnoses, such as arthritis, idiopathic thrombocytopenic purpura, or simply failure to thrive. Monotherapy with prednisone could negatively impact DFS owing the development of steroid-resistant clones before the initiation of ALL-directed therapy.

3. Undernutrition is prevalent among children in LMICs, and especially so in children with cancer at diagnosis. In a large sample in Central America approximately two-thirds of such children were classified as severely malnourished and had a notably lower survival than those who were not so deprived nutritionally.[38] However. It was demonstrated subsequently, in a cohort with ALL in Guatemala, that restoration of normal nutritional status within 6 months of the initiation of treatment was associated with a survival rate similar to that in children who had maintained a normal nutritional status throughout.[39]

4. Inadequate supportive care measures: In the United States, treatment-related mortality is less than 5% in children with ALL. This number is significantly higher in resource-poor settings and can account for up to one-fourth of deaths.[34,40] The main causes of mortality are infection and bleeding. Provision of better antibiotic therapy and more rapid access to transfusion support are thus needed. However, improved education of providers, written supportive care guidelines, and the identification and treatment of malnutrition and concurrent infection may also decrease the proportion of deaths owing to treatment-related complications.[41]

5. Delays in therapy: There are many reasons for delays in therapy, including missed appointments, patient-specific medical complications (fever, prolonged neutropenia), and drug unavailability. One study of ALL in Colombia found that delays

between starting induction and beginning maintenance therapy (a 24-week period according to protocol), regardless of whether owing to medical issues or other reasons, was associated with a significantly inferior DFS.[42]

6. Abandonment: There have been many attempts to address the intertwined issues of refusal (refusing treatment), noncompliance (lack of cooperation with recommended therapy), and abandonment (termination of therapy prematurely).[43] Key components of successful intervention strategies include family education about therapy duration, side effects, and the potential curability of cancer[44,45] in addition to increased social support systems including housing, transportation, and stipends to cover loss of income.[44]

Core resources required to treat acute lymphoblastic leukemia in low- and middle-income countries

- Adequate pathology capacity that allows for rapid diagnosis, as well as determination of immunophenotype (B- vs T-cell disease) and other features necessary for risk stratification at diagnosis and at the end of induction therapy.
- Access to a safe and reliable supply of red cells and platelets for transfusional support, particularly during induction.
- Ability to adequately diagnose and treat bacterial, fungal, and viral infections during periods of prolonged neutropenia.
- Adequate family supports (transportation, outpatient housing near the hospital, community health worker involvement) so that maintenance chemotherapy can be administered consistently.

Future directions

Changes in care delivery Safety initiatives: The delivery of oncologic care is a complex, high-risk, multidisciplinary endeavor. In LMICs, there are often no systems in place to support this type of care delivery. Standardization of protocols and supportive care interventions can help prevent errors across centers and providers. A safety checklist has been shown to decrease surgical morbidity and mortality in a diverse group of hospitals around the world.[46] A similar approach could be particularly effective in the oncology setting where teamwork is similarly critical to improving outcomes.

Risk stratification: Much of the progress in ALL in HICs has been the result of adjusting the intensity of therapy based on prognostic factors determined at the time of presentation (age, initial white cell blood count, for example) or based on response to induction therapy. Ideally, patients determined to be at the lowest risk of treatment failure could receive therapy that is not only less intense, but also of shorter duration given the hardships of protracted frequent care in LMICs. However, a recent Japanese study showed that shortening the duration of maintenance therapy from 2 years to 6 months decreased DFS in standard risk ALL patients despite the addition of early intensification[47] and thus any truncation of therapy would need to be studied carefully before being implemented. To successfully treat patients who are designated as high risk, a broader array of chemotherapeutic agents, radiation therapy, and more advanced supportive care needs to be available than currently exists in the majority of LMICs.

Minimal residual disease assessment: Failure to attain morphologic remission (<5% lymphoblasts in the marrow) is known to confer a poor prognosis but the presence of even minimal residual disease has been shown to be important as well. One interesting approach that may be applicable to middle income countries is the use of a simplified flow cytometry technique using a 4 marker assay for minimal residual disease detection.[48] This would allow a broader definition of poor initial response and allow for appropriate upstaging of therapy.

Improved parent/child support systems Parental and patient education regarding the importance of consistent delivery of outpatient medication and excellent compliance with medical visits will be crucial to improving outcomes in ALL. Advances in this area are challenging to operationalize and it is difficult to identify which interventions have a positive impact, given the many variables affecting DFS. A study in Indonesia where mothers of children with ALL were assigned randomly to receive a journal in which future appointments and medication times were outlined resulted in improved compliance in families from higher socioeconomic strata, but had no effect on outcome in the poorest families.[49] Use of an educational video in Indonesia, however, decreased treatment refusal and increased DFS in the poorest families, highlighting the necessity of tailored approaches depending on the target audience.[50]

Acute Myelogenous Leukemia

Incidence
Acute myelogenous leukemia (AML) accounts for approximately 15% of acute pediatric leukemia in HICs. In comparison with ALL, there seems to be no difference in the incidence between HICs and LMICs.[26]

Treatment and outcomes
There is much less published data on treating AML versus ALL in LMICs. Compared with ALL, therapy is of much shorter duration but of correspondingly greater intensity. The overall duration of therapy is 4 to 6 months, and the majority of that time is spent in the hospital receiving systemic and intrathecal chemotherapy and intensive blood product and antimicrobial support and use of granulocyte colony-stimulating factor is routine. Radiation therapy is not used routinely. Reports are scarce from LMIC settings, although it seems that between 0% and 40% of children are long-term survivors.[33,51–53] Treatment related deaths are reported to occur in more than 20% of patients, reflecting the problems encountered in HICs before the routine use of antimicrobial and antifungal prophylaxis.[54,55] Predicting those at greatest risk of treatment-related mortality remains problematic, although it is assumed that comorbidities such as malnutrition are important and this remains an area requiring more investigation.[56] Bone marrow transplantation is the therapy of choice for refractory or recurrent AML in HICs; in the resource-limited setting, treatment may be best directed toward palliation. Children with late relapses (>18 months from diagnosis) are a possible exception because they can experience a prolonged period of remission with salvage chemotherapy; cure, however, remains very unlikely.[57]

Core resources required to treat acute myelogenous leukemia in low- and middle-income countries

- Adequate pathology capacity that allows for rapid diagnosis, as well as identification of other features (FLT3 positivity, monosomy 7) necessary for risk stratification at diagnosis and at the end of induction therapy.
- Ability to manage leukostasis, bleeding, and tumor lysis syndrome that can occur at presentation and during induction therapy.
- Access to a safe and reliable supply of red cells and platelets for transfusional support.
- Availability of growth factors as well as broad spectrum antimicrobials for prophylaxis and treatment of infection with Gram-positive organisms and fungus.

Chronic Myelogenous Leukemia

The incidence of chronic myelogenous leukemia (CML) is relatively rare in children, accounting for less than 5% of pediatric leukemias. For the vast majority of patients who present in chronic phase, daily and likely life-long therapy with the oral tyrosine kinase inhibitor (TKI) imatinib (Gleevac) can provide normalization of blood counts and very good quality of life with tolerable side effects, although younger patients seem to experience both more medical and emotional consequences of therapy.[58] This treatment is expensive, however, with a 1-year supply costing almost 100,000 USD.[59] In many resource-restricted countries, imatinib is provided free of charge through the Glivac International Patient Assistance Program. Access to medication requires only physician oversight and confirmation of the diagnosis of CML; the latter is most commonly accomplished through molecular testing for the presence of the bcr-abl protein product arising from translocation between chromosomes 9 and 11. Testing can be done relatively easily, even in low-resource settings, using an automated technology initially developed to test for multidrug-resistant tuberculosis and yields results comparable with the polymerase chain reaction testing done in HICs.[60] There are minimal data on outcomes using imatinib in LMICs. The most extensive experience is in 3188 pediatric patients with CML treated through the Glivac International Patient Assistance Program. Outcomes are comparable with those reported in the United States with a 3-year overall survival of almost 90%. Increased time between diagnosis and commencement of imatinib therapy was associated with an increased risk of death.[61] However, the frequency of acquisition of mutations leading to imatinib resistance is not known and this is of particular concern in children who will require decades of therapy. The biggest challenge—regardless of resource level—is ensuring continued compliance with a daily medication in patients often having no obvious signs of illness. A recent study in the United States identified medication noncompliance as the most important contributor to imatinib failure.[62] Use of a community health worker model as first described with antiretroviral therapy may be a useful approach to this pervasive issue. If drug resistance does develop, few LMICs have access to second- and third-generation TKI or stem cell transplantation for salvage therapy.

Future directions

Standard therapy for CML treated with TKIs involves routine assessment of quantitative levels of bcr-abl from the peripheral blood throughout the course of treatment. Patients who have evidence of early disease progression are switched to another TKI. Currently, few countries have the infrastructure to monitor patients consistently in this fashion and even fewer have access to the expensive subsequent generation TKIs.

Hodgkin Lymphoma

Incidence

HL seems to occur more commonly in LMICs perhaps owing to the high incidence of Epstein–Barr virus (EBV) infection in the population. Latent EBV can be found in Reed–Sternberg cells, the malignant cell type in HL, in 50% of patients in LMICs, although it does not seem to impact on prognosis.[63,64] HL also occurs at a younger age in this setting with a peak incidence of 5 to 9 years, which also may be related to the role of EBV infection in this disease.[63,65]

Treatment and outcome

Accurate staging is critical because it directs both the components and duration of therapy. Evaluation of chest, neck, abdomen and pelvis with computed tomography is the minimum assessment needed. It remains difficult to distinguish normal from pathologic nodes without functional imaging such as F-labeled 2-deoxyglucose PET. This imaging modality is rarely available in resource-poor settings and as a result patients are at risk for being assigned a stage that is either higher or lower than that reflected by the actual burden of disease. Most children present with stage III or IV disease in LMICs.[65,66] Treatment has been adapted from HICs and most often involves 4 to 6 cycles of combined chemotherapy that can usually be administered in the outpatient setting. Most approaches include radiation therapy to sites of previous disease. Radiation almost always occurs at a different facility and often in a different city or country. Difficulties in coordination of care across settings is always a challenge and can negatively impact outcome as a result of many factors, including treatment delays, loss of disease control, and abandonment of therapy.[66] However, in general, HL is a very treatable malignancy and using a variety of standard published approaches reported DFS is between 60% and 90%, in many settings approaching that reported in HICs.[65–68]

Non-Hodgkin Lymphoma

The non-Hodgkin lymphomas include lymphoblastic lymphoma, BL, and large cell lymphoma.

Incidence

Lymphoblastic lymphoma can be of either a pre-B or T-cell phenotype and is treated identically to ALL.

BL is the most common subtype of pediatric non-Hodgkin lymphoma and is particularly prevalent in sub-Saharan Africa, where it accounts for almost 50% of all childhood cancers.[35] This is thought to be related to endemic EBV infection because more than 90% of cases contain the ebv genome in tumor tissue. Malaria transmission may be an additional factor. T-cell control of EBV is impaired during attacks of malaria[69] and Plasmodium falciparum may also interact directly with B-cell receptors stimulating proliferation of EBV-infected lymphocytes.[70] The incidence varies by region but can be as high as 22 per 100,000 children and account for up to 70% of all new childhood cancers in parts of Tanzania.[71] It does not seem that human immunodeficiency virus has made an impact on the incidence of the disease, although patients with BL coinfected with human immunodeficiency virus seem to have a worse survival.[72] In the African setting, the disease presents most often as a jaw mass, although a recent report suggests that obtaining abdominal ultrasound in addition to a physical examination improves staging accuracy and the incidence of abdominal involvement then becomes similar to that in HIC.[57] The incidence of B-cell large cell lymphoma is not described in LMICs and can be difficult to distinguish clinically and pathologically from BL; these patients can be treated effectively on BL protocols.

Treatment and outcomes

In HICs, B-cell lymphomas can be cured in 90% of children but therapy is very myelosuppressive and requires a prolonged hospital stay and availability of a broad range of antimicrobial agents. Historically, oral cytoxan (cyclophosphamide) alone has been reported to cure a small number of cases of BL and low-dose combination chemotherapy regimens up to one-third of children. Currently in LMICs, risk stratification has improved survival to greater than 50%. The least intense approach for those with low risk disease, as assessed by stage and clinical response to initial therapy, consists only of cytoxan and intrathecal (IT) therapy. Intravenous methotrexate is added for higher risk patients and total duration of therapy is less than 3 months for all groups.[73] Unfortunately, the time to diagnosis is often delayed in resource-poor settings, particularly when children present with findings such as cervical adenopathy, which usually reflects a benign self-limited process.[70] Thus, the vast majority present with nonlocalized disease[74,75] and require the more aggressive regimen. A consortium of 8 African countries have adopted modified protocols used in HIC by lowering the dosages of drugs most associated with profound myelosuppression. This resulted in an overall survival of 84%, including a 76% overall survival for stage II patients. Of import, treatment-related mortality decreased by 50% (from 26% to 12%) over the 3-year study period, likely related to quality improvement initiatives including regular meetings and review of adverse events.[74] Relapsed/resistant disease remains problematic, although in a small series of patients, retreatment with cytoxan and IT therapy and the addition of vincristine provided disease control in more than one-third of those treated. Patients whose relapse occurred after more than 6 months off therapy and who presented with limited disease were most likely to respond.[76]

Core resources required to treat B-cell lymphoma in low- and middle income countries

Management of tumor lysis syndrome: Tumor lysis syndrome is a frequent problem in patients with advanced stage BL and can lead to severe electrolyte abnormalities, renal failure, and death. Frequent clinical and laboratory monitoring is essential but difficult to ensure in the setting of limited staffing. The use of allopurinol, intravenous hydration, and involvement of caretakers in monitoring urine output has been suggested as a feasible approach to the management of this complication.[73]

Future directions

Improvements in supportive care are key to better survival. Currently almost one-third of those on protocols of moderate intensity succumb to treatment related complications.[75] As in AML, broad spectrum antibiotics and antifungal drugs must be available in addition to growth factor support.

Rituximab, a monoclonal antibody directed against the CD20 antigen found on mature B cells, has been incorporated into many B-cell lymphoma regimens in HICs. It has been shown repeatedly to improve survival in adults but definitive evidence assessing its role in pediatric B-cell lymphomas is lacking.[77] It is expensive and requires close monitoring during administration but may allow for incremental improvement in DFS when combined with the less intense regimens often used in LMICs for these diseases.

REFERENCES

1. Hunger SP, Sung L, Howard SC. Treatment strategies and regimens of graduated intensity for childhood acute lymphoblastic leukemia in low-income countries: a proposal. Pediatr Blood Cancer 2009;52(5):559–65.
2. Yeoh AE, Tan D, Li CK, et al. Management of adult and paediatric acute lymphoblastic leukaemia in Asia: resource-stratified guidelines from the Asian Oncology Summit 2013. Lancet Oncol 2013;14(12):508–23.
3. Israels T, Ribeiro RC, Molyneux EM. Strategies to improve care for children with cancer in Sub-Saharan Africa. Eur J Cancer 2010;46(11):1960–6.
4. Ddungu H. Palliative care: what approaches are suitable in developing countries? Br J Haematol 2011;154:728–36.

5. Knapp C, Woodworth L, Wright M, et al. Pediatric palliative care provision around the world: a systematic review. Pediatr Blood Cancer 2011;57(3):361–8.

6. Liu Y, Chen J, Tang J, et al. Cost of childhood acute lymphoblastic leukemia care in Shanghai, China. Pediatr Blood Cancer 2009;53(4):557–62.

7. Bhakta N, Martiniuk AL, Gupta S, et al. The cost effectiveness of treating paediatric cancer in low-income and middle-income countries: a case-study approach using acute lymphocytic leukaemia in Brazil and Burkitt lymphoma in Malawi. Arch Dis Child 2013;98(2):155–60.

8. Mostert SS, Sitaresmi MN, Gundy CM, et al. Attitude of health-care providers toward childhood leukemia patients with different socio-economic status. Pediatr Blood Cancer 2008;50(5):1001–5.

9. Rodriguez-Galindo C, Friedrich P, Alcasabas P, et al. Towards the cure of all children with cancer through collaborative efforts: pediatric oncology as a global challenge. J Clin Oncol 2015;33(27):3065–73.

10. Denburg AE, Joffe S, Gupta S, et al. Pediatric oncology research in low income countries: ethical concepts and challenges. Pediatr Blood Cancer 2012;58(4):492–7.

11. Barr RD, Antillón Klussmann F, Baez F, et al. Asociación de Hemato-Oncología Pediátrica de Centro América (AHOPCA): a model for sustainable development in pediatric oncology. Pediatr Blood Cancer 2014;61(2):345–54.

12. Ayoub L, Fú L, Peña A, et al. Implementation of a data management program in a pediatric cancer unit in a low income country. Pediatr Blood Cancer 2007;49(1):23–7.

13. Denburg AE, Knaul FM, Atun R, et al. Beyond the bench and the bedside: economic and health systems dimensions of global childhood cancer outcomes. Pediatr Blood Cancer 2014;61(3):572–6.

14. Pan-American Health Organization (PAHO). Pan-American Health Organization (PAHO) HHS strategic fund. 2014. Available at: http://www.paho.org/hq/index.php?option=com_content&view=category&layout=blog&id=1159&Itemid=588. Accessed May 25, 2015.

15. World Health Organization (WHO), W.H.O. Access to essential medicines. World health assembly 2014. Available at: http://apps.who.int/medicinedocs/documents/s21453en/s21453en.pdf. Accessed May 24, 2015.

16. Van den Hamm RB, Lisa B, Laing R. The world medicines situation 2011; selection of essential medicines. 2011. Available at: http://apps.who.int/medicinedocs/documents/s18770en/s18770en.pdf. Accessed May 24, 2015.

17. Robertson J, Magrini N, Barr R, et al. Medicines for cancers in children: the WHO model for selection of essential medicines. Pediatr Blood Cancer 2015;62:1–5.

18. Mehta PS, Wiernikowski JT, Petrilli JA, et al, Working Group on Essential Medicines of the Pediatric Oncology in Developing Countries committee of SIOP. Essential medicines for pediatric oncology in developing countries. Pediatr Blood Cancer 2013;60(5):889–91.

19. World Health Organization (WHO), W.H.O. 18th expert committee on the selection and use of essential medicines: review of medicines for the treatment of common tumours in children. 18th expert committee on the selection and use of essential medicines. 2011. Available at: http://www.who.int/selection_medicines/committees/expert/18/applications/Binder1.pdf. Accessed May 24, 2015.

20. World Health Organization (WHO), W.H.O. Cost effectiveness and strategic planning (WHO-CHOICE). Available at: http://www.who.int/choice/cost-effectiveness/en/. Accessed May 24, 2015.

21. Sala A, Barr RD, Masera G, MISPHO Consortium. A survey of resources and activities in the MISPHO families of institutions in Latin America: a comparison of two eras. Pediatr Blood Cancer 2004;43(7):758–64.
22. Howard SC, Campana D, Coustan-Smith E, et al. Development of a regional flow cytometry center for diagnosis of childhood leukemia in Central America. Leukemia 2005;19(3):323–5.
23. Harif M, Traoré F, Hessissen L, et al. Challenges for paediatric oncology in Africa. Lancet Oncol 2013;14(4):279–81.
24. Day SW, McKeon LM, Garcia J, et al. Use of Joint Commission international standards to evaluate and improve pediatric oncology nursing in Guatemala. Pediatr Blood Cancer 2013;60(5):810–5.
25. International Society of Oncology Pharmacy Practitioners Standards Committee. ISOPP standards of practice for oncology pharmacy. J Oncol Pharm Pract 2007; 13:1–81.
26. Demanelis K, Sriplung H, Meza R, et al. Differences in childhood leukemia incidence and survival between Southern Thailand and the United States: a population-based analysis. Pediatr Blood Cancer 2015;62(10):1790–8.
27. Valsecchi MG, Steliarova-Foucher E. Cancer registration in developing countries: luxury or necessity? Lancet Oncol 2008;9(2):159–67.
28. Supriyadi E, Widjajanto PH, Purwanto I, et al. Incidence of childhood Leukemia in Yogyakarta, Indonesia, 1998-2009. Pediatr Blood Cancer 2011;57(4):588–93.
29. Petridou ET, Sergentanis TN, Perlepe C, et al. Socioeconomic disparities in survival from childhood leukemia in the United States and globally: a meta-analysis. Ann Oncol 2015;26(3):589–97.
30. Chagaluka G, Carey P, Banda K, et al. Treating childhood acute lymphoblastic leukemia in Malawi. Haematologica 2013;98(1):e1–3.
31. Pacheco C, Lucchini G, Valsecchi MG, et al. Childhood acute lymphoblastic leukemia in Nicaragua: long-term results in the context of an international cooperative program. Pediatr Blood Cancer 2014;61(5):827–32.
32. Yadav SP, Ramzan M, Lall M, et al. Childhood acute lymphoblastic leukemia outcome in India: progress on all fronts. J Pediatr Hematol Oncol 2012; 34(4):324.
33. Kersten E, Scanlan P, Dubois SG, et al. Current treatment and outcome for childhood acute leukemia in Tanzania. Pediatr Blood Cancer 2013;60(12):2047–53.
34. Gunes AM, Oren H, Baytan B, et al. The long-term results of childhood acute lymphoblastic leukemia at two centers from Turkey: 15 years of experience with the ALL-BFM 95 protocol. Ann Hematol 2014;93(10):1677–84.
35. Magrath I, Shanta V, Advani S, et al. Treatment of acute lymphoblastic leukaemia in countries with limited resources; lessons from use of a single protocol in India over a twenty year period [corrected]. Eur J Cancer 2005;41(11):1570–83.
36. Iqbal Z. Molecular genetic studies on 167 pediatric ALL patients from different areas of Pakistan confirm a low frequency of the favorable prognosis fusion oncogene TEL-AML1 (t 12; 21) in underdeveloped countries of the region. Asian Pac J Cancer Prev 2014;15(8):3541–6.
37. Chukwu BF, Ezenwosu OU, Ikefuna AN, et al. Diagnostic delay in pediatric cancer in Enugu, Nigeria: a prospective study. Pediatr Hematol Oncol 2015; 32(2):164–71.
38. Sala A, Rossi E, Antillon F, et al. Nutritional status at diagnosis is related to clinical outcomes in children and adolescents with cancer: a perspective from Central America. Eur J Cancer 2012;48(2):243–52.

39. Antillon FR, Rossi E, Molina AL, et al. Nutritional status of children during treatment for acute lymphoblastic leukemia in Guatemala. Pediatr Blood Cancer 2013;60(6):911–5.
40. Kulkarni KP, Arora RS, Marwaha RK. Survival outcome of childhood acute lymphoblastic leukemia in India: a resource-limited perspective of more than 40 years. J Pediatr Hematol Oncol 2011;33(6):475–9.
41. Howard SC, Pedrosa M, Lins M, et al. Establishment of a pediatric oncology program and outcomes of childhood acute lymphoblastic leukemia in a resource-poor area. JAMA 2004;291(20):2471–5.
42. Suarez A, Piña M, Nichols-Vinueza DX, et al. A strategy to improve treatment-related mortality and abandonment of therapy for childhood ALL in a developing country reveals the impact of treatment delays. Pediatr Blood Cancer 2015;62(8): 1395–402.
43. Spinetta JJ, Masera G, Eden T, et al. Refusal, non-compliance, and abandonment of treatment in children and adolescents with cancer: a report of the SIOP Working Committee on Phychosocial Issues in Pediatric Oncology. Med Pediatr Oncol 2002;38(2):114–7.
44. Israels T, Chirambo C, Caron H, et al. The guardians' perspective on paediatric cancer treatment in Malawi and factors affecting adherence. Pediatr Blood Cancer 2008;51(5):639–42.
45. Wang YR, Jin RM, Xu JW, et al. A report about treatment refusal and abandonment in children with acute lymphoblastic leukemia in China, 1997-2007. Leuk Res 2011;35(12):1628–31.
46. Haynes AB, Weiser TG, Berry WR, et al. A surgical safety checklist to reduce morbidity and mortality in a global population. N Engl J Med 2009;360(5): 491–9.
47. Toyoda Y, Manabe A, Tsuchida M, et al. Six months of maintenance chemotherapy after intensified treatment for acute lymphoblastic leukemia of childhood. J Clin Oncol 2000;18(7):1508–16.
48. Coustan-Smith E, Ribeiro RC, Stow P, et al. A simplified flow cytometric assay identifies children with acute lymphoblastic leukemia who have superior clinical outcome. Blood 2006;108(1):97–102.
49. Sitaresmi MN, Mostert S, Gundy CM, et al. A medication diary-book for pediatric patients with acute lymphoblastic leukemia in Indonesia. Pediatr Blood Cancer 2013;60(10):1593–7.
50. Mostert S, Sitaresmi MN, Gundy CM, et al. Comparing childhood leukaemia treatment before and after the introduction of a parental education programme in Indonesia. Arch Dis Child 2015;95(2):20–5.
51. Chan L, Abdel-Latif ME, Ariffin WA, et al. Treating childhood acute myeloid leukaemia with the AML-BFM-83 protocol: experience in a developing country. Br J Haematol 2004;126(6):799–805.
52. Xu X, Tang YM, Song H, et al. Long-term outcome of childhood acute myeloid leukemia in a developing country: experience from a children's hospital in China. Leuk Lymphoma 2010;51(12):2262–9.
53. Gallegos-Castorena S, Medina-Sanson A, Gonzalez-Ramella O. Improved treatment results in Mexican children with acute myeloid leukemia using a Medical Research Council (MRC)-acute myeloid leukemia 10 modified protocol. Leuk Lymphoma 2009;50(7):1132–7.
54. Gupta S, Bonilla M, Valverde P, et al. Treatment-related mortality in children with acute myeloid leukaemia in Central America: incidence, timing and predictors. Eur J Cancer 2012;48(9):1363–9.

55. Yadav SP, Ramzan M, Lall M, et al. Pediatric acute myeloid leukemia: final frontier for pediatric oncologists in developing world. Pediatr Hematol Oncol 2011;28(8):647–8.
56. Gupta S, Bonilla M, Fuentes SL, et al. Incidence and predictors of treatment-related mortality in paediatric acute leukaemia in El Salvador. Br J Cancer 2009;100(7):1026–31.
57. Marjerrison S, Antillon F, Bonilla M, et al. Outcome of children treated for relapsed acute myeloid leukemia in Central America. Pediatr Blood Cancer 2014;61(7):1222–6.
58. Efficace F, Baccarani M, Breccia M, et al. Health-related quality of life in chronic myeloid leukemia patients receiving long-term therapy with imatinib compared with the general population. Blood 2011;118(17):4554–60.
59. Experts in Chronic Myeloid Leukemia. The price of drugs for chronic myeloid leukemia (CML) is a reflection of the unsustainable prices of cancer drugs: from the perspective of a large group of CML experts. Blood 2013;121(22):4439–42.
60. Lopez-Jorge CE, Gómez-Casares MT, Jiménez-Velasco A, et al. Comparative study of BCR-ABL1 quantification: Xpert assay, a feasible solution to standardization concerns. Ann Hematol 2012;91(8):1245–50.
61. Sadak KT, Fultz K, Mendizabal A, et al. International patterns of childhood chronic myeloid leukemia: comparisons between the United States and resource-restricted nations. Pediatr Blood Cancer 2014;61(10):1774–8.
62. Ganesan P, Sagar TG, Dubashi B, et al. Nonadherence to imatinib adversely affects event free survival in chronic phase chronic myeloid leukemia. Am J Hematol 2011;86(6):1–4.
63. Lee JH, Kim Y, Choi JW, et al. Prevalence and prognostic significance of Epstein-Barr virus infection in classical Hodgkin's lymphoma: a meta-analysis. Arch Med Res 2014;45(5):417–31.
64. Souza EM, Baiocchi OC, Zanichelli MA, et al. Impact of Epstein-Barr virus in the clinical evolution of patients with classical Hodgkin's lymphoma in Brazil. Hematol Oncol 2010;28(3):137–41.
65. Sherief LM, Elsafy UR, Abdelkhalek ER, et al. Hodgkin lymphoma in childhood: clinicopathological features and therapy outcome at 2 centers from a developing country. Medicine (Baltimore) 2015;94(15):e670.
66. Hessissen L, Khtar R, Madani A, et al. Improving the prognosis of pediatric Hodgkin lymphoma in developing countries: a Moroccan Society of Pediatric Hematology and Oncology study. Pediatr Blood Cancer 2013;60(9):1464–9.
67. Alebouyeh M, Moussavi F, Haddad-Deylami H, et al. Successful ambulatory treatment of Hodgkin's disease in Iranian children based on German-Austrian DAL-HD 85-90: single institutional results. Ann Oncol 2005;16(12):1936–40.
68. Büyükpamukçu M, Varan A, Akyüz C, et al. The treatment of childhood Hodgkin lymphoma: improved survival in a developing country. Acta Oncol 2009;48(1):44–51.
69. Whittle HC, Brown J, Marsh K, et al. T-cell control of Epstein-Barr virus-infected B cells is lost during P. falciparum malaria. Nature 1984;312(5993):449–50.
70. Cecen E, Gunes D, Mutafoglu K, et al. The time to diagnosis in childhood lymphomas and other solid tumors. Pediatr Blood Cancer 2011;57(3):392–7.
71. Aka P, Kawira E, Masalu N, et al. Incidence and trends in Burkitt lymphoma in Northern Tanzania from 2000-2009. Pediatr Blood Cancer 2012;59(7):1234–8.
72. Walusansa V, Okuku F, Orem J. Burkitt lymphoma in Uganda, the legacy of Denis Burkitt and an update on the disease status. Br J Haematol 2012;156(6):757–60.
73. Hesseling P, Israels T, Harif M, et al. Practical recommendations for the management of children with endemic Burkitt lymphoma (BL) in a resource limited setting. Pediatr Blood Cancer 2013;60(3):357–62.

74. Harif M, Barsaoui S, Benchekroun S, et al. Treatment of B-cell lymphoma with LMB modified protocols in Africa–report of the French-African Pediatric Oncology Group (GFAOP). Pediatr Blood Cancer 2008;50(6):1138–42.
75. Moleti ML, Al-Hadad SA, Al-Jadiry MF, et al. Treatment of children with B-cell non-Hodgkin lymphoma in a low-income country. Pediatr Blood Cancer 2011;56(4): 560–7.
76. Hesseling PB, Molyneux E, Kamiza S, et al. Rescue chemotherapy for patients with resistant or relapsed endemic Burkitt's lymphoma. Trans R Soc Trop Med Hyg 2008;102(6):602–7.
77. Attias D, Weitzman S. The efficacy of rituximab in high-grade pediatric B-cell lymphoma/leukemia: a review of available evidence. Curr Opin Pediatr 2008; 20(1):17–22.

Hematological Practice in India

Reena Das, MD, DNB*, Jasmina Ahluwalia, MD, Man Updesh Singh Sachdeva, MD

KEYWORDS

- Iron deficiency anemia • Beta thalassemia trait • Hemophilia • Thrombophilia
- Leukemia • Lymphoma

KEY POINTS

- Globally, India contributes significantly to the burden of hematological disorders because of the large population and inadequate resources for diagnosis and management.
- Iron deficiency anemia in children is commonly nutritional, whereas in women, menorrhagia and pregnancy contribute significantly. Thalassemia major (TM) and hemophilias are common genetic disorders with increased morbidity, and preventive strategies are required to contain the disorders.
- Factor v leiden prevalence in inherited thrombophilias ranges between 3% to 20%, and PT G20210A is absent.
- Non hodgkin lymphoma and acute leukemias are common with presentation at 10 years younger median ages for chronic myeloid leukemia, chronic lymphocytic leukemia and multiple myeloma than the west. Limited finances restrict use of standard treatment protocols in the majority.

INTRODUCTION

Hematological practice ranges from availability of advanced diagnostic facilities and treatment to unavailability of basic medical services to rural India. Problems include a huge population (1.21 billion in the 15th national census survey www.census2011.co.in), socioeconomic disparity, minimal coverage of health insurance schemes, and the government's inability to provide universal health coverage. Therefore India contributes significantly to global disease burden for hematological disorders. Lack of national registries contributes to inaccurate epidemiologic data and nonavailability of micromapping of diseases. Health services are offered nationally as a public (Government of India–Ministry of Health and Family Welfare) and private service; however, most patients have to arrange personal finances for diagnosis and treatment.[1]

The authors have nothing to disclose.
Department of Hematology, Postgraduate Institute of Medical Education and Research, Sector 12, Chandigarh 160012, India
* Corresponding author.
E-mail addresses: reenadaspgi@hotmail.com; das.reena@pgimer.edu.in

Nutritional iron deficiency anemia (IDA) is common in pediatric practice, whereas anemia caused by bleeding disorders and anemia of chronic disorders (ACD) are more common in adults. Nationally, the most common genetic disorder is thalassemia major (TM), and other genetic red cell disorders include sickle cell anemia, glucose-6-phosphate dehydrogenase (G6PD) deficiency, and hereditary spherocytosis. Among acquired conditions, autoimmune hemolytic anemia, severe aplastic anemia, and paroxysmal nocturnal hemoglobinuria are encountered.[2]

Coagulation disorders encountered include bleeding and thrombotic disorders. Patients on oral anticoagulants, hepatic dysfunction, or disseminated intravascular coagulation also require close monitoring in coagulation laboratories. Genetic bleeding disorders like hemophilia A (HA) and B (HB) occur in similar frequencies to global figures. Consanguinity is prevalent in few endogamous communities where autosomal recessive disorders like von Willebrand disease (vWD) are more common.[3–5] Complexity of coagulation testing, need for expert laboratory staff, high cost of reagents, and equipment are common difficulties for wider availability of coagulation tests.

The National Cancer Registry Program (NCRP) was launched in 1981 by the Indian Council of Medical Research (ICMR) for obtaining epidemiologic data on hematological malignancies. A 3-year report (2009–2011) of the Population Based Cancer Registry (PBCR) from 25 registries determined non-Hodgkin lymphoma (NHL) to be the most frequent, followed by lymphoid and myeloid leukemias.[6] Difficulties in complete characterization include unavailability of diagnostic and prognostic facilities like flow cytometry, karyotyping, and molecular genetics. Prohibitive cost of therapy leads to inability of treating physicians to use standard recommended protocols, and hence interprotocol comparative merits are difficult to assess.

DISORDERS OF RED CELLS
Nutritional Anemias

India has the largest number of anemic persons worldwide, and common etiologies are nutritional deficiency of iron, folic acid, and vitamin B12 in descending order of frequency.[7] The National Nutritional Anaemia Prophylaxis Programme (NNAPP) was started in 1972 for iron and folic acid supplementation to pregnant women and children. Screening for anemia, iron–folate therapy, and route of administration for prevention and management of anemia was incorporated. The national prevalence of IDA in children younger than 5 years, women 15 to 49 years, and pregnant women are 75%, 51%, and 87%, respectively. Estimates on maternal deaths from anemia/year are 22,000, which contribute to 20% to 40% of maternal deaths and low birth weight. Anemia increases susceptibility to infections, reduced work capacity, and poor concentration. The National Rural Health Mission was launched in 2005 to educate mothers on health and nutrition in villages. Despite continued efforts, anemia continues to be a major problem affecting all population strata (http://www.mohfw.nic.in).

Plausible reasons include adverse effects of iron pills, improper utilization of health service, and personal beliefs. Poor iron (<20 mg/d) and folic acid intake (<70 μg/d), poor bioavailability of iron (3%–4%) in a phytate fiber-rich Indian diet, and chronic blood loss due to malaria and hookworm infestations contribute to continued high prevalence of IDA.[8] Oral iron therapy is useful, as ferrous ascorbate and intravenous colloidal preparations are reserved only after inadequate response to oral preparation.[9]

Thalassemias and Hemoglobinopathies

These constitute a heterogeneous group of autosomal-recessive disorders caused by globin gene defects causing quantitative reduction (thalassemias) or qualitative defects (hemoglobinopathies) in globin chains. Thalassemias are classified based on defective globin chain, as α-thalassemia, β-thalassemia, δ-thalassemia, and. Symptomatic hemoglobinopathies include sickling syndromes like homozygous HbS, HbS/BTT, and rarely HbS/HbD Punjab. Double heterozygosity of HbE with beta thalassemia causes symptomatic thalassemia syndrome in eastern states.[10]

Identification of asymptomatic β-thalassemia traits (BTT) has led to screening of partners and offered prenatal diagnosis to at-risk pregnancies.[11] Hypochromic microcytosis with raised red blood cell count is encountered in BTT and α-thalassemia trait. The diagnostic hallmark of BTT is HbA2 of between 4% and 8%, which remains normal (2.2%–3.5%) in α-thalassemia trait. The national average frequency of BTT is 3.5% (range 0.3%–15%) and greater than 10,000 infants affected with TM are born each year.[12] Estimates of α-thalassemia traits are limited, because DNA-based molecular tests are required. The average frequency ranges from 12.5% in the general population to 78.4% in endogamous tribal population.[13,14] Management of TM includes 3 weekly blood transfusions and iron chelation. Currently, 3 centers are offering bone marrow transplantation (BMT) to TM patients nationally.

Molecular analysis to detect causative mutations for β-thalassemia shows regional differences. There are 64 mutations reported nationally, and the most common 5 traits, namely IVSI-5(G→C), 619 bpdel, IVSI-1(G→T), Codon 41/42(-TCCT), and Codon 8/9(-G) account for 82.5% of alleles. Uncommon mutations like Codon 15(G→A), Codon 30(G→C), Cap+1(A→C), Codon 5(-CT), and Codon 16(-C) account for an additional 11% of mutations.[15–18] Ten centers perform prenatal diagnosis for reducing the burden of TM.

Other Anemias

ACD is encountered because of disorders like tuberculosis, rheumatoid arthritis, and chronic renal failure. ACD causes increased morbidity and can coexist with IDA. Serum ferritin with soluble transferrin receptor (sTfR/log ferritin ratio) levels can distinguish between ACD and IDA; however, few laboratories perform sTfR. Physicians need to distinguish these disorders to decide treatment with iron supplementation or erythropoietin.[19,20] Genetic hemolytic anemias like G6PD deficiency are common and present as neonatal hyperbilirubinemia or sporadic infection-related hemolysis. Hereditary spherocytosis, sideroblastic anemia, and congenital dyserythropoieticanemias are seen uncommonly. Recently, homozygosity mapping revealed a founder SEC23B–Y462C mutation in Indian CDA type II patients.[21] Acquired anemias include aplastic anemia, paroxysmal nocturnal hemoglobinuria, and pure red cell aplasia, but there are no documented epidemiologic studies to indicate that the frequencies are different to the West.

Hereditary Hemochromatosis

Hereditary hemochromatosis, a common genetic disorder in the West, is rare in Indians. Low index of suspicion and a high prevalence of IDA could contribute to late presentation of the disorder. The HFE gene mutation c.845G→A; p.C282Y, which accounts for 90% to 95% of cases in Northern Europeans, is absent in Indians.[22,23] Recently, the authors have found novel mutations in the hemojuvelin gene (HJV; Barjinder Kaur, Reena Das, unpublished 2013), and private mutations have been reported from Pakistan and Bangladesh.[24]

DISORDERS OF HEMOSTASIS AND COAGULATION
Inherited Coagulation Disorders

Hemophilias (HA and HB) are the most common inherited bleeding disorders. The Hemophilia Federation India, a nongovernment organization, was established in 1983 and has 76 chapters and provides data on bleeding disorders. In 2013, there were 16,800 registered HA patients, compared with 3000 in 2003. The registry is incomplete, and most patients are registered from west India.[25] India reported 462 vWD cases and 458 cases with platelet function disorders and rare coagulation factor deficiencies.[26] Among the latter, data from 54 hemophilia treatment centers showed FXIII (30%) to be the most common deficiency, followed by deficiencies of FX (15.6%), FVII (15%), and fibrinogen (12.1%).[4] Automation in coagulation in referral hospitals has made tests standardized and reproducible.

Confirmatory tests for vWD (eg, von Willebrand Factor antigen assay, Ristocetin Cofactor assay, and multimer analysis) are available in specialized laboratories, leading to inaccurate diagnosis of type 2vWD.[27,28] The Indian Society of Hematology and Blood Transfusion and the Christian Medical College, Vellore run an External Quality Assessment Scheme (EQAS) program for hemostasis with more than 100 participants. Prenatal diagnostic facilities for hemophilias are available nationally in five centers.

Qualitative Disorders of Platelets

Platelet function analyzers and aggregometers are not in common use, and therefore the estimates for qualitative disorders of platelets are inaccurate. Bernard Soulier Syndrome and Glanzmann thrombasthenia are uncommonly encountered. Confirmatory flow cytometry has facilitated early diagnosis but is restricted in availability.

Management of Bleeding Disorders

The chronic nature of the bleeding disorders requires comprehensive care involving replacement of deficient coagulation factor, preventing further bleeds, reducing disability, orthopedic support, and rehabilitation programs including psychosocial support to the family. Suboptimal management is reflected by presentation with joint deformities. Currently only 16 of 29 Indian states provide free FVIII and IX replacement to patients during a major bleed (on-demand situations). In other states, patients are dependent on fresh frozen plasma or cryoprecipitate. Financial constraints limit prophylactic replacement therapy. Plasma-derived factor products available are Immunate P and Immunine, whereas, recombinant factors available are Recombinate and Advate. There exists a large gap between the recommended 1 IU/capita usage of FVIII for optimal survival and the available 0.023 IU/capita.[26,29] Bleeds in vWD are managed with 10 to 20 IU/kg of FVIII concentrates or 1 to 2 cryobags/10 kg weight. Supportive therapy includes topical tranexamic acid (30–40 mg/kg/d) for oral mucosal bleeds or epistaxis. Desmopressin is used in mild vWD with minor bleeds and menorrhagia. Females with vWD require hormonal preparations for regulating menstruation and iron supplementation.[30,31] Use of rest, ice, compression, and elevation is beneficial and inexpensive supportive therapy. Need for compliance with hormonal therapy for control of ovulation may be overlooked with disastrous consequences. Indian patients have been managed with lower doses of FVIII replacement (35 IU/kg preoperatively and 10–20 IU/kg postoperatively in major surgery) without undue excess of serious bleeding in the setting of major and minor surgical procedures.[32] Development of inhibitors is less frequent in Indians, possibly due to late initiation of replacement therapy. Inhibitors were seen in 6.07% of 1285 HA patients, with highest frequencies from

South India (20.99%).[33] Activated prothrombin complex concentrates and recombinant FVII are needed, but the high cost becomes a limiting factor. Immune tolerance is rarely attempted.

Thrombotic Disorders

Hospital-based studies on medical patients and postoperative surgical situations are available on the prevalence of deep vein thrombosis (DVT) and pulmonary embolism (PE). The DVT rate in a retrospective study from South India was 17.46 cases per 10,000 admissions, with 64% of cases in nonsurgical settings.[34] A north Indian study found the incidence of DVT as 2.7/1000 person–days of hospital stay in medically ill patients with grade 1 to 2 mobility.[35] Compression ultrasonography and color Doppler imaging are used for the diagnosis of limb DVT. Angiography, MRI and D-dimer assay are available. Risk factors like factor V Leiden (FVL; G1691A) mutation, deficiencies of protein C, S and antithrombin, and antiphospholipid antibodies are encountered. The prevalence of FVL ranges between 3% and 20% in patients with thrombosis at various sites.[36] In contrast to the western population, prothrombin mutation G20210A is absent.[37]

For thromboprophylaxis, unfractionated heparin is popular because of the low cost of therapy. The low molecular weight heparins (LMWH) available in India are dalteparin, enoxaparin, nadroparin, fondaparin, parnaparin, and fondaparinux.[38] Monitoring of LMWH is mostly empirical, because anti-Xa assay is largely unavailable. The oral anticoagulants available are warfarin and acenocoumarol. Close monitoring of dosage is challenging, as point-of-care instruments are sparsely available. Becuse Indians are predominantly vegetarian, high consumption of green leafy vegetables can lead to variation in anticoagulant effect of the drugs, and good patient education and counseling are required. Experience with the newer anticoagulants is limited.

HEMATOLOGIC MALIGNANCIES

Launched by ICMR in 1981, collected national epidemiologic data on hematological malignancies. PBCR from 2009 to 2011 (included 25 centers) found NHL in the top 10 frequent cancers,[6] and Hospital Based Cancer Registries (HBCRs), involving 7 hospitals, showed myeloid and lymphoid leukemia to be among thetop 10 common neoplasms (**Table 1**).[39]

Myeloproliferative Disorders

Chronic myeloid leukemia (CML) accounts for 30% to 60% of adult leukemias, with the median age at diagnosis being 38 to 40 years, which is a decade earlier than the West.[40] Most cases are symptomatic secondary to splenomegaly, compared with Western patients, in whom approximately 40% of cases are detected incidentally. FISH and reverse transcriptase polymerase chain reaction (RT-PCR)-based detection of breakpoint cluster region-abelson (BCR-ABL) transcripts are used for confirmation in major hospitals. The treatment evolution of CML in India resembles the world with use of radiotherapy, busulphan, hydroxyurea, interferon α, cytarabine in the preimatinib era. Early imatinib treatment has resulted in improved survival and quality of life (**Table 2**) through the Glivec International Patient Assistance Program, which provides free Glivec to developing countries. A generic drug is available as a cheaper option and has shown comparable results to Glivec.[41] Data on MPN showed that 89.6% of cases were CML, and 4.7% of cases were polycythemia vera. Three percent of cases were primary myelofibrosis, and 2.6% of cases

Table 1
Relative proportion (%) and rank (R) of non-Hodgkins lymphoma, myeloid and lymphoid leukemias among common cancer listed in seven hospital based registries during period of January 2007 to December 2011

Center	Gender	NHL		Myeloid Leukemia		Lymphoid Leukemia	
		%	R	%	R	%	R
Mumbai (2006–07)	Males	6.1	4	3.9	6	2.9	10
	Females	3.5	6	2.2	a		b
Bengaluru (2007–09)	Males	4.6	7	3.9	9	3.5	a
	Females	1.9	10	2.6	7		b
Chennai (2007–10)	Males	4.2	8	4.5	7	2.9	a
	Females	1.7	a	2.7	7		b
Thiruvananthapuram (2007–10)	Males	5	4	4.9	5	3.8	9
	Females	2.7	10	3.8	6		b
Dibrugarh (2007–11)	Males	2.9	9	1.6	a	0.9	a
	Females	1.4	a	0.8	a		b
Guwahati (2010–11)	Males	1.9	a	0.5	a	0.4	a
	Females	1.3	a	0.5	a		b
Chandigarh (2011)	Males	4.3	7	4.3	8	5.9	5
	Females	2.2	10	2.6	8		b

[a] Rank not within first ten.
[b] Data not mentioned.
From National Cancer Registry Programme. Consolidated report of hospital based cancer registries: 2007-2011. New Delhi (India): ICMR; 2013; with permission.

were essential thrombocythemia.[42] Recently, the MPN-Working Group formulated consensus recommendations for management of patients with BCR-ABL negative MPNs for India.[43] The diagnostic workup and the treatment algorithms for BCR-ABL negative MPNs are shown in **Fig. 1.**

Table 2
Overall and disease-free survival rates of chronic myeloid leukemia patients from 11 centers in India

Sr. No.	Center	OAS	DFS
1.	NIMS, Hyderabad	100% CCR; 94% others	77
2.	TMH, Mumbai	86	NA
3.	SL Raheja Hospital, Mumbai	81	NA
4.	Sterling Ahmedabad, Gujarat	82	NA
5.	IGIMS, Patna	89	NA
6.	Action Cancer Hospital, Delhi	92	NA
7.	Kidwai, Bangalore	86.85	NA
8.	WIA, Chennai	88	65
9.	Ashirwad, Mumbai	87	72
10.	N.S.C. Bose, Kolkata	81.5	75.5
11.	GCRI Ahmedabad, Gujarat	86	NA

Abbreviations: CCR, complete cytogenetic response; DFS, disease-free survival; OAS, overall survival.
From Bansal S, Prabhash K, Parikh P. Chronic myeloid leukemia data from India. Indian J Med Paediatr Oncol 2013;34:154–8; with permission.

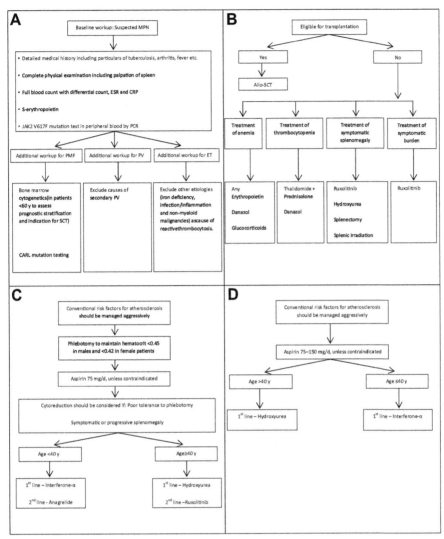

Fig. 1. (*A*) Baseline workup for classical Philadelphia chromosome negative MPNs, and treatment algorithms for (*B*) primary myelofibrosis, (*C*) polycythemia vera, (*D*) and essential thrombocythemia. (*Adapted from* Agarwal MB, Malhotra H, Chakrabarti P, et al. Myeloproliferative neoplasms working group consensus recommendations for diagnosis and management of primary myelofibrosis, polycythemia vera, and essential thrombocythemia. Indian J Med Paediatr Oncol 2015;36(1):3–16; with permission.)

Acute Leukemias

A hospital-based study from north India revealed that 60.5% of acute leukemias were acute lymphoblastic leukemia (ALL); 36.5% were acute myeloid leukemia (AML), and 3% were mixed phenotypic acute leukemia (MPAL).[44] Few tertiary care centers follow NCI risk stratification or perform immunophenotyping or cytogenetics/molecular testing (BCR-ABL, MLL gene rearrangements, and hypodiploidy) to identify high-risk patients and perform minimal residual disease analysis on follow-up. Favorable genotypes like TEL-AML1 and hyperdiploidy are lower, and the frequency of unfavourable genotypes like BCR-ABL1 are higher than the West.[45–47] The outcome of childhood ALL is inferior to developed countries, with survival rates of approximately 70%. The recently formulated Childhood Collaborative Leukemia Group for Multicentre Trial for ALL aims to establish national protocols for diagnostic workup, MRD assessment, and treatment.

AML is more common in adults than ALL. Major oncology centers classify and prognosticate AMLs according to World Health Organization (WHO) 2008 using cytogenetic and molecular tests. However, FAB classification is still practised at many centers. Most physicians require categorization into acute promyelocytic leukemia (APML) and non-promyelocytic leukemia (non-APML) to plan therapy. APML is treated with combinations of ATRA with anthracyclins, and a study showed postinduction complete response in 82% of cases, febrile neutropenia in 64% of cases, and ATRA syndrome in 33% of cases. Fifty-eight percent of cases developed bleeding episodes during induction.[48] Single-agent arsenic trioxide was given to 72 PML-RARA positive patients, in whom long term follow-up showed complete remission (CR) in 86% of cases and overall survival of 74.2%.[49] Management of the non-APML group is comprised of induction with cytosine arabinoside (100–200 mg/m^2) for 7 days and daunorubicin (45–60 mg/m^2) for 3 days. Inadequate finances are the major reasons for incomplete treatment in almost 80% of AMLs.[50]

Multiple Myeloma

The median age of presentation of multiple myeloma (MM) is 55 years, which is 10 years lower than in the United States.[40] Patients present with malaise, backache, anemia, renal failure, soft tissue masses, neurologic symptoms, and recurrent bacterial infections.[51] In large oncology centers, diagnostic work-up includes routine biochemistry, M-band quantification, immunofixation, serum free light chain assay, and FISH. In eligible patients younger than 65 years of age, chemotherapy with autologous BMT is used. Novel agents like bortezomib, thalidomide, and lenalidomide are used in combinations with melphalan, dexamethasone, prednisone, vincristine, adriamycin, and cyclophosphamide. Supportive care includes bisphosphonates, erythropoietin, and prophylactic antibiotics. Prognosis of MM has improved in the last decade, and data on patients with advanced disease who received high-dose melphalan with BMT showed CR in 54%.[52]

Lymphoproliferative Neoplasms

Data on 2773 lymphoma patients showed B-NHL in 79% and T-NHL in 16%. Diffuse large cell lymphoma (DLBCL) was the most common subtype at 34%.[53] A multicentrer study on 1723 lymphoma patients from 13 centers (2005–2009) found 83.16% NHL (DLBCL at 55%) and 16.83% Hodgkin lymphoma (HL).[54] Chronic lymphocytic leukemia (CLL) constitutes 3% of adult leukemia, compared with approximately 30% in the West, with a lower median age than the Surveillance, Epidemiology, and End Results Program (SEER) data. Data on 285 patients showed that 33% presented in clinical Rai stage II, and 22% were asymptomatic.[55,56]

National incidence of NHL is increasing, possibly because of improved diagnosis, changes in classification, and acquired immunodeficiency syndrome-related lymphoma.[57,58] Histopathology and immunohistochemistry are used to subcategorize NHLs. Few centers perform flow cytometry for lymphomas infiltrating bone marrow/leukemic phase and molecular studies for diagnostic evaluation. Fluorodeoxyglucose–positron emission tomography–computed tomography (FDG-PET/PET-CT) scans at baseline and follow-up are used in referral hospitals.

Low-grade asymptomatic NHLs are not treated. Indian patients with DLBCL have lower median age, higher male preponderance, and higher frequency of B symptoms in comparison to Western data. Indian lymphoma registry data on 1733 patients showed cyclophosphamide, hydroxydaunarubicin, oncovin, prednisolone (CHOP) was administered to 84% of DLBCL and rituximab in 42.7%. At a median follow-up of 31 months, 47% of patients had no evidence of disease, and deaths were reported in 14% of cases.[54] Few metropolitan cities offer BMT for therapeutic cure.

Analysis on 262 HL patients with a median age of 30 years showed stage III/IV disease in 70% and B symptoms in 64% of patients. Mixed cellularity (52.3%) was the most common histology, followed by nodular sclerosis (38%). ABVD-based chemotherapy was used in 85% of patients, and 50% of patients received radiotherapy at consolidation, with CR in 92% and OS of 86.6% of patients.[59] Similar data were obtained from another center on 125 patients; that study showed CR in 76% of patients.[60]

SUMMARY

The burden of hematological disorders in India is considerable, being contributed by the huge population and inadequate resources for patient management. Lack of registries contributes to inadequate data for the country. IDA is a common nutritional anemia, and despite efforts by the government, the incidence is not decreasing. TM is a common genetic disorder, for which preventive strategies can reduce the number of births with affected children. Hemophilias also need genetic counseling and prenatal diagnosis to reduce the burden in affected families. Among genetic causes of thrombophilia, FVL frequencies are similar to the European populations, and PT G20210A is absent in Indians. Most leukemias and lymphomas have an earlier age of presentation by a decade. As treatment is not provided by insurance coverage or by the government, most patients are unable to receive appropriate therapy, and many are forced to withdraw therapy, causing increased frequencies of morbidity and mortality compared with the West.

REFERENCES

1. Balarajan Y, Selvaraj S, Subramanian SV. Health care and equity in India. Lancet 2011;377(9764):505–15.
2. Weatherall DJ. The inherited diseases of hemoglobin are an emerging global health burden. Blood 2010;115(22):4331–6.
3. Bittles AH. Endogamy, consanguinity and community genetics. J Genet 2002; 81(3):91–8.
4. Shetty S, Shelar T, Mirgal D, et al. Rare coagulation factor deficiencies: a countrywide screening data from India. Haemophilia 2014;20(4):575–81.
5. Srivastava A, Rodeghiero F. Epidemiology of von Willebrand disease in developing countries. Semin Thromb Hemost 2005;31(5):569–76.
6. National Cancer Registry Programme. Three year report of population based cancer registries 2009–2011. New Delhi (India): Indian Council of Medical Research; 2013.
7. Chellan R, Paul L. Prevalence of iron-deficiency anaemia in India: results from a large nationwide survey. Journal of Population and Social Studies 2010;19:59–80.
8. Galloway R, McGuire J. Determinants of compliance with iron supplementation: supplies, side effects, or psychology? Soc Sci Med 1994;39(3):381–90.

9. Yewale VN, Dewan B. Treatment of iron deficiency anemia in children: a comparative study of ferrous ascorbate and colloidal iron. Indian J Pediatr 2013;80(5): 385–90.

10. Das R. The management of inherited blood diseases in the Indian subcontinent. In: Kumar D, editor. Genomics and health in the developing world; Oxford monographs on medical genetics. United Kingdom: Oxford University Press; 2012. p. 1082–95.

11. WHO Working Group Report. Community control of hereditary anemias. Bull World Health Organ 1982;60:643–60.

12. Weatherall DJ, Clegg JB. Inherited haemoglobin disorders: an increasing global health problem. Bull World Health Organ 2001;79(8):704–12.

13. Nadkarni A, Phanasgaonkar S, Colah R, et al. Prevalence and molecular characterization of alpha-thalassemia syndromes among Indians. Genet Test 2008; 12(2):177–80.

14. Tehran U, Garewal G, Kaul D, et al. Alpha thalassemia and alpha gene triplications in Punjabis, with and without beta thalassemia trait. Hematology 2000;6: 153–60.

15. Garewal G, Das R. Spectrum of beta thalassemia mutations in north India. Int J Hum Genet 2003;3:217–9.

16. Garewal G, Fearon CW, Warren TC, et al. The molecular basis of beta thalassaemia in Punjabi and Maharashtran Indians includes a multilocus aetiology involving triplicated alpha-globin loci. Br J Haematol 1994;86(2): 372–6.

17. Edison ES, Shaji RV, Devi SG, et al. Analysis of beta globin mutations in the Indian population: presence of rare and novel mutations and region-wise heterogeneity. Clin Genet 2008;73(4):331–7.

18. Sinha S, Black ML, Agarwal S, et al. Profiling beta-thalassaemia mutations in India at state and regional levels: implications for genetic education, screening and counseling programmes. Hugo J 2009;3(1–4):51–62.

19. Goyal R, Das R, Bambery P, et al. Serum transferrin receptor-ferritin index shows concomitant iron deficiency anemia and anemia of chronic disease is common in patients with rheumatoid arthritis in north India. Indian J Pathol Microbiol 2008; 51(1):102–4.

20. Jairam A, Das R, Aggarwal PK, et al. Iron status, inflammation and hepcidin in ESRD patients: the confounding role of intravenous iron therapy. Indian J Nephrol 2010;20(3):125–31.

21. Singleton B, Bansal D, Varma N, et al. Homozygosity mapping reveals founder SEC23B-Y462C mutations in Indian congenital dyserythropoietic anemia type II. Clin Genet 2015;88(2):195–7.

22. Camaschella C, DeGoobi M, Rotteo A. Hereditary hemochromatosis: progress and perspective. Rev Clin Exp Hematol 2000;4:302–21.

23. Dhillon BK, Das R, Garewal G, et al. Frequency of primary iron overload and HFE gene mutations (C282Y, H63D and S65C) in chronic liver disease patients in north India. World J Gastroenterol 2007;13(21):2956–9.

24. Lok CY, Merryweather-Clarke AT, Viprakasit V, et al. Iron overload in the Asian community. Blood 2009;114(1):20–5.

25. Annual report of the hemophilia federation of India. 2013.

26. World Federation of Hemophilia report of the annual global survey, 2013. (Canada): World Federation of Hemophilia.

27. Trasi S, Shetty S, Ghosh K, et al. Prevalence and spectrum of von Willebrand disease from western India. Indian J Med Res 2005;121(5):653–8.

28. Gupta PK, Ahmed RP, Sazawal S, et al. Relatively high frequency of VWD types 3 and 2 in a cohort of Indian patients: the role of multimeric analysis. J Thromb Haemost 2005;3(6):1321–2.

29. Srivastava A, You SK, Ayob Y, et al. Hemophilia treatment in developing countries: products and protocols. Semin Thromb Hemost 2005;31(5):495–500.

30. Nair SC, Viswabandya A, Srivastava A. Diagnosis and management of von Willebrand disease: a developing country perspective. Semin Thromb Hemost 2011; 37(5):587–94.

31. Viswabandya A, Mathews V, George B, et al. Successful surgical haemostasis in patients with von Willebrand disease with Koate DVI. Haemophilia 2008;14(4): 763–7.

32. Badyal RK, Jain K, Mandrelle K, et al. Recurrent hemoperitoneum secondary to haemorrhage from the corpus luteum unmasks factor V deficiency. Blood Coagul Fibrinolysis 2015;26(6):703–6.

33. Pinto P, Shelar T, Nawadkar V, et al. The Epidemiology of FVIII Inhibitors in Indian Haemophilia A Patients. Indian J Hematol Blood Transfus 2014;30(4):356–63.

34. Lee AD, Stephen E, Agarwal S, et al. Venous thrombo-embolism in India. Eur J Vasc Endovasc Surg 2009;37(4):482–5.

35. Sharma SK, Gupta V, Kadhiravan T, et al. A prospective study of risk factor profile & incidence of deep venous thrombosis among medically-ill hospitalized patients at a tertiary care hospital in northern India. Indian J Med Res 2009;130(6): 726–30.

36. Garewal G, Das R, Varma S, et al. Heterogeneous distribution of factor V Leiden in patients from north India with venous thromboembolism. J Thromb Haemost 2003;1(6):1329–30.

37. Garewal G, Das R, Ahluwalia J, et al. Prothrombin G20210A is not prevalent in North India. J Thromb Haemost 2003;1(10):2253–4.

38. Parakh R, Kakkar VV, Kakkar AK, Venous Thromboembolism (VTE) Core Study Group. Management of venous thromboembolism. J Assoc Physicians India 2007;55:49–70.

39. National Cancer Registry Programme. Consolidated report of hospital based cancer registries: 2007-2011. New Delhi (India): Indian Council of Medical Research; 2013.

40. Bhutani M, Vora A, Kumar L, et al. Lympho-hemopoietic malignancies in India. Med Oncol 2002;19(3):141–50.

41. Bansal S, Prabhash K, Parikh P. Chronic myeloid leukemia data from India. Indian J Med Paediatr Oncol 2013;34(3):154–8.

42. Varma S, Naseem S, Malhotra P, et al. Incidence rates of myeloproliferative neoplasms in India: a hospital based based study. Anchorage (AK): International Epidemiological Association (IEA) World Congress of Epidemiology; 2014.

43. Agarwal MB, Malhotra H, Chakrabarti P, et al. Myeloproliferative neoplasms working group consensus recommendations for diagnosis and management of primary myelofibrosis, polycythemia vera, and essential thrombocythemia. Indian J Med Paediatr Oncol 2015;36(1):3–16.

44. Sharma M, Sachdeva MUS, Bose P, et al. Hematological profile of cases of mixed-phenotype acute leukemia from a tertiary care centre of north India. Indian J Med Res, in press.

45. Siraj AK, Kamat S, Gutierrez MI, et al. Frequencies of the major subgroups of precursor B-cell acute lymphoblastic leukemia in Indian children differ from the West. Leukemia 2003;17(6):1192–3.

46. Amare P, Gladstone B, Varghese C, et al. Clinical significance of cytogenetic findings at diagnosis and in remission in childhood and adult acute lymphoblastic leukemia: experience from India. Cancer Genet Cytogenet 1999;110(1):44–53.
47. Kulkarni KP, Arora RS, Marwaha RK. Survival outcome of childhood acute lymphoblastic leukemia in India: a resource-limited perspective of more than 40 years. J Pediatr Hematol Oncol 2011;33(6):475–9.
48. Bajpai J, Sharma A, Kumar L, et al. Acute promyelocytic leukemia: an experience from a tertiary care centre in north India. Indian J Cancer 2011;48(3):316–22.
49. Mathews V, George B, Chendamarai E, et al. Single-agent arsenic trioxide in the treatment of newly diagnosed acute promyelocytic leukemia: long-term follow-up data. J Clin Oncol 2010;28(24):3866–71.
50. Philip C, George B, Ganapule A, et al. Acute myeloid leukaemia: challenges and real world data from India. Br J Haematol 2015;170(1):110–7.
51. Kumar L, Vikram P, Kochupillai V. Recent advances in the management of multiple myeloma. Natl Med J India 2006;19(2):80–9.
52. Kumar L, Raju GM, Ganessan K, et al. High dose chemotherapy followed by autologous haemopoietic stem cell transplant in multiple myeloma. Natl Med J India 2003;16(1):16–21.
53. Naresh KN, Srinivas V, Soman CS. Distribution of various subtypes of non-Hodgkin's lymphoma in India: a study of 2773 lymphomas using R.E.A.L. and WHO Classifications. Ann Oncol 2000;11(Suppl 1):63–7.
54. Aggarwal S, Apte S, Bhurani D, et al. Histopathological pattern of lymphomas and clinical presentation and outcomes of diffuse large B cell lymphoma: a multicentric registry based study from India. Indian J Med Paediatr Oncol 2013;34(4):299–304.
55. Gogia AS, Raina V, Kumar L, et al. Clinico-hematological characteristics and outcome assessment of patients with chronic lymphocytic leukemia: a single-institution study of 285 cases. J Clin Oncol 2011;29(Suppl) [abstr: 6584].
56. Dighiero G, Hamblin TJ. Chronic lymphocytic leukaemia. Lancet 2008;371(9617):1017–29.
57. Yeole BB. Trends in the incidence of Non-Hodgkin's lymphoma in India. Asian Pac J Cancer Prev 2008;9(3):433–6.
58. Sachdeva RK, Sharma A, Wanchu A, et al. Hematological malignancies in human immunodeficiency virus-positive individuals in North India. Leuk Lymphoma 2011;52(8):1597–600.
59. Ganesan P, Lalit K, Raina V, et al. Hodgkins lymphoma-long-term outcome: an experience from a tertiary care cancer center in north India. Ann Hematol 2011;90(10):1153–60.
60. Jain H, Sengar M, Nair R, et al. Treatment results in advanced stage Hodgkin's lymphoma: a retrospective study. J Postgrad Med 2015;61:88–91.

Hematological Practice in Hong Kong and China

Yok-Lam Kwong, MD[a], Shau-Yin Ha, FHKAM (Paediatrics)[b], Vivian Chan, PhD, FRCPath[a],*

KEYWORDS

- Thalassemia • Hemophilia • Glucose-6-phosphate dehydrogenase deficiency
- Arsenic trioxide • Acute promyelocytic leukemia • Natural killer cell lymphoma

KEY POINTS

- Prenatal diagnoses of thalassemia, the most important inherited hematological disease in Hong Kong and Southern China, and hemophilia A and B have very significantly decreased the burden of these disorders.
- Adequate transfusion and iron chelation therapy for thalassemia major patients, and optimal factor replacement for hemophilia patients, have dramatically improved the outlook of these disorders.
- Arsenic trioxide is an active drug for acute promyelocytic leukemia on presentation and at relapse; the availability of an oral formulation means that long-term consolidation of remission with this drug can be achieved.
- Natural killer cell lymphomas, prevalent in Hong Kong and parts of China, have much better prognosis when treated with combination chemotherapy containing non-P-glycoprotein-dependent drugs and L-asparaginase.

INTRODUCTION

China has a population of 1.3 billion. Hong Kong is a special administrative region in China, with a population of 7.5 million. The Han ethnic group accounts for about 92% of the population in both places. Disease patterns in Hong Kong therefore closely reflect those in China.

The first major hematology center combining clinical and laboratory research was established in China in 1958.[1] In Hong Kong, research in blood diseases also started in the late 1950s. Allogeneic hematopoietic stem cell transplantation (HSCT) was first performed in 1981 in China,[2] and in 1990 in Hong Kong.

Disclosure Statement: The authors have nothing to disclose.
[a] Department of Medicine, Queen Mary Hospital, University of Hong Kong, Pokfulam Road, Hong Kong, China; [b] Department of Paediatrics and Adolescent Medicine, Queen Mary Hospital, Pokfulam Road, Hong Kong, China
* Corresponding author.
E-mail address: vnychana@hku.hk

Hematol Oncol Clin N Am 30 (2016) 445–456
http://dx.doi.org/10.1016/j.hoc.2015.11.010
0889-8588/16/$ – see front matter © 2016 Elsevier Inc. All rights reserved.

hemonc.theclinics.com

Health Care Systems in China and Hong Kong

For a long time, patients or their employers were responsible for medical expenses in China. Recently, 3 systems of government-subsidized insurance schemes have been introduced, which cover up to 95% of the population. Hong Kong adopted a model similar to a national health care system, with patients paying a nominal daily fee of less than 15 US dollars even for complicated treatment such as HSCT.

However, with rising medical costs, such systems are becoming difficult to maintain. Whether the soaring fees should be met by increasing government expenditure or higher insurance premiums is hotly debated.

Burden of Hematological Diseases

Nonmalignant diseases including hemoglobin and bleeding disorders were predominant hematological problems in China and Hong Kong. However, malignant diseases now constitute the major burden, owing to an aging population and improvement in patient survivals.

NONMALIGNANT HEMATOLOGICAL DISEASES: GENETIC DISORDERS

The most common genetic diseases in this region are thalassemias (α- and β-thal) and glucose-6-phosphate dehydrogenase (G6PD) deficiency.

Thalassemias

The combined carrier rates for α^+- and α^0-thalassemia in Hong Kong are 4% and 3.5% for β-thalassemia minor.[3] In China, thalassemias are mainly restricted to the southern provinces of Guangxi and Guangdong, with α-thalassemia much more prevalent in Guangxi, with a carrier rate of up to 15%. In Guangdong, incidences of both types of thalassemias are similar to those in Hong Kong.[4] In Northern China, thalassemias are uncommon.

Prenatal Diagnosis for Thalassemias

Couples with the same thalassemia trait (α^0-thal or β-thal minor) carry a 25% risk of having a homozygous child. The homozygous α^0-thal fetus (Hb Barts hydrops fetalis) is incompatible with life. Early termination of pregnancy prevents maternal morbidity or even mortality. The homozygous β-thalassemia child (β-thalassemia major) lives, but is transfusion-dependent and suffers from the consequences of iron overload. Screening of at-risk couples in early pregnancy and subsequent prenatal diagnosis (PND) are advocated. Since 2000, screening is offered to all pregnant women on antenatal booking at every public hospital and maternity center in Hong Kong. A maternal mean corpuscular volume of less than 80 fl and a normal serum iron level necessitates investigation of the couple. In Hong Kong, PND was first performed in 1975 by globin-chain analysis of fetal blood. With the establishment of a DNA-based PND program in 1982, the detection of α-globin genes in fetal DNA excludes homozygous α^0-thal, but misses the occurrence of nondeletion Hb-H hydrops fetalis.[5] The various common nondeletion α-globin gene defects can be detected by reverse dot-blot or by microarray based on an allele-specific arrayed primer-extension technology[6]; this is important because nondeletion Hb-H accounts for 22.8% of Hb-H disease,[7] with at least 4 types giving rise to hydrops fetalis. However, α-Quong Sze (QS) and α-Constant Spring (CS), highly prevalent in Guangxi province and Southeast Asia, respectively, rarely cause hydrops fetalis. Most Hb-H patients are not transfusion-dependent and have a long lifespan.[7] Their only morbidity is increasing iron overload with age, which may then benefit from short-term iron chelation therapy.[8] Hence, termination of pregnancy is not justified for nonhydropic Hb-H fetus.

An alternative strategy is noninvasive ultrasound diagnosis by measurement of the placental thickness or cardiothoracic ratio (CTR) and/or middle cerebral artery systolic velocity (MCA-PSV) of the fetus at 12 to 15 weeks of gestation.[9] Transient and marginal increases in CTR and MCA-PSV have been reported in 2 fetuses affected by Hb-H-QS, but both were delivered alive.[10] Hence, in cases of marginal increase in CTR, serial follow-up will be necessary and fetal DNA analysis is needed to confirm a positive ultrasound diagnosis.

In β-thalassemia, each ethnic group has its own specific gene mutations. For ethnic Chinese (constituting 95% of the Hong Kong population), 12 mutations of the β-globin gene have been characterized, with 4 common ones accounting for 87% of cases. A reverse dot-blot or microarray with allele-specific sequences for β-globin gene mutations provides a convenient means of PND.[6] Noninvasive techniques with array-based detection of the paternal-derived mutation and informative paternal-derived single-nucleotide polymorphisms in maternal plasma-DNA have been explored.[11] This method potentially achieves a diagnosis in 40% of cases, thus obviating invasive procedures.

In China, PND has been available in Guangzhou, Beijing, and Shanghai since the 1990s, but is mainly self-financed. Recent government funding is available to encourage PND among ethnic minorities in the Guangxi province.

Preimplantation Genetic Diagnosis

Since 2002, preimplantation genetic diagnosis (PGD) is offered to thalassemia couples with fertility problems, or a history of repeated elective terminations following PND of affected pregnancies. Only embryos diagnosed as unaffected are transferred to establish pregnancy.

Preimplantation Genetic Diagnosis of α-Thalassemia

Single-cell multiplex polymerase chain reaction (PCR) of the normal and α^0-thal alleles is performed. The use of duplicate blastomeres prevents misdiagnosis due to allele dropout (ADO), and a second seminested PCR ensures specific amplification.[12] The use of whole genome amplification, before allele-specific PCR, has decreased ADO.

Preimplantation Genetic Diagnosis of β-Thalassemia

For couples with a previous β-thalassemia major child, PGD is performed to select embryos that are either normal or have β-thalassemia minor, and when available, HLA-identical to the affected elder sibling, with a view to obtaining cord blood stem cells for HSCT.

Transfusion and Iron Chelation Therapy for Thalassemia Major

In 2009, it was estimated that 9.5% of the blood supply in Hong Kong (13,460 units) was used by about 380 transfusion-dependent thalassemia patients, with a predicted annual consumption increment of 0.8%.[13] Blood safety has progressively improved, from the introduction of serologic testing for hepatitis C in 1991 to the implementation of rapid nucleic acid testing for infectious agents and full compliance with the ISO (International Organization for Standardization) international standards in the late 2000s. Thalassemia patients have been provided with prestorage filtered blood as a standard for the past 15 years. Iron chelation with subcutaneous desferrioxamine started in the late 1970s. Since then, regular blood transfusion and subcutaneous desferrioxamine have become the standard management. However, complications due to iron overload, including cardiomyopathy and endocrinopathy, still occur in some patients. Infections by *Klebsiella* spp in different sites were commonly encountered, which may be associated with significant morbidity and mortality.[14] Other desferrioxamine-associated complications such as skeletal dysplasia are occasionally observed. Deferiprone was shown in a randomized control study to significantly reduce ferritin levels in poorly chelated Chinese patients when combined with desferrioxamine.[15] Therefore, combination therapy of desferrioxamine with deferiprone is frequently used in poorly chelated patients, with benefits validated by MRI T2*.[16] The oral iron chelator deferasirox is recommended for first-line treatment in children aged between 2 and 6 years, and for second-line treatment for children older than 6 years, who are not responding optimally to combined desferrioxamine with deferiprone. Renal tubular dysfunction has been observed to be a frequent but reversible adverse effect.[17]

Hematopoietic Stem Cell Transplantation for Thalassemia Major

In Hong Kong, HLA-matched sibling HSCT for thalassemia started initially with marrow in 1991 and with cord blood in 1994.[18] Using conditioning regimens containing antithymocyte globulin, HSCT results in transfusion independence in more than 90% of recipients. HSCT is a curative treatment that may be suitable for centers unable to meet the demands of lifelong transfusion and chelation and is increasingly adopted in Southern China.[19] Because of a one-child policy, unrelated donor HSCT is predominant in China, with good results reported.[20]

Hemophilia

The incidences of hemophilias A and B in China have not been well-defined. In a global study of hemophilia A, the incidence in China was reported to be merely 0.3 to 0.5/100,000 males, as compared with 7.6 to 8.0/100,000 males in the United States and 17.4 to 22.6/100,000 males in the United Kingdom.[21] This low incidence was likely due to underreporting. Given the vast population in China, hemophilias are important inherited diseases. Although patients with hemophilias may lead a normal life with adequate coagulation factor support, the consequent enormous economic and emotional costs make PND necessary to communities where termination of pregnancy is acceptable.

Prenatal Diagnosis for Hemophilias

In Hong Kong, PND for hemophilia A has been available since 1989. Except those with intron 18 or 22 inversions in the *F8* gene, 3 common restriction fragment length polymorphisms provide informativeness for 98% of Chinese families[22]; this is further enhanced by analysis of dinucleotide repeats in introns 13 and 22. For hemophilia B, the genetic aberrations are heterogeneous and more than 900 mutations of the *F9* gene have been characterized. A microarray that examines simultaneously 69 common mutations of the *F9* gene has been devised, covering 53% of the 2891 mutation entries in the *F9* database.[23]

Treatment of Hemophilias

In Hong Kong, plasma-derived factor VIII and IX concentrates are manufactured from plasma of normal blood donors. This local source of factor concentrates, while adequate for hemophilia B patients, is inadequate for the bigger population of hemophilia A patients, so that plasma-derived factor VIII concentrates are needed from other suppliers. Before the implementation of prophylactic use of factor concentrates in 2004, a significant portion of patients developed chronic joint problems. This complication has much decreased since. Recombinant factor VIII is not reimbursed.

In China, the establishment of the Hemophilia Treatment Centre Collaborative Network of China, in conjunction with the World Federation of Hemophilia, has improved the identification and treatment of hemophilia patients.[24]

Glucose-6-Phosphate Dehydrogenase Deficiency

G6PD deficiency occurs in approximately 4% to 6% of males in South China and Hong Kong, The gene is X-linked. As well as hemizygous male patients, heterozygote female patients (mosaic for normal and G6PD-deficient red cells due to variable X-inactivation of the normal chromosome) may also suffer from mild hemolysis.[25] Neonatal screening of the genetic trait has been implemented in all public hospitals in Hong Kong since the 1980s. Mothers of babies carrying the genetic trait are given a list of offending drugs and agents to avoid.[26]

The most serious clinical manifestation of G6PD deficiency is massive intravascular hemolysis, which can occur as an idiosyncratic reaction to multiple drugs and chemicals (primaquine, sulfonamide, nitrofurantoin, naphthalene, and aniline dye), after ingestion of fava bean (favism) or herbs, and as a complication of febrile illnesses (particularly typhoid fever and viral hepatitis). In the neonatal period, hemolysis may lead to kernicterus. A useful hallmark of severe oxidative injury in G6PD-deficient erythrocytes is the appearance of hemighost.[27] Furthermore, the percentage of hemighosts also indicates the severity of hemolysis within the next 1 to 2 days, providing a useful guide to the necessity of prophylactic measures needed to avert renal shutdown.

MALIGNANT HEMATOLOGICAL DISEASES

Malignancies are the major problems in clinical hematology in Hong Kong and China and are the most rapidly evolving area in service and research.

Different Patterns of Lymphomas

The epidemiology of lymphomas is different in China as compared with Europe and North America,[28] with significant disparities being observed in follicular lymphoma (6%–10% vs 20%–35%) and mature T-cell and natural killer (NK) cell lymphomas (20%–25% vs 5%–10%). These differences are likely genetic, because Chinese migrants to foreign countries retain similar patterns of lymphomas.

Epidemiology and Pathology of Natural Killer/T-cell Lymphomas

Mature T-cell lymphomas were regarded to be more frequent in Asia. With advances in diagnostics, it is now realized that the apparent prevalence is due to a higher frequency of NK/T-cell lymphomas,[29] with other T-cell lymphomas being found at frequencies comparable with those of Western countries.

NK/T-cell lymphomas show a geographic predilection, occurring predominantly in Asia and South America.[29] Lymphoma cells are derived putatively from NK cells and are typically negative for surface CD3, but positive for cytoplasmic CD3ε, cytotoxic molecules, and CD56. Clonal episomal Epstein-Barr virus (EBV) is invariably present. Clinically, the nose, nasopharynx, and upper airways are most commonly involved. In about 10% of cases, nonnasal sites, including skin, salivary glands, and testes, are involved. Very occasionally, the lymphoma is disseminated with a leukemic phase. In some cases, lymphomas may be derived from cytotoxic T cells, accounting for the notation of NK/T-cell lymphoma.[29]

Advances in Natural Killer/T-cell Lymphomas

NK/T-cell lymphoma is conventionally regarded as aggressive with a poor prognosis. Studies performed in the 1980s to 1990s showed that survivals were only achieved in about 30% of patients.[29] However, this dismal outlook has been totally reversed in the last decade, during which significant advances have been made in this lymphoma.[29]

Treatment of Natural Killer/T-cell Lymphomas

NK cells express very high concentrations of P-glycoprotein and therefore the multidrug-resistance phenotype. Hence, anthracycline-containing regimens designed for B-cell lymphomas are ineffective, with remissions achieved in only about 30% to 50% of patients, and long-term survival ranging from 10% to 30%.[29,30] Early observations showed that L-asparaginase was efficacious for relapsed/refractory NK/T-cell lymphomas. Many protocols have subsequently been designed, combining L-asparaginase with drugs unaffected by P-glycoprotein.[30] These protocols are useful in both newly diagnosed and relapsed/refractory cases, achieving overall response rates (ORR) of up to 80%.[30]

Among L-asparaginase-containing protocols, only SMILE (steroid, methotrexate, ifosfamide, L-asparaginase, etoposide) has been tested in multicenter trials. In a phase II study, an ORR of 79% (complete remission, CR: 45%; partial remission, PR: 34%) was achieved in relapsed/refractory and stage III/IV NK/T-cell lymphomas.[31] These results were validated in Hong Kong, Seoul, and Singapore, where an ORR of 81% (CR: 66%; PR: 15%) was demonstrated in newly diagnosed and relapsed/refractory patients. Importantly, a 5-year overall survival (OS) of 50% and a disease-free survival (DFS) of 64% were achieved, clearly demonstrating that a significant proportion of NK/T-cell lymphoma patients is curable.[32]

Monitoring of Treatment Outcome

When lymphoma cells undergo apoptosis, EBV DNA fragments are released into the circulation. Circulating EBV DNA constitutes a sensitive surrogate biomarker of lymphoma load. Plasma is the preferred starting material. Whole blood is unsuitable, because it may contain EBV-infected memory B cells. Furthermore, quantifying EBV DNA per unit mass of total DNA in whole blood (to adjust for different leukocyte counts) renders the results difficult to be replicated or compared between different laboratories. These issues are overcome by quantifying plasma EBV DNA, now considered the standard methodology. Plasma EBV DNA has been shown to correlate with standard parameters of tumor load, including stage and lactate dehydrogenase (LDH).[33]

Prognostication of Natural Killer/T-cell Lymphomas

Conventional prognostic indicators including the International Prognostic Index (IPI) and the Korean Prognostic Index (KIPI) rely on presentation features (including stage, LDH, number of nodes, or extranodal sites involved),[29] which reflect tumor load. An emerging concept is that sensitivity to treatment is prognostically more important than tumor load, making interim assessment of response to treatment necessary.

This hypothesis has been validated in 2 seminal studies. In the first study, serial plasma EBV DNA was quantified in patients treated with SMILE.[34] Although presentation EBV DNA correlated with conventional parameters of lymphoma load, such as IPI and KIPI, it had no impact on survivals. However, interim assessment of plasma EBV DNA was highly prognostic. Patients achieving undetectable EBV DNA after one course of SMILE had OS far superior to those still having detectable EBV DNA. More-over, patients with persistently undetectable EBV DNA had DFS significantly superior to that of patients never achieving undetectable EBV DNA.

In the second study, interim positron emission tomography/computed tomography (PET/CT) scan was performed in patients treated with SMILE.[35] The results were remarkably similar to plasma EBV DNA. Patients with negative interim PET/CT scan (defined as a Deauville score of 1–3) after 2 to 3 courses of SMILE had OS and DFS significantly superior to those of patients still having a positive scan (Deauville score of 4–5).

Therefore, interim plasma EBV DNA or PET/CT scan provide a powerful way of iden-tifying patients who do not fare well with SMILE, currently the best regimen available for NK/T-cell lymphomas. These assessments offer the possibility of early intervention in order to improve the final outcome in these poor-risk patients.

Other T-cell Lymphoid Malignancies

Most mature T-cell lymphomas occur with similar frequencies and clinical manifesta-tions in China and Hong Kong as compared with other countries. However, 2 entities are notably different.

T-cell large granular lymphocyte (T-LGL) leukemia is a rare T-cell lymphoproliferative disease.[36] The main manifestations are neutropenia and infections. In Western patients, an association with rheumatoid arthritis is seen in about 30% of cases.[36] Treatment with low-dose methotrexate is recommended. Methotrexate does not induce molecular remission, so long-term treatment is necessary. Interestingly, in Chinese patients with T-LGL leukemia, the predominant manifestation is pure red cell aplasia, with neutrope-nia found only in about 30% of cases. Moreover, there is no association with rheumatoid arthritis. Treatment with cyclosporine is highly efficacious and may induce molecular re-missions. In patients not responding to cyclosporine, the purine analogue fludarabine has been shown to induce molecular remission in up to 60% of patients.[37]

Enteropathy-associated T-cell lymphoma (EATL) accounts for less than 5% of all T-cell lymphomas. In Western countries, EATL is almost invariably associated with celiac disease and is referred to as type I. Because celiac disease rarely exists in Chinese peo-ple, type I EATL is not observed. Instead, a monomorphic intestinal T-cell lymphoma, positive for CD8 and CD56 and often referred to as type II, is observed. Patients present with abdominal pain, intestinal hemorrhage, or perforation.[38] A history of enteropathy is absent. Prognosis is poor, with patients who are able to undergo chemotherapy, partic-ularly SMILE, having a slightly better outcome. This lymphoma is distinct from type I EATL and will be renamed monomorphic epitheliotropic intestinal T-cell lymphoma in the upcoming revised World Health Organization lymphoma classification.

Acute Promyelocytic Leukemia: The Chinese Revolution

APL used to be one of the most lethal leukemias, with up to 30% of patients dying from bleeding due to disseminated intravascular coagulopathy (DIC) within the first week. However, the discovery by Chinese hematologists of the clinical efficacy of all-trans retinoic acid (ATRA) and later arsenic trioxide (As_2O_3) completely revolutionized the treatment of APL.[39] It is now the most curable acute leukemia, with at least 90% of newly diagnosed patients expecting a durable remission.

All-Trans Retinoic Acid in Induction Treatment of Newly Diagnosed Acute Promyelocytic Leukemia: The Shanghai Connection

The extraordinary efficacy of ATRA in APL was first reported by Shanghai hematolo-gists in 1988.[40] ATRA induces partial maturation of the APL cells, thereby abrogating the development of DIC.[39] These observations were made before the reciprocal fusion of the *PML* and *RARA* genes characteristic of APL was known, making the discovery even more remarkable. Remission was achieved with ATRA alone, its efficacy much improved if concomitant chemotherapy was used. These results were soon validated worldwide.

Relapse of Acute Promyelocytic Leukemia After All-Trans Retinoic Acid Therapy

Relapse occurs in up to 30% of newly diagnosed patients, even with ATRA maintenance. Most relapsed patients fail to respond to ATRA again. Treatment with conventional chemotherapy supplemented with high-dose chemotherapy and HSCT resulted at best in survivals of only 50%, clearly indicating that better treatment strategies were needed.

As$_2$O$_3$ in Relapsed Acute Promyelocytic Leukemia: The Harbin Connection

The efficacy of As$_2$O$_3$ in APL was first discovered in a remote village in Harbin, a Northern Chinese city near Russia. The initial success was published in Chinese and unknown to the rest of the world.[38] The same group of Shanghai hematologists who discovered the efficacy of ATRA validated these early observations. Intravenous (iV) As$_2$O$_3$ induced remissions in practically every case of relapsed APL.[41] Elemental arsenic is the active drug, as tetraarsenic tetrasulphide is also effective,[42] although its poor solubility limits its general application. Arsenic binds to cysteine residues in the PML part of the PML-RARA fusion protein, increasing its sumoylation and degradation in proteasomes.[43] As$_2$O$_3$ is now the standard treatment for relapsed APL.

Role of As$_2$O$_3$ in Newly-Diagnosed Acute Promyelocytic Leukemia

As$_2$O$_3$ has also been tested in newly diagnosed APL. With quantitative PCR, an early Chinese study had shown that ATRA + As$_2$O$_3$ induced a deeper CR for newly diagnosed APL, with a greater reduction of *PML-RARA* fusion transcript than when ATRA was used with chemotherapy.[44] Single-agent As$_2$O$_3$ also induces CR in a high proportion of APL patients, but such remissions are short-lived, and up to 30% to 40% of patients relapse. Recently, ATRA + As$_2$O$_3$ has been shown to induce a high CR rate and durable remission in good-risk newly diagnosed APL patients, thereby validating the earlier Chinese observations.[45]

Oral As$_2$O$_3$: The Hong Kong Connection

Because the early Harbin and Shanghai studies used iV-As$_2$O$_3$, all subsequent studies used this administration route. Hong Kong investigators experimented on an oral formulation of As$_2$O$_3$ and showed that intestinal absorption of oral-As$_2$O$_3$ achieved an area-under-the-curve bioavailability reaching 90% to 95% of that of iV-As$_2$O$_3$.[46] Oral-As$_2$O$_3$ is as efficacious as iV-As$_2$O$_3$, inducing remissions in practically every patient with relapsed APL.[47]

Oral-As$_2$O$_3$ Maintenance of Acute Promyelocytic Leukemia in CR1 (First Complete Remission) Decreases Relapses

About 30% of patients treated with ATRA and chemotherapy relapse. Risk-adopted protocols decrease relapses, but they are cumbersome and entail the use of multiple chemotherapies.

The availability of oral-As$_2$O$_3$ makes it possible to be administered as an outpatient maintenance. This strategy has been shown by Hong Kong investigators to be safe and efficacious, reducing relapses to less than 10%.[48]

DEVELOPING STRATEGIES

Oral-As_2O_3 will soon be tested in trials worldwide. For the first time, it may be possible to cure APL by an entirely oral regimen. Future strategies should also examine the best timing of As_2O_3 therapy in the consolidation and maintenance of APL.

HAPLOIDENTICAL ALLOGENEIC HEMATOPOIETIC STEM CELL TRANSPLANTATION: SCIENCE DRIVEN BY CLINICAL NEED

Owing to a one-child policy, HLA-identical sibling donors are not available for most patients in China. However, haploidentical family donors (including both parents and 50% of siblings) are readily available. HSCT with haploidentical donors had sporadically been described. Beijing investigators were the first to report in a large series of patients that haploidentical HSCT might give results comparable with those of HLA-identical sibling HSCT.[49] In a recent review of 1210 haploidentical HSCTs, young male donors (father or son) were shown to be associated with less nonrelapse mortality, less acute graft-versus-host disease, and better survivals.[50] These results have established convincingly haploidentical HSCT as a standard procedure, now adopted in virtually all major transplantation centers.

SUMMARY

China is the most populous country in the world, and her research and service in hematology therefore arguably affect the largest number of patients. Future collaboration of China and Hong Kong with the international medical community is necessary to effect the largest impact in the global hematology arena.

REFERENCES

1. Institute of Hematology and Blood Diseases Hospital, Chinese Academy of Medical Sciences and Peking Union Medical College. Available at: http://www.chinablood.com.cn/english/. Accessed June 29, 2015.
2. Wu T, Lu DP. Blood and marrow transplantation in the People's Republic of China. Bone Marrow Transplant 2008;42(Suppl 1):S73–5.
3. Chan V, Chan TK, Cheng MY, et al. Organisation of the zeta-alpha genes in Chinese. Br J Haematol 1986;64:97–105.
4. Zeng YT, Huang SZ. Disorders of haemoglobin in China. J Med Genet 1987;24:578–83.
5. Chan V, Chan TK, Liang ST, et al. Hydrops fetalis due to an unusual form of Hb H disease. Blood 1985;66:224–8.
6. Chan K, Wong MS, Chan TK, et al. A thalassaemia array for Southeast Asia. Br J Haematol 2004;124:232–9.
7. Chen FE, Ooi C, Ha SY, et al. Genetic and clinical features of hemoglobin H disease in Chinese patients. N Engl J Med 2000;343:544–50.
8. Chan JC, Chim CS, Ooi CG, et al. Use of the oral chelator deferiprone in the treatment of iron overload in patients with Hb H disease. Br J Haematol 2006;133(2):198–205.
9. Leung KY, Lee CP, Tang MHY, et al. Detection of increased middle cerebral artery peak systolic velocity in foetuses affected by Hemoglobin H Quong Sze disease. Ultraosond Obstet Gynecol 2004;23:523–6.
10. Leung KY, Cheong KB, Lee CP, et al. Ultrasonographic prediction of homozygous alpha⁰-thalassemia using placental thickness, fetal cardiothoracic ratio and middle cerebral artery Doppler: alone or in combination? Ultrasound Obstet Gynecol 2010;35(2):149–54.

11. Chan K, Yam I, Leung KY, et al. Detection of paternal alleles in maternal plasma for non-invasive prenatal diagnosis of beta-thalassemia: a feasibility study in southern Chinese. Eur J Obstet Gynecol Reprod Biol 2010;150(1):28–33.

12. Chan V, Ng EH, Yam I, et al. Experience in preimplantation genetic diagnosis for exclusion of homozygous alpha^0 thalassemia. Prenat Diagn 2006;26(11): 1029–36.

13. Lau EH, He XQ, Lee CK, et al. Predicting future blood demand from thalassemia major patients in Hong Kong. PLoS One 2013;8(12):e81846.

14. Chung BH, Ha SY, Chan GC, et al. Klebsiella infection in patients with thalassemia. Clin Infect Dis 2003;36(5):575–9.

15. Ha SY, Chik KW, Ling SC, et al. A randomized controlled study evaluating the safety and efficacy of deferiprone treatment in thalassemia major patients from Hong Kong. Hemoglobin 2006;30(2):263–74.

16. Ha SY, Mok AS, Chu WC, et al. Intermediate-term evaluation of a practical chelation protocol based on stratification of thalassemic patients by serum ferritin and magnetic resonance imaging cardiac T2*. Hemoglobin 2011;35(3): 199–205.

17. Dee CM, Cheuk DK, Ha SY, et al. Incidence of deferasirox-associated renal tubular dysfunction in children and young adults with beta-thalassaemia. Br J Haematol 2014;167(3):434–6.

18. Li CK, Shing MM, Chik KW, et al. Haematopoietic stem cell transplantation for thalassaemia major in Hong Kong: prognostic factors and outcome. Bone Marrow Transplant 2002;29(2):101–5.

19. Xu LH, Fang JP. The current status of β-thalassemia major in Mainland China. Hemoglobin 2013;37(4):307–14.

20. Li C, Wu X, Feng X, et al. A novel conditioning regimen improves outcomes in β-thalassemia major patients using unrelated donor peripheral blood stem cell transplantation. Blood 2012;120(19):3875–81.

21. Stonebraker JS, Bolton-Maggs PH, Soucie JM, et al. A study of variations in the reported haemophilia A prevalence around the world. Haemophilia 2010;16(1):20–32.

22. Chan V, Tong TM, Chan TP, et al. Multiple Xbal polymorphisms for carrier detection and prenatal diagnosis of haemophilia A. Br J Haematol 1989;73(4): 497–500.

23. Chan K, Sasanakul W, Mellars G, et al. Detection of known haemophilia B mutations and carrier testing by microarray. Thromb Haemost 2005;94(4):872–8.

24. Ozelo MC, Matta MA, Yang R. Meeting the challenges of haemophilia care and patient support in China and Brazil. Haemophilia 2012;18(Suppl 5):33–8.

25. Beutler E, Yeh M, Fairbanks VF. The normal human female as a mosaic of X-chromosome activity: studies using the gene for G-6-PD-deficiency as a marker. Proc Natl Acad Sci U S A 1962;48:9–16.

26. Chan TK. Glucose-6-phosphate dehydrogenase (G6PD) deficiency: a review. HK J Paediatr 1996;1:23–30. Available at: http://www.hkjpaed.org/details.asp?id=436&show=1234. Accessed June 29, 2015.

27. Chan TK, Chan WC, Weed RI. Erythrocyte hemighosts: a hallmark of severe oxidative injury in vivo. Br J Haematol 1982;50:575–82.

28. Yang QP, Zhang WY, Yu JB, et al. Subtype distribution of lymphomas in Southwest China: analysis of 6,382 cases using WHO classification in a single institution. Diagn Pathol 2011;6:77.

29. Kwong YL. Natural killer-cell malignancies: diagnosis and treatment. Leukemia 2005;19(12):2186–94.

30. Tse E, Kwong YL. How I treat NK/T-cell lymphomas. Blood 2013;121(25):
    4997–5005.
31. Yamaguchi M, Kwong YL, Kim WS, et al. Phase II study of SMILE chemotherapy
    for newly diagnosed stage IV, relapsed, or refractory extranodal natural killer
    (NK)/T-cell lymphoma, nasal type: the NK-Cell Tumor Study Group study. J Clin
    Oncol 2011;29(33):4410–6.
32. Kwong YL, Kim WS, Lim ST, et al. SMILE for natural killer/T-cell lymphoma: anal-
    ysis of safety and efficacy from the Asia Lymphoma Study Group. Blood 2012;
    120(15):2973–80.
33. Au WY, Pang A, Choy C, et al. Quantification of circulating Epstein-Barr
    virus (EBV) DNA in the diagnosis and monitoring of natural killer cell and
    EBV-positive lymphomas in immunocompetent patients. Blood 2004;104(1):
    243–9.
34. Kwong YL, Pang AW, Leung AY, et al. Quantification of circulating Epstein-Barr
    virus DNA in NK/T-cell lymphoma treated with the SMILE protocol: diagnostic
    and prognostic significance. Leukemia 2014;28(4):865–70.
35. Khong PL, Huang B, Phin Lee EY, et al. Midtreatment 18F-FDG PET/CT scan
    for early response assessment of SMILE therapy in natural killer/T-cell lym-
    phoma: a prospective study from a single center. J Nucl Med 2014;55(6):
    911–6.
36. Kwong YL, Au WY, Leung AY, et al. T-cell large granular lymphocyte leukemia: an
    Asian perspective. Ann Hematol 2010;89(4):331–9.
37. Tse E, Chan JC, Pang A, et al. Fludarabine, mitoxantrone and dexamethasone as
    first-line treatment for T-cell large granular lymphocyte leukemia. Leukemia 2007;
    21(10):2225–6.
38. Tse E, Gill H, Loong F, et al. Type II enteropathy-associated T-cell lymphoma: a
    multicenter analysis from the Asia Lymphoma Study Group. Am J Hematol
    2012;87(7):663–8.
39. Wang ZY, Chen Z. Acute promyelocytic leukemia: from highly fatal to highly
    curable. Blood 2008;111(5):2505–15.
40. Huang ME, Ye YC, Chen SR, et al. Use of all-trans retinoic acid in the treatment of
    acute promyelocytic leukemia. Blood 1988;72(2):567–72.
41. Shen ZX, Chen GQ, Ni JH, et al. Use of arsenic trioxide (As_2O_3) in the treatment of
    acute promyelocytic leukemia (APL): II. Clinical efficacy and pharmacokinetics in
    relapsed patients. Blood 1997;89(9):3354–60.
42. Lu DP, Qiu JY, Jiang B, et al. Tetra-arsenic tetra-sulfide for the treatment of acute
    promyelocytic leukemia: a pilot report. Blood 2002;99(9):3136–43.
43. Zhang XW, Yan XJ, Zhou ZR, et al. Arsenic trioxide controls the fate of the
    PML-RARalpha oncoprotein by directly binding PML. Science 2010;328(5975):
    240–3.
44. Shen ZX, Shi ZZ, Fang J, et al. All-trans retinoic acid/As_2O_3 combination yields a
    high quality remission and survival in newly diagnosed acute promyelocytic
    leukemia. Proc Natl Acad Sci U S A 2004;101(15):5328–35.
45. Lo-Coco F, Avvisati G, Vignetti M, et al, Gruppo Italiano Malattie Ematologiche
    dell'Adulto, German-Austrian Acute Myeloid Leukemia Study Group, Study
    Alliance Leukemia. Retinoic acid and arsenic trioxide for acute promyelocytic
    leukemia. N Engl J Med 2013;369(2):111–21.
46. Kumana CR, Au WY, Lee NS, et al. Systemic availability of arsenic from oral
    arsenic-trioxide used to treat patients with hematological malignancies. Eur J
    Clin Pharmacol 2002;58(8):521–6.

47. Au WY, Kumana CR, Kou M, et al. Oral arsenic trioxide in the treatment of relapsed acute promyelocytic leukemia. Blood 2003;102(1):407–8.
48. Au WY, Kumana CR, Lee HK, et al. Oral arsenic trioxide-based maintenance regimens for first complete remission of acute promyelocytic leukemia: a 10-year follow-up study. Blood 2011;118(25):6535–43.
49. Lu DP, Dong L, Wu T, et al. Conditioning including antithymocyte globulin followed by unmanipulated HLA-mismatched/haploidentical blood and marrow transplantation can achieve comparable outcomes with HLA-identical sibling transplantation. Blood 2006;107(8):3065–73.
50. Wang Y, Chang YJ, Xu LP, et al. Who is the best donor for a related HLA haplotype-mismatched transplant? Blood 2014;124(6):843–50.

Hematology in Africa

Julie Makani, MD, PhD, FRCP, FTAAS[a],
David J. Roberts, DPhil, MRCP, FRCPath[b],*

KEYWORDS

- Sub-Saharan Africa • Hematology • Sickle cell disease • Iron deficiency anemia
- Transfusion • Laboratory hematology • Leukemia • Lymphoma

KEY POINTS

- Hematology practice in Africa is rapidly evolving to encompass the growing and changing demands in clinical and laboratory services and blood transfusion.
- Anemia is the most common hematological disorder, with iron deficiency the most common form, and is more prevalent in children (secondary to nutritional deficiency) and women (secondary to menorrhagia and pregnancy).
- The global burden of sickle cell disease (SCD) is highest in Africa, with significant birth prevalence, morbidity, and mortality. There are increasing efforts to introduce effective interventions.
- There is growing need for specialist services for bleeding and coagulation disorders, with increased incidence of thromboembolic disorders and an increase in the use of anticoagulation therapy.
- Hematological malignancies, such as leukemias and lymphomas, seem more prevalent and aggressive. The poor prognosis may be compounded by the late diagnosis and limited resources available to provide basic treatment protocols.

INTRODUCTION

The practice of hematology and blood transfusion (BT) is rapidly evolving in many countries in sub-Saharan Africa (SSA). Although SSA covers an enormous and diverse geographic area with a considerable range of economic and social circumstances, there are common themes that run through much of the medical and hematological practice of the continent. This review addresses the major topics of common concern, based on epidemiologic burden, existing programs and opportunities for addressing some of the major challenges in this field.

Disclosure Statement: The authors have nothing to disclose.
[a] Department of Haematology and Blood Transfusion, Muhimbili University of Health and Allied Sciences, PO Box 65001, Dar-es-Salaam, Tanzania; [b] Radcliffe Department of Medicine, University of Oxford, National Health Service Blood and Transplant, John Radcliffe Hospital, Oxford OX3 9BQ, UK
* Corresponding author.
E-mail address: david.roberts@ndcls.ox.ac.uk

Hematol Oncol Clin N Am 30 (2016) 457–475
http://dx.doi.org/10.1016/j.hoc.2015.12.002
0889-8588/16/$ – see front matter © 2016 Elsevier Inc. All rights reserved.

hemonc.theclinics.com

Many countries in SSA are going through similar socioeconomic changes that are influencing hematology practice. First, there is the epidemiologic transition that is occurring, with reduction in burden of infectious disease and increase in burden of noncommunicable diseases. This is accompanied by increased childhood survival and longer life expectancy. Hematological diseases are increasingly common and form a major part of everyday medicine across all specialties. Health systems (in both the public and private sectors) are growing stronger, leading to improvement in the diagnosis and management of hematological disorders. In many health facilities, hemoglobin concentration and blood counts from automated analyzers are available and are the most frequently requested laboratory tests. There has been strengthening of BT services with provision of safe blood components as an emergency, life-saving intervention or as part of planned interventions, for example, elective surgery.

The overwhelming focus of development of health services and training of health personnel has been to develop primary and secondary health services. Understandably, everyday hematological practice has fallen within the scope of primary health care workers. At secondary health care facilities, this has been provided by general medical staff in adult and pediatric departments. This provision of care has been necessary and sufficient to deal with common conditions, but it is now apparent that greater expertise is required, not only for the treatment of hematological diseases, but also for the wider development of hematological services. Over the past 2 decades, most of the hematological conditions requiring monitoring and follow-up have been occurring at tertiary-level health facilities. There is an increasing need, however, to improve the capacity to provide hematology services at primary-level and secondary-level health facilities. This is critical to decentralize and ensure that services are more accessible to a wider population and not limited to urban hospitals.

Furthermore, aspects of prevention and management of blood diseases require knowledge and improvement in practice in the community. As a consequence, many governments are investing in improving the capacity of the health care system to enable prompt recognition and referral of suspected cases from primary-level and secondary-level health facilities to tertiary-level hospitals as well as strengthening the development of specialist centers for diagnosis and treatment. Although there has previously been a limitation in human resources and infrastructure, many centers now have a critical mass of both clinical and laboratory hematological expertise and experience from national, regional and global partnerships.

Given this background of the current position of hematology in Africa and the extensive coverage of anemia, iron deficiency, infection, SCD, glucose 6-phosphate dehydrogenase deficiency, and BT in other articles in this issue, this review highlights some of the other areas of hematological diseases and also the scope for further development of hematological practice in SSA.

RED CELL DISORDERS
Anemia

Anemia is widespread throughout SSA and is frequently multifactorial in origin, but the major contributing factors are iron deficiency, malaria, anemia of chronic disease, and disorders of red cell, both hemoglobinopathies and enzymopathies. It has been estimated that more than 50% of preschool children, more than 60% of pregnant women and more than 40% of nonpregnant women are anemic.[1]

The burden of disease caused by chronic anemia on individuals has been difficult to estimate. It is widely recognized that those with a hemoglobin of greater than 70 g/L can compensate for reduced levels of hemoglobin by increasing oxygen delivery through increasing red cell 2,3-diphosphoglycerate and increasing blood flow. Mild chronic anemia in children, however, typically due to iron deficiency and malaria, is associated with reduced growth and development, reduced neurocognitive function and learning and in many diseases with increased mortality and morbidity. The challenges are not only to improve treatment of severe acute anemia but also to understand and reduce the enormous burden of disease associated with chronic anemia.

Heart failure is recognized as a common complication of anemia that results in hospitalization and emergency BT. In many hospitals, a hemoglobin of less than 50 g/L is considered an indication for BT. Due to the rapidly life-threatening nature of severe anemia, however, the presence of clinical features of severe anemia and heart failure is often an indication of BT, even without the laboratory result of the hemoglobin. This practice has been critical to reduce mortality but has led to difficulty in understanding the causes of anemia. There are now an increasing number of studies, however, that are reporting on the etiology of anemia that have highlighted the contribution of bacterial infection to severe anemia[2] and the contribution of anemia, in particular iron deficiency anemia (IDA), to heart failure.[3]

Malaria

Falciparum malaria causes acute and chronic anemia. Severe malarial anemia due to *Plasmodium falciparum* carries low mortality when it appears in isolation but significantly contributes to increased mortality in those children where severe anemia (hemoglobin <50 g/L) is accompanied by cerebral malaria or respiratory distress.[4]

The burden of anemia due to malaria is considerable and may account for 60% of episodes of anemia in young children.[5] Where transmission is intense, younger children under 3 years of age present with isolated anemia.[6] In areas of lower transmission, older children develop severe anemia and, for reasons not well understood, often accompanied by other syndromes of severe disease, such as cerebral malaria or respiratory distress. In many areas, older children with partial immunity to malaria may have chronic anemia with low parasitemia and marked dyserythropoiesis.

The complex etiology of malarial anemia has been described elsewhere (see David J. Roberts: Hematologic Changes Associated with Specific Infections in the Tropics, in this issue). The mainstays of therapy are now artemisinin derivatives for acute disease and oral artemisinin in combination with mefloquine (ASMQ), lumefantrine (Coartem), amodiaquine (ASAQ), piperaquine (Duo-Cotecxin), and pyronaridine (Pyramax) for oral therapy for less severely ill patients. The detailed chemotherapy of disease is beyond the scope of this article but is well described in a recent review from the World Health Organization (WHO).[7]

The guidelines for blood transfusion in malaria are that transfusion should be given for those with hemoglobin less than 50 g/L or if there is evidence of respiratory distress at higher levels of hemoglobin concentration. There is little high-quality evidence, however, for more detailed guidance in complicated malaria, but transfusion is commonly given for anemic children (hemoglobin <100 g/L) with cerebral malaria with or without respiratory distress.

There is increasing evidence of the contribution of severe malaria and anemia to morbidity and mortality in SCD,[8–10] despite the protection against malaria in the presence of sickle cell hemoglobin (HbS), particularly in individuals with heterozygous state of HbS.[11,12] There is high mortality due to malaria in the homozygous state (HbSS). It is likely that this high mortality is a result of worsening hemolysis and anemia in individuals who already have a low steady state of hemoglobin.

Pregnancy

The maternal mortality rate is high in many African countries, making this one of the health-related millennium development goals. Tanzania reported that anemia and antepartum/postpartum hemorrhage account for up to 13% of maternal mortality. Maternal mortality rises rapidly when the hematocrit falls below 0.20, and low birthweight and perinatal and infant mortality rise if the hematocrit falls below 0.3.[13] Reports from most BT services show that the highest demand for blood in terms of volume is from obstetrics and gynecology, whereas the highest demand in terms of numbers is from pediatrics. It is, therefore, critical to improve hematology and BT services to improve the diagnosis and management of the different hematological complications that result in morbidity and mortality during pregnancy.

Anemia is common in pregnancy and is associated with major morbidity and mortality (**Fig. 1**). In malarial areas, pregnancy is associated with increased parasitemia and severity of acute malaria.[14] The particular susceptibility factors to malaria include altered systemic immune responses and also specific local factors, including the ability of infected red cells to adhere to the syncytiotrophoblast in the placenta.[15,16]

In nonimmune women, malaria infection is associated with severe complications, including anemia and cerebral malaria. Severe malarial anemia causes prematurity, intrauterine growth retardation, and increased maternal and infant mortality. In areas of high transmission, clinical malaria is increased with a peak instance in the second trimester.[17] Multigravida women are less commonly symptomatic, reflecting the

Burden of Disease Profile 2001
SMI Addressable Conditions

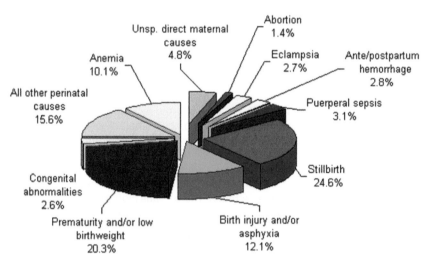

Fig. 1. The maternal and early childhood causes of mortality addressed by the Safe Motherhood Initiative (SMI). Anemia is a significant problem that can be addressed by the SMI. (*Data from* National Mortality Burden Estimates for 2001, Ministry of Health, Dar-es-Salaam, Tanzania. 2001. Available at: http://research.ncl.ac.uk/ammp/site_files/public_html/nationalest2001.pdf.)

acquired immunity to specific malarial antigens that mediate adherence of infected cells to the placenta.

Diagnosis of malaria in pregnancy is difficult because the peripheral parasitemia may be low, even if placental vessels are heavily parasitized. Presumptive treatment of malaria is recommended for all severely anemic women exposed to malaria.[13] Furthermore, most countries in Africa recommend intermittent treatment of malaria during pregnancy and in infants.[18]

Iron Deficiency Anemia

Iron deficiency is the most common cause of anemia. This is more prevalent in pregnancy, particularly in multigravida women because iron stores are depleted by successive confinements. The treatment of IDA and supplementation of pregnant women to avoid iron deficiency is part of the recommended maternal and child health services.[19] Given the links between pregnancy and malaria, presumptive treatment of malaria and/or intermittent preventive treatment of malaria is central to effective antenatal care.

Supplementation with folic acid (5 mg/d) and ferrous sulfate (200 mg/d) and antimalarial prophylaxis form the backbone of treatment of malarial anemia in pregnancy. If maternal anemia is corrected at least 6 months before delivery, nearly normal neonatal outcomes ensue.[20]

Hyperreactive Malarial Splenomegaly

Hyperreactive malarial splenomegaly (HMS) is characterized by chronic splenomegaly greater than 10 cm below the costal margin, elevated IgM (>2 SD above the mean), high titers of antimalarial antibodies, and lymphocytic infiltration of hepatic sinusoids.[21] Treatment requires a curative course of chemotherapy for malaria and lifelong antimalarial prophylaxis. Splenectomy carries significant immediate perioperative and long-term infective risks and is not recommended.

Inherited Red Cell Disorders

The care and management of SCD dominate acute and chronic hematological diseases seen in Africa, but the distribution and severity of disease vary considerably. The disease distribution severity depends on the co-inheritance of ameliorating α^+-thalassemia traits (in homozygous or heterozygous forms), the beta-globin haplotype, and other as-yet poorly characterized genetic and possibly environmental differences.

The level of fetal hemoglobin (HbF) has a substantial outcome on reducing the severity of disease. Polymorphisms at several loci are known to raise HbF, including genetic variants at 3 major genetic loci: Xmn1-HBG2, HMIP-2, and BCL11A. Recently, the influence of variants at these loci on the phenotype of SCD in Africa was shown in Tanzania, Cameroon, and Benin.[22–24] The presence of the T allele at Xmn1-HBG2 led to a significant increase in hemoglobin ($P = 9.8 \times 10[-3]$); the BCL11A variant (rs11886868-'C') increases hemoglobin ($P = 2 \times 10[-3]$); and one of the HBS1L-MYB variants decreases white blood cell count values selectively ($P = 2.3 \times 10[-4]$). The distinct pattern of effects of each variant suggests that disease alleviation may occur, not only through increased HbF production, but also by indirect effects on blood cells through a variety of pathways.[23]

The hemoglobin C allele is common in the Sahel region of West Africa and people with hemoglobin C disease (HbCC) and HbS hemoglobins present with chronic hemolytic anemia with a mild form of SCD with a marked predisposition to exacerbations during pregnancy (**Box 1**).

Box 1
Features of hemoglobin C disease

- Homozygous HbCC causes mild hemolytic anemia.
- Steady state hemoglobin varies between 100 g/L and 120 g/L.
- Hemoglobin levels may fall to 90 g/L to 100 g/L in pregnancy.
- Folate deficiency may be severe.
- Iron deficiency is not uncommon.
- Peripheral blood shows target cells and microspheres.
- HbCC is readily diagnosed by mobility of a hemogolobin equivalent to hemoglobin A_2 on alkaline hemoglobin electrophoresis.

α^+-Thalassemia trait in Africa is almost always due to the 1 gene deletion and even when inherited as a homozygous α^+-thalassemia causes only mild asymptomatic microcytic anemia.

Sickle Cell Disease

The principal pathology and management of SCD is discussed elsewhere (see Thomas Williams: Sickle Cell Disease in Sub-Saharan Africa, in this issue). Rather than review the well-described clinical features, the focus in this article is on key factors that enhance the care of SCD in Africa.

First, newborn screening (NBS) for SCD would allow early prophylaxis and vaccination to prevent infection and prompt diagnosis and treatment of crises when children present to hospital. Reports from high-income countries have reported a 70% reduction in mortality in the 0- to 3-year age group that is thought to be a result of NBS and comprehensive care.[25,26] Because most African countries do not have NBS for SCD as part of national health care program, this has been highlighted as a priority intervention to improve childhood survival in SCD.[27,28]

Laboratory investigations for confirmation of diagnosis for SCD are not available in most hospitals in Africa. Therefore, efforts are being made to strengthen the diagnostic facilities in secondary and tertiary hospitals, particularly in areas with high prevalence of disease. NBS for SCD is being done using isoelectronic focusing or high-performance liquid chromatography to detect HbS. Due to the high prevalence of SCD in Africa and the absence of NBS for SCD in many countries, there is a strong justification for rapid diagnostic tests to detect hemoglobin variants by the bedside or at least at the point of care. There are increasing efforts being made to develop rapid point-of-care diagnostic tests[29,30] and if protein-based or DNA-based assays cost less than $1, mass screening would be cost-effective.[31]

The provision of comprehensive care for SCD has been found effective in reducing morbidity and mortality, and many African counties have been able to establish SCD services.[25,32] Although the management of SCD requires a broad range of skilled specialist services, a minimum set of interventions can be introduced and provided at primary and secondary health care facilities.[27] As such, the strategy in some African countries has been to develop SCD services as part of a package of noncommunicable disease services, for example, in Tanzania.[33] This addresses the challenge that is faced by regional hospitals, and developing guidelines, training and staff to reach across the smaller towns and rural areas will require thoughtful and targeted training of clinical and laboratory staff. Such services will have to be delivered by nonspecialist medical or dedicated, trained nursing staff. Reaching out to spread SCD services across countries is a challenging, but achievable, goal.

Realizing these possibilities requires considerable raising of public awareness to promote such services. Public awareness of the nature of this inherited disease as a chance event and the treatable conditions associated with SCD will allow increased sympathy for patients and their families and allocation of more resources targeted at the diagnosis and care of patients with SCD. SCD societies exist in many countries and SCD awareness events are promoted across Africa. Support for patient societies can catalyze the allocation of resources and increase public awareness for SCD and should be an important aspect of hematological work.

Recent advances in the care of SCD include the use of hydroxyurea and long-term transfusion.[34] Although there are barriers to implementing these strategies in Africa, there is increasing evidence that these interventions can be introduced.[35–37] Most African countries should be able to provide penicillin prophylaxis for SCD in children under age 5.[28]

There is increasing use of hydroxyurea for management of SCD in Africa.[37,38] Extension of guidelines in North America or Europe suggests that chronic, if not lifelong, hydroxyurea would benefit patients with 1 life-threatening episode of complication of SCD or frequent hospitalizations with less severe disease. The safety and monitoring of patients on hydroxyurea have not been established in Africa. There are issues with compliance, cost and the increased incidence of invasive bacterial disease and malaria in African countries. Baseline data for such policy decisions, however, may soon be forthcoming, because several SCD centers have started to evaluate the use of hydroxyurea as well as beginning clinical trials.[39] The cost of hydroxyurea at $0.66 per day is expensive when this is a high proportion of daily family income. Bulk purchases and international support could, however, overcome these problems, as has been proved for support for HIV, tuberculosis and malaria treatment by the Global Fund.

Chronic transfusion therapy for primary or secondary prevention of stroke is well established. It is possible that such therapy may be extended if the recent trials that demonstrated a reduction in silent infarcts by chronic transfusion therapy is confirmed. The implications of such transfusion therapy are considerable. These regimes require not only an adequate supply of blood but also sophisticated grouping, antibody screening, and identification and extended donor and recipient screening to reduce or manage alloimmunization after multiple transfusions. Developing transfusion services is a high priority because few centers at present could cope with such chronic transfusion regimes. Nevertheless, developing a program for the management of acute crises is essential.

The development of long-term hydroxyurea programs and transfusion therapy will require an extensive and robust evidence base from Africa and a wider health economic analysis.

With survival in SCD, the number of women with SCD requiring obstetric services is increasing. This is critical, because evidence shows that pregnancy in SCD is associated with poor fetal and maternal outcome.[40,41] Further aspects of the obstetric care and treatment of the crises have been thoroughly reviewed, but specific guidance on key clinical scenarios have been given to highlight the salient parts in the management of sickle cell patients.

It is particularly evident when reviewing these guidelines that good clinical care depends on a wide range of services. Establishing, training and managing such teams at larger and at smaller hospital centers is critical.

Nutritional Anemia

Iron, folate, and vitamin B_{12} deficiency are common in Africa and the diagnosis and treatment are often straightforward.

Iron Deficiency Anemia

The high prevalence of iron deficiency is due to several interacting factors. Diets are poor in iron, particularly in those in poverty who eat little animal protein; demand for iron is increased in infancy, in adolescence, and by menstruation and pregnancy, especially after multiple and/or closely spaced births. Iron loss may be increased by hookworm, schistosomiasis, *Schistosoma haematobium*, and *Schistosoma mansoni* in their respective geographic distributions. Finally, infection (in particular malaria) may contribute to raised hepcidin levels as part of a broad protective acute-phase response, which unfortunately also restricts iron absorption and mobilization of iron to developing erythroid cells. In many African countries, hookworm is considered the most common cause of IDA in children. Therefore, antihelminthic agents, such as mebendazole, are routinely prescribed for presumptive treatment.

The side effects of iron deficiency are not limited to anemia and fatigue but include impaired concentration, memory and attention. These neurocognitive effects are of great importance and one of many reasons for a focus on providing iron supplements to children on a large scale. In addition, there is increasing evidence that iron deficiency can cause heart failure, even in the absence of anemia.[3]

The physiology of iron absorption and its diagnosis and management has been described elsewhere (see Pasricha, Drakesmith: Iron Deficiency Anemia – Problems in Diagnosis and Prevention at the Population Level, in this issue). Pivotal trials in Africa, however, have shown increased overall mortality in a community-wide iron supplementation trial in young children in Pemba, Tanzania.[42] It seems that iron, particularly when given to non–iron-deficient children, remains unabsorbed and can be predisposed to increased bacterial infection, hospitalization, and mortality, possibly through alteration of the microbiome and promotion of pathogenic strains of commensal organisms.[43] Moreover, iron deficiency may be protective from malaria infection,[44,45] and the reticulocytosis in iron-deficient children receiving iron supplementation may increase malarial parasitemia.[46]

The diagnosis of IDA in most African countries is challenging. Iron studies, such as serum iron, serum ferritin, transferrin saturation, and total iron-binding capacity, are not available in most facilities and when available, are expensive. Serum ferritin is the test that is the most available but its value is limited in individuals who have evidence of infection and inflammation because it is an acute-phase protein. As a consequence, the diagnosis of IDA is often made on the basis of a microcytic, hypochromic anemia.

Management of IDA is with oral formulations, although parenteral iron is used in the third trimester of pregnancy when rapid repletion of iron stores is required. Due to the high prevalence of iron and folate deficiency anemia, pregnant women are empirically prescribed supplementation.[47]

After the risk of adverse outcomes after iron supplementation became clear, the WHO issued additional guidance that "caution (for iron and folate supplementation) should be exercised in settings where the prevalence of malaria and other infectious diseases is high."[48] Evidence-based guidance for the optimal rate and route of community-wide iron supplementation remains, however, unclear, in spite of widespread implementation of micronutrient powders that include iron.

Folate Deficiency

Active forms of folic acid form an essential component of 1-carbon metabolism that, among other things, is required for the conversion of uridine to thymidine for DNA synthesis and for the conversion of homocysteine to methionine.

Although many foods, in particular leaves (*folium* is Latin for leaf), contain folic acid, it is easily destroyed by cooking, and body stores are not at all extensive, only sufficient for 3 to 6 weeks' supply. Folate deficiency can, therefore, develop rapidly and be profound. Folate deficiency is commonly increased when cell turnover is enhanced, such as in hemolytic anemia and pregnancy and for much of normal development.

The diagnosis of folate deficiency is relatively easy, recognized by the features of macrocytic, megaloblastic anemia that may be accompanied by pancytopenia and mild hemolysis. There are challenges, however, with diagnosis in African countries where there may be mixed microcytic and macrocytic anemia due to iron deficiency and folate deficiency, respectively. In this instance, the red cell distribution width, which gives an indication of the heterogeneity of cell size, is a useful parameter. In the absence of red cell distribution width, which is available from most automated hematology analyzers, a blood film is used in the diagnosis, where the presence of hypersegmented neutrophils form a prominent part of the blood morphology in this condition. The measurement of serum or red cell folate is available in some African countries, but only in tertiary care hospitals, and is limited by the cost.

The management of folate deficiency is oral folic acid, given 5 mg per day. This is available and accessible in most African countries. Oral chemoprophylaxis for prevention of folate deficiency is recommended in neonates, in pregnant women and for chronic hemolytic anemia, such as SCD. In South Africa, co-ordination of cereal production has allowed straightforward fortification of maize flour. Such community-wide action may reduce neural tube defects in children, particularly because high levels of folic acid are required in the first trimester and, therefore, not amenable to improvement through attendance at antenatal clinics after the first trimester. Folate deficiency can also cause intrauterine growth retardation, prematurity and low birthweight.

Vitamin B₁₂ Deficiency

Vitamin B_{12} deficiency is as common as folic acid deficiency.[49] There is an overlap of the function of vitamin B_{12} with folate in 1-carbon metabolism, thus the similarity of the clinical hematological syndromes. Vitamin B_{12} is also needed, however, for myelination and is so severe that vitamin B_{12} deficiency may present with subacute combined degeneration of the spinal cord.

Vitamin B_{12} deficiency is not usually caused by dietary insufficiency but usually by autoimmune disease, leading to impairment of the absorption of vitamin B_{12} by the intrinsic fact or chronic inflammation in the bowel. The diagnosis of vitamin B_{12} deficiency often relies on clinical features, macrocytic hypochromic red cell indices and a megaloblastic blood film. As with diagnosis of folate deficiency, the laboratory tests for vitamin B_{12} are not easily available due to access and costs. Management of vitamin B_{12} deficiency is with parenteral injections. Although most hospitals do not have this available, it is readily available in private pharmacies.

BONE MARROW DEPRESSION OR APLASIA

Infection or inflammation may be a cause of a variety of cytopenias. Infections, including malaria, HIV, hepatitis B or C, and parvovirus B19, may cause acute profound cytopenias, whereas chronic infection and inflammation, such as that found in tuberculosis, may result in a chronic cytopenia. Disseminated infections, such as tuberculosis, or parasitic infections, such as leishmaniasis, can cause infiltration and fibrosis of the bone marrow, resulting in cytopenia.[50–52]

In Africa, most children are infected early in life with parvovirus B19. The virus binds to the P blood group carbohydrate antigen and enters and multiplies in developing erythroid cells. It, therefore, causes transient hypoplasia and precipitates acute anemia in those children with a previously compensated hemolytic anemia most commonly due to SCD. In immunocompromised patients, parvovirus infection can cause profound pancytopenia.[53]

The management of cytopenias is challenging in Africa. Intrinsic bone marrow failure is a diagnosis of exclusion, and it is a challenge to make this diagnosis in Africa where there are limitations in diagnostic capacity. In hospitals where investigations are available, diagnosis is often made by reduced reticulocyte count and cytopenia on bone marrow examination. Symptomatic treatment of cytopenias is made with transfusion of the appropriate blood components. Immunosuppression therapy is given with steroids and in some centers cyclosporine is prescribed, but most centers do not have antithymocyte globulin, which is currently recommended for management of aplastic anemia.[54]

WHITE BLOOD CELL DISORDERS

Normal ranges for white blood cell counts vary with age and in pregnancy and may be different in African populations compared with North American and European populations, due to both genetic and environmental factors. The markedly lower neutrophil count in Africans is due, at least in part, to the low or absent expression of the interleukin-8 chemokine receptor that carries the Duffy blood group antigen.[55]

Eosinophilia is common in African populations and the normal range in adults is considerably wider than in European populations, almost certainly a reflection of widespread helminth infections in the community. The difference in normal ranges behooves all laboratories to develop their own reference ranges for different age groups using randomly selected, healthy members of the local community. In adults, blood donors may provide a suitable source of samples.

The common causes of leukocytosis and leukopenia in Africans have been well described. HIV remains an important cause of neutropenia and lymphopenia and should be excluded as a cause in the first line of investigation of any cytopenia.[53]

Malignant White Cell Disorders

Acute lymphoblastic anemia (ALL), acute myeloid leukemia and the chronic myeloid and lymphatic leukemias (CMLs) all occur in Africa, although almost certainly the incidence of these diseases is underestimated because diagnosis requires some degree of hematological expertise.

Published literature suggests that the incidence of ALL is much less in Africa than in Europe and is only less than $1/10^6$ per year compared with approximately $10/10^6$ per year in a recent survey in the United Kingdom. This may be due to environmental factors and gives a tantalizing clue to the etiology of this malignancy. Good protocols for the treatment of ALL are used across the specialist hematology and oncology services in Africa.

A tiered system of chemotherapy allowing greater intensity of treatment in relation to the predicted severity of the disease and the resources available has been developed. This is a wonderful model for the development of cost-effective and medically effective protocols, and these initiatives are likely to be replicated (for further discussion, see Lehmann L, El-Haddad A, Barr RD: Global Approach to Hematologic Malignancies, in this issue).

Comprehensive treatment of hematological malignancies requires a range of supportive medical, nursing care and laboratory facilities. Medical and nursing expenditure is provided at specialist centers and laboratory techniques for diagnostics can be effectively centralized or even outsourced (eg, in diagnosis of the bcr-abl mutation for diagnosis of CML).

The most pressing needs across all medical services, however, are to strengthen diagnostic facilities and provide quality care that needs to be accompanied by good palliative care. Sympathetic care and pain relief are essential components of humane medical care. The evidence is that palliative care has been given a low priority in the face of pressures of acute illness and urgent preventive measures. Recent initiatives, however, have addressed establishing and supporting these services.

Chronic Myeloid Leukemia

A diagnosis of CML is easily made in Africa from the clinical presentation, high white blood cell count, and morphology on blood film and bone marrow examination. Management is with hydroxyurea or busulphan, which are agents used to maintain low white blood cell counts. The treatment with imatinib (Glivec), however, a specific bcr-abl tyrosine kinase inhibitor, has a selective effect on proliferation of CML blasts and provides prolonged disease survival and possibly even cure. It is now provided pro bono by the Glivec International Patient Assistance Program (http://www.themaxfoundation.org/gipap/Default.aspx), if a patient has a confirmed molecular diagnosis. The challenge in many African countries is laboratory confirmation of the molecular diagnosis.

Chronic Lymphocytic Leukemia

CLL is common in Africa and presents with a bimodal distribution, more common in women under the age of 45, but more common in men over the age of 45. Prolonged exposure to malaria may predispose to B-cell proliferation, which can develop into HMS or predispose to CLL. The pathology of development of CLL on the background of malaria and/or HMS is not well established.[56]

The presentation of CLL is often an insidious onset of significant hepatosplenomegaly and lymphadenopathy in adults, although lymphadenopathy is not marked in children. Later anemia and bone marrow failure supervene. The course of the disease may be complicated by autoimmune hemolytic anemia and/or immune thrombocytopenic purpura. The high count of circulating mature lymphocytes with abundant smear cells is well described. CLL is pathologically distinguished from HMS with lymphocytosis by the blood film morphology and characteristic high antimalarial antibodies in HMS. Age less than 40 years, however, and absolute lymphocyte count ($<10 \times 10^9$/L) are the only useful and widely available discriminators for distinguishing patients with HMS from those with lymphoproliferative disorders.[56]

The treatment of CLL is with alkylating agents (chlorambucil) or hydroxyurea and also prednisolone to reduce symptomatic lymphadenopathy and to treat autoimmune hemolytic anemia or immune thrombocytopenic purpura. Antimalarial prophylaxis may improve anemia and reduce the size of the spleen.[57]

Adult T-Cell Leukemia and Lymphoma

Human T-lymphotropic virus 1 (HTLV-1) is common in some parts of Africa and may reach a seroprevalence of 10% to 15% in West Central Africa and 5% elsewhere in West Africa. There are other clusters of high seroprevalence of up to 3% to 4% in South Africa.[58] Transmission of the virus occurs by sexual contact, BT, or contaminated needles after intravenous drug abuse. It is more common in sex workers where it is often associated with HIV-1 and HIV-2.[59]

People carrying HTLV-1 carry a lifetime risk of adult T-cell leukemia of 5% if infected in childhood, although the disease may take decades to develop. Carriers may also develop tropical spastic paraparesis and be at increased risk of opportunistic parasitic infections, such as *Strongyloides* spp. Adult T-cell leukemia/lymphoma may present as a leukemia or lymphoma with lymphadenopathy, hepatosplenomegaly, skin lesions, and potentially life-threatening hypocalcemia. There may also be extensive osteolysis and central nervous system involvement. Seropositive patients developing the disease usually have a white blood cell count of 30 to 120 × 10^9/L with the characteristic morphology of polylobulated lymphocytes. The lymph node histology resembles a diffuse non-Hodgkin lymphoma with CD4$^+$ and is probably commonly misdiagnosed as a non-Burkitt non-Hodgkin lymphoma.[60]

Treatment is difficult and prevention of infections may provide some relief. Mother-to-child transmission may be largely prevented by avoiding breastfeeding and limited to a transmission risk of less than 5% if breastfeeding is less than 6 months' duration. Blood donors should be tested for HTLV-1 and seropositive donors should be excluded.

PLATELET DISORDERS

The normal reference ranges for platelets are lower in adult African populations than in European populations, typically 70 to 170 × 10^9/L.[61] It seems this is environmentally determined. Platelet aggregation may also be weaker in Africa, although it is unclear if this is an effect of plasma or platelet differences.[61,62] Fibrinogen levels, factor VIII, and factor VIII–related antigens and fibrinolysis are higher and the platelet count and ristocetin-induced aggregation of platelets are lower in Africans.[62] Establishing local reference ranges is crucial for laboratory tests where these assays are available.

Thrombocytopenia may accompany many other viral and also bacterial infections and is an outstanding feature of malaria infection. Immune thrombocytopenia is well described in African populations[61,63] and low platelets may also be caused by a variety of herbal remedies.

Vascular Purpura

Vascular purpuras may occur through a variety of causes in Africa. Viral hemorrhagic fevers can cause hemostatic problems and Lassa fever virus can cause platelet dysfunction and consumption. Ebola and Marburg viruses cause hepatic failure, thrombocytopenia and disseminated intravascular coagulation (DIC), secondary to both reduce production and increase consumption of clotting factors.

A specific form of thrombocytopenia associated with florid blood blisters is known as *onyalai*, described in southern Angola and northern Namibia. It seems common, with an incidence of 50/10^5 per year, although the cause is unclear. It has been suggested this is due to fungal contamination of millet. Extensive hemorrhagic bullae may present all over the body.[64] The mortality associated with this mystifying illness without treatment is as high as 10%. It has been treated with supportive care and blood and platelet transfusion and splenectomy. More promising results have been seen with high-dose methylprednisolone.[65]

HEMOSTASIS AND THROMBOSIS
Coagulopathies

Acquired disorders of coagulation dominate hematological practice but present considerable difficulties in their management without specialized blood products. DIC may follow a wide variety of systemic infections or insults and cause massive uncontrolled consumption of clotting factors, leading to prolonged clotting times and clinically to widespread bleeding. DIC is recognized by the failure of blood to clot and prolongation of the prothrombin time (PT), activated partial thromboplastin time (APTT) and thrombin time (TT), with reduced fibrinogen and high products of fibrin degradation.

The treatment is principally by reversal of the cause of disturbed coagulation and supported as far as possible by fresh frozen plasma, cryoprecipitate and platelet transfusion to restore normal clotting parameters and maintain fibrinogen greater than 1 g/L and platelets to greater than 50×10^9/L or greater.[66]

Thromboembolic Disease

Deep vein thrombosis (DVT) is increasingly recognized in African countries, and the approach has been to exclude etiologic or risk factors associated with DVTs reported from Western settings. There is limited knowledge on whether these factors have different prevalence and impact in African settings.

The diagnosis of DVTs in the lower limb can be made in most specialized hospitals using Doppler ultrasonography and sometimes venograms. The diagnosis of pulmonary embolism remains, however, a challenge. Laboratory tests to confirm DVTs and to monitor response to treatment are only available in a few specialist hospitals.

Anticoagulation Therapy

The management of individuals who require anticoagulation therapy is often the responsibility of hematology. A majority of individuals requiring anticoagulation therapy are those with prosthetic heart valves. Management is with oral warfarin.

The other common indication for anticoagulation therapy is thromboembolic disease, frequently presenting with DVT. Intravenous heparin is available and there is increasing availability of low-molecular-weight heparin in the market.

Snake Bite

Several venomous snakes have poisons that activate coagulation and represent a significant public health hazard, particularly in rural areas. *Echis ocellatus* (carpet viper) and *Dispholidus typus* (boomslang) are found north and south of the equator, respectively, and the venoms from these snakes may cause widespread activation and ultimately failure of the coagulation system.[67–69] *Naja* spp (cobras) and *Bitis arietans* (puff adder) also have poisons that may indirectly disturb the hemostasis. *E ocellatus* (carpet viper) represents a significant proportion of fatal snake bites a year in Africa and specific antivenoms may significantly reduce morbidity and mortality.[70]

Low Prothrombin and Vitamin K–Dependent Coagulation Factors

Vitamin K is essential for α-hydroxylation of glutamate residues in the modification of factors II, VII, IX, and X and the antithrombotic factors, proteins C and S. Acquired deficiency of the factors follows hepatic failure or vitamin K deficiency or the use or potentiation of warfarin or other coumarin anticoagulants.

Vitamin K deficiency is frequently seen in neonates and newborns who have low vitamin K levels of half that of adults. Vitamin K levels increase as the gut is colonized. Hemorrhagic disease of the newborn is thought common in Africa and may be associated with prematurity or maternal antituberculosis treatment. It can present early in the neonatal period or later in breastfed children treated with antibiotics at 1 to 3 months of age.[71] Bleeding can occur in the skin, mucous membranes, or gastrointestinal tract; at the umbilical stump; or after circumcision.[72] Intracranial bleeds may be fatal. Diagnosis is straightforward because the PT is prolonged whereas other coagulation tests are normal.

The disease is treated by vitamin K, 10 mg or 5 mg in children weighing less than 2500 g, and the response may be seen within 30 minutes.[72] It is prevented by vitamin K, 1 g intramuscularly, to newborn children.[73] Oral prophylaxis at birth with lipid-soluble forms of vitamin K may prevent late-onset hemorrhagic disease. The epidemiology of hemorrhagic disease of the newborn in Africa is poorly documented but a survey of biochemical evidence of vitamin K deficiency by measuring undercarboxy-lated prothrombin (PIVKA-II) showed severely reduced vitamin K may occur in up to 20% of newborns.[74] Programs for administration of routine vitamin K are not well formulated in Africa, but further study of the cost-effectiveness and efficacy of such a simple public health measure may be worthwhile.

Hemophilia

Hemophilia A (factor VIII deficiency) and hemophilia B (factor IX deficiency) are believed to have the same incidence in African as in European populations, but there is good evidence that both are grossly underdiagnosed.[75,76] It is likely that many children with severe hemophilia die before diagnosis is made and specific treatment instituted. Hemorrhage after circumcision and intracranial bleeding are common presentations, whereas repeated joint bleeds lead to substantial deformity and disability.

The APTT is prolonged, but specific factor assays are required for definitive diagnosis and are rarely available. More than 80% of individuals with hemophilia in the world are in low-income and middle-income countries and only rarely have access to modern therapy and comprehensive care.[66]

Transfusion services can provide cryoprecipitate if they have a refrigerated centrifuge and adequate cold storage. Cryoprecipitate can provide factor VIII for treatment of hemophilia but must be supplied from HIV-screened, hepatitis B–screened and hepatitis C–screened donors.[77] Nevertheless, hepatitis B vaccination should be given to all groups of patients likely to have repeated exposure to blood products. Viral inactivation methods should be applied if possible to prepare fresh frozen plasma.

The World Federation of Hemophilia has recommended the use of viral inactivated and/or recombinant factors VIII and IX, although it is not apparent what level of subsidy or resource could be provided for the administration of these products across Africa. Development of local capacity to develop more simple products may have wider benefits.

von Willebrand Disease

von Willebrand disease presents with a combination of epistaxis, prolonged wound bleeding and, in women, menorrhagia. Both bleeding time and APTT are usually prolonged and patients can be treated with desmopressin (DDAVP) (Ferring Pharmaceuticals (UK)) infusion to increase factor VIII–related antigen. More immediate and simple measures include local or systemic tranexamic acid to reduce fibrinolysis. Cryoprecipitate may be given for severe bleeding.

BLOOD TRANSFUSION

In Africa, when blood is needed, it is often required urgently. Even in well-equipped and staffed units, delays in sourcing, preparing and cross-matching blood can be substantial and be many hours. This delay is sometimes associated with increased mortality.

There has been considerable improvement in blood transfusion services in many African countries. This has been mainly due to investment by governments to improve blood safety after the HIV epidemic. Enormous efforts have been made to ensure blood safety is optimal in Africa in the face of significant HIV and hepatitis B carriage in donors.

In many countries, the rapid supply of adequate volumes of blood remains a pressing problem. The initial approach taken to improve blood donation was to motivate and encourage voluntary, regular, nonremunerated blood donors and to discourage replacement blood donors. There have been challenges, however, with this strategy and the current approach is to encourage replacement donors to become regular donors.

With improvement in diagnosis of hematological disorders, there is a change in the requirements to transfusion services. The management of stroke in SCD is with chronic transfusion, which requires adequate volumes of blood as well as exchange transfusion. In addition, the challenges of alloimmunization and iron overload need to be addressed. There is every reason to believe that these challenges will be addressed and, through partnerships, that there will be an improvement in transfusion services in Africa.

SUMMARY

This review of hematology in Africa highlights areas of current practice and the immediate needs for development and clinical research. There are many areas of medical practice where straightforward measures would result in better outcomes for patients. There is also an urgent need for good clinical research to describe the epidemiology, natural history and management of hematological diseases in Africa. Developing hematological practice requires all the efforts of a new generation of hematologists who are now beginning to practice. The gains for patient welfare are considerable and it can only be hoped that a new era of medicine will soon be ushered into Africa.

REFERENCES

1. WHO. The global anaemia prevalence in 2011. Geneva (Switzerland): World Health Organization; 2015.
2. Calis JC, Phiri KS, Faragher EB, et al. Severe anemia in Malawian children. N Engl J Med 2008;358(9):888–99.
3. Makubi A, Hage C, Lwakatare J, et al. Prevalence and prognostic implications of anaemia and iron deficiency in Tanzanian patients with heart failure. Heart 2015; 101(8):592–9.
4. Marsh K, Forster D, Waruiru C, et al. Indicators of life-threatening malaria in African children. N Engl J Med 1995;332(21):1399–404.
5. Menendez C, Kahigwa E, Hirt R, et al. Randomised placebo-controlled trial of iron supplementation and malaria chemoprophylaxis for prevention of severe anaemia and malaria in Tanzanian infants. Lancet 1997;350(9081):844–50.
6. Snow RW, Omumbo JA, Lowe B, et al. Relation between severe malaria morbidity in children and level of Plasmodium falciparum transmission in Africa. Lancet 1997;349(9066):1650–4.
7. WHO. Guidelines for the treatment of Malaria. Geneva (Switzerland): World Health Organization; 2015.
8. Komba AN, Makani J, Sadarangani M, et al. Malaria as a cause of morbidity and mortality in children with homozygous sickle cell disease on the coast of Kenya. Clin Infect Dis 2009;49(2):216–22.
9. Makani J, Komba AN, Cox SE, et al. Malaria in patients with sickle cell anemia: burden, risk factors, and outcome at the outpatient clinic and during hospitalization. Blood 2010;115(2):215–20.
10. McAuley CF, Webb C, Makani J, et al. High mortality from Plasmodium falciparum malaria in children living with sickle cell anemia on the coast of Kenya. Blood 2010;116(10):1663–8.

11. Allison AC. Protection afforded by sickle-cell trait against subtertian malareal infection. Br Med J 1954;4857:290–4.

12. Aidoo M, Terlouw DJ, Kolczak MS, et al. Protective effects of the sickle cell gene against malaria morbidity and mortality. Lancet 2002;359(9314):1311–2.

13. Shulman CE, Dorman EK, Bulmer JN. Malaria as a cause of severe anaemia in pregnancy. Lancet 2002;360(9331):494.

14. Menendez C, Todd J, Alonso PL, et al. The response to iron supplementation of pregnant women with the haemoglobin genotype AA or AS. Trans R Soc Trop Med Hyg 1995;89(3):289–92.

15. Rogerson SJ, Hviid L, Duffy PE, et al. Malaria in pregnancy: pathogenesis and immunity. Lancet Infect Dis 2007;7(2):105–17.

16. Fried M, Duffy PE. Designing a VAR2CSA-based vaccine to prevent placental malaria. Vaccine 2015;33(52):7483–8. [Epub ahead of print].

17. Diagne N, Rogier C, Sokhna CS, et al. Increased susceptibility to malaria during the early postpartum period. N Engl J Med 2000;343(9):598–603.

18. Aponte JJ, Schellenberg D, Egan A, et al. Efficacy and safety of intermittent preventive treatment with sulfadoxine-pyrimethamine for malaria in African infants: a pooled analysis of six randomised, placebo-controlled trials. Lancet 2009; 374(9700):1533–42.

19. WHO. Essential nutrition actions: improving maternal, newborn, infant and young child health and nutrition. Geneva (Switzerland): World Health Organization; 2013.

20. Fleming AF. Tropical obstetrics and gynaecology. 1. Anaemia in pregnancy in tropical Africa. Trans R Soc Trop Med Hyg 1989;83(4):441–8.

21. Bryceson A, Fakunle YM, Fleming AF, et al. Malaria and splenomegaly. Trans R Soc Trop Med Hyg 1983;77(6):879.

22. Menzel S, Rooks H, Zelenika D, et al. Global genetic architecture of an erythroid quantitative trait locus, HMIP-2. Ann Hum Genet 2014;78(6):434–51.

23. Mtatiro SN, Singh T, Rooks H, et al. Genome wide association study of fetal hemoglobin in sickle cell anemia in Tanzania. PLoS One 2014;9(11):e111464.

24. Bitoungui VJ, Ngogang J, Wonkam A. Polymorphism at BCL11A compared to HBS1L-MYB loci explains less of the variance in HbF in patients with sickle cell disease in Cameroon. Blood Cells Mol Dis 2015;54(3):268–9.

25. Rahimy MC, Gangbo A, Ahouignan G, et al. Effect of a comprehensive clinical care program on disease course in severely ill children with sickle cell anemia in a sub-Saharan African setting. Blood 2003;102(3):834–8.

26. Yanni E, Grosse SD, Yang Q, et al. Trends in pediatric sickle cell disease-related mortality in the United States, 1983-2002. J Pediatr 2009;154(4):541–5.

27. WHO. Sickle cell disease: a strategy for the WHO African region. 2010. Available at: http://www.who.int/mediacentre/factsheets/fs308/en/. Accessed October 20, 2015.

28. Makani J, Soka D, Rwezaula S, et al. Health policy for sickle cell disease in Africa: experience from Tanzania on interventions to reduce under-five mortality. Trop Med Int Health 2015;20(2):184–7.

29. Kumar AA, Patton MR, Hennek JW, et al. Density-based separation in multiphase systems provides a simple method to identify sickle cell disease. Proc Natl Acad Sci U S A 2014;111(41):14864–9.

30. Kanter J, Telen MJ, Hoppe C, et al. Validation of a novel point of care testing device for sickle cell disease. BMC Med 2015;13:225.

31. Williams TN. An accurate and affordable test for the rapid diagnosis of sickle cell disease could revolutionize the outlook for affected children born in resource-limited settings. BMC Med 2015;13:238.

32. Galadanci N, Wudil BJ, Balogun TM, et al. Current sickle cell disease management practices in Nigeria. Int Health 2014;6(1):23–8.

33. Ministry of Health and Social Welfare. National Strategy for Non-Communicable Diseases 2009-2015. Division of Preventative Health Services, Tanzania Food and Nutrition Centre: Government publication; 2009.

34. Yawn BP, Buchanan GR, Afenyi-Annan AN, et al. Management of sickle cell disease: summary of the 2014 evidence-based report by expert panel members. JAMA 2014;312(10):1033–48.

35. De Montalembert M, Tshilolo L. Is therapeutic progress in the management of sickle cell disease applicable in sub-Saharan Africa? Med Trop (Mars) 2007; 67(6):612–6 [in French].

36. Tshilolo L, Kafando E, Sawadogo M, et al. Neonatal screening and clinical care programmes for sickle cell disorders in sub-Saharan Africa: lessons from pilot studies. Public Health 2008;122(9):933–41.

37. Lagunju I, Brown BJ, Sodeinde O. Hydroxyurea lowers transcranial Doppler flow velocities in children with sickle cell anaemia in a Nigerian cohort. Pediatr Blood Cancer 2015;62(9):1587–91.

38. Obaro SK. Hydroxyurea for sickle-cell anaemia in Africa: mind the gap. Lancet Glob Health 2015;3(3):e124–5.

39. McGann PT, Tshilolo L, Santos B, et al. Hydroxyurea therapy for children with sickle cell anemia in sub-Saharan Africa: rationale and design of the REACH trial. Pediatr Blood Cancer 2016;63:98–104.

40. Muganyizi PS, Kidanto H. Sickle cell disease in pregnancy: trend and pregnancy outcomes at a tertiary hospital in Tanzania. PLoS One 2013;8(2):e56541.

41. Alayed N, Kezouh A, Oddy L, et al. Sickle cell disease and pregnancy outcomes: population-based study on 8.8 million births. J Perinat Med 2014;42(4):487–92.

42. Sazawal S, Black RE, Ramsan M, et al. Effects of routine prophylactic supplementation with iron and folic acid on admission to hospital and mortality in preschool children in a high malaria transmission setting: community-based, randomised, placebo-controlled trial. Lancet 2006;367(9505):133–43.

43. Jaeggi T, Kortman GA, Moretti D, et al. Iron fortification adversely affects the gut microbiome, increases pathogen abundance and induces intestinal inflammation in Kenyan infants. Gut 2015;64(5):731–42.

44. Jonker FA, Calis JC, van Hensbroek MB, et al. Iron status predicts malaria risk in Malawian preschool children. PLoS One 2012;7(8):e42670.

45. Gwamaka M, Kurtis JD, Sorensen BE, et al. Iron deficiency protects against severe Plasmodium falciparum malaria and death in young children. Clin Infect Dis 2012;54(8):1137–44.

46. Clark MA, Goheen MM, Fulford A, et al. Host iron status and iron supplementation mediate susceptibility to erythrocytic stage Plasmodium falciparum. Nat Commun 2014;5:4446.

47. Manzi F, Schellenberg J, Hamis Y, et al. Intermittent preventive treatment for malaria and anaemia control in Tanzanian infants; the development and implementation of a public health strategy. Trans R Soc Trop Med Hyg 2009;103(1): 79–86.

48. WHO. Iron supplementation of young children in regions where malaria transmission is intense and infectious disease highly prevalent. Geneva (Switzerland): World Health Organization; 2006.

49. Ingram CF, Fleming AF, Patel M, et al. Pregnancy- and lactation-related folate deficiency in South Africa–a case for folate food fortification. S Afr Med J 1999; 89(12):1279–84.

50. van Schalkwyk WA, Opie J, Novitzky N. The diagnostic utility of bone marrow biopsies performed for the investigation of fever and/or cytopenias in HIV-infected adults at *Groote Schuur Hospital, Western Cape, South Africa*. Int J Lab Hematol 2011;33(3):258–66.

51. Grewal R, Abayomi EA. Bone marrow morphological features and diagnostic value in paediatric disseminated tuberculosis in the setting of increased HIV prevalence. S Afr Med J 2013;103(5):326–9.

52. Silva JM, Zacarias DA, de Figueirêdo LC, et al. Bone marrow parasite burden among patients with New World kala-azar is associated with disease severity. Am J Trop Med Hyg 2014;90(4):621–6.

53. Bain BJ. The haematological features of HIV infection. Br J Haematol 1997;99(1): 1–8.

54. Scheinberg P, Young NS. How I treat acquired aplastic anemia. Blood 2012; 120(6):1185–96.

55. Thobakgale CF, Ndung'u T. Neutrophil counts in persons of African origin. Curr Opin Hematol 2014;21(1):50–7.

56. Bedu-Addo G, Bates I. Causes of massive tropical splenomegaly in Ghana. Lancet 2002;360(9331):449–54.

57. Fleming AF. Chronic lymphocytic leukaemia in tropical Africa: a review. Leuk Lymphoma 1990;1(3–4):169–73.

58. Bhigjee AI, Thaler D, Madurai S, et al. Seroprevalence of HTLV-I in Natal/KwaZulu. S Afr Med J 1994;84(6):368.

59. Weber T, Hunsmann G, Stevens W, et al. Human retroviruses. Baillieres Clin Haematol 1992;5(2):273–314.

60. Williams CK, Alexander SS, Bodner A, et al. Frequency of adult T-cell leukaemia/lymphoma and HTLV-I in Ibadan, Nigeria. Br J Cancer 1993;67(4):783–6.

61. Essien EM. Platelets and platelet disorders in Africa. Baillieres Clin Haematol 1992;5(2):441–56.

62. Dupuy E, Fleming AF, Caen JP. Platelet function, factor VIII, fibrinogen, and fibrinolysis in Nigerians and Europeans in relation to atheroma and thrombosis. J Clin Pathol 1978;31(11):1094–101.

63. Mukiibi JM. Autoimmune thrombocytopenic purpura (AITP) in Zimbabwe. Trop Geogr Med 1989;41(4):326–30.

64. Hesseling PB. Onyalai. Baillieres Clin Haematol 1992;5(2):457–73.

65. Hesseling PB, Smith S, Oosthuizen O, et al. High dose methylprednisolone therapy in children with onyalai. Ann Trop Paediatr 1994;14(3):239–43.

66. WHO/GPA, Global Blood Safety Initiative. Guidelines on the appropriate use of blood. Geneva (Switzerland): World Health Organization; 1989. p.18.

67. Habib AG, Gebi UI, Onyemelukwe GC. Snake bite in Nigeria. Afr J Med Med Sci 2001;30(3):171–8.

68. Weinstein SA, White J, Keyler DE, et al. Non-front-fanged colubroid snakes: a current evidence-based analysis of medical significance. Toxicon 2013;69:103–13.

69. Habib AG. Public health aspects of snakebite care in West Africa: perspectives from Nigeria. J Venom Anim Toxins Incl Trop Dis 2013;19(1):27.

70. Habib AG, Warrell DA. Antivenom therapy of carpet viper (Echis ocellatus) envenoming: effectiveness and strategies for delivery in *West Africa*. Toxicon 2013;69:82–9.

71. Elalfy MS, Elagouza IA, Ibrahim FA, et al. Intracranial haemorrhage is linked to late onset vitamin K deficiency in infants aged 2-24 weeks. Acta Paediatr 2014; 103(6):e273–6.

72. Plank RM, Steinmetz T, Sokal DC, et al. Vitamin K deficiency bleeding and early infant male circumcision in Africa. Obstet Gynecol 2013;122(2 Pt 2):503–5.

73. Canadian Agency for Drugs and Technologies in Health. Neonatal vitamin K administration for the prevention of hemorrhagic disease: a review of the clinical effectiveness, comparative effectiveness, and guideline. Ottawa (Canada): 2015.

74. Santorino D, Siedner MJ, Mwanga-Amumpaire J, et al. Prevalence and Predictors of Functional Vitamin K Insufficiency in Mothers and Newborns in Uganda. Nutrients 2015;7(10):8545–52.

75. Adewuyi JO, Coutts AM, Levy L, et al. Haemophilia care in Zimbabwe. Cent Afr J Med 1996;42(5):153–6.

76. WFH. WFH Annual Global Survey 2014. Québec, (Canada): World Federation of Hemophilia; 2014.

77. Lloyd S. The preparation of single donor cryoprecipitate. World Federation of Hemophilia; 2004.

Problems and Approaches for Blood Transfusion in the Developing Countries

David J. Roberts, DPhil, MRCP, FRCPath[a],*,
Stephen Field, MMed(Path) (SA), FCPath (SA)[b],
Meghan Delaney, DO, MPH[c], Imelda Bates, FRCP, FRCPath[d]

KEYWORDS

- Blood transfusion • Blood donor • Transfusion-transmitted infection • Use of blood

KEY POINTS

- In the last 5 years, nearly all African states had a national blood policy; but just more than half have been able to implement their policies.
- The main obstacles to implementation are a lack of trained staff, the high cost of blood in relation to the health care budgets and recruitment of donors. In the absence of centralized services, facilities rely on blood collected by hospitals from family or replacement donors.
- The high rate of chronic viral infections in the populations implies that the residual risk of infection of human immunodeficiency virus and hepatitis B infection remains substantial with enzyme immunoassay testing, but there is evidence that the residual risks for these infections are decreasing.
- Several initiatives are being trialed to improve the supply, safety and use of blood by encouraging repeat voluntary donors, developing systems that rely more on local resources, establishing international networks across Africa for research and education and improving clinical practice through guidelines and audits of the use of blood.

INTRODUCTION

Blood transfusion is life saving and life enhancing, not only directly in emergency situations and acute or chronic illness, but also in facilitating surgery and chemotherapy that would not be possible without blood components. In high-income countries, the

The authors have nothing to disclose.
[a] Department of Haematology, NHS Blood and Transplant, John Radcliffe Hospital, University of Oxford, Level 2, Oxford OX3 9BQ, UK; [b] Welsh Blood Service, Talbot Green, Pontyclun CF72 9WB, Wales, UK; [c] Department of Laboratory Medicine, Bloodworks NW, University of Washington, 921 Terry Avenue, Seattle 98102, WA 98102, USA; [d] International Public Health Department, Liverpool School of Tropical Medicine, Pembroke Place, Liverpool L3 5QA, UK
* Corresponding author.
E-mail address: david.roberts@ndcls.ox.ac.uk

Hematol Oncol Clin N Am 30 (2016) 477–495
http://dx.doi.org/10.1016/j.hoc.2015.11.011
0889-8588/16/$ – see front matter © 2016 Elsevier Inc. All rights reserved.

safety and availability of blood transfusion and the human and material resources to use blood are largely taken for granted. However, in many parts of the world the reliable supply of safe blood is far from secure.

For many reasons, blood has to be collected and used locally. It is far from being a simple medicinal product that can be ordered from a catalog. A blood transfusion for a child with malarial anemia or a woman with severe postpartum hemorrhage requires a complex social, technical, and medical infrastructure, including a pool of donors, organization of collection, testing processing of blood, and the clinical and laboratory skills to use blood. Given the complexity of this process, it is not perhaps so surprising that strengthening this chain is not a trivial exercise and by its very nature cannot be completely solved by addressing only one aspect of this process. Here, the authors examine the elements required for the most effective use of blood and how they are being developed across the world.

SAFETY AND SUPPLY

A safe supply of blood is an essential part of medical services. An unsafe blood supply is costly in both human and economic terms. Transfusion of infected blood not only causes direct morbidity and mortality, but also undermines confidence in modern health care. Those who become infected through blood transfusion may also contribute to a secondary wave of infections. Investment in safe supplies of blood is cost-effective for every country, even those with few resources. At the same time, an insufficient supply costs lives because severely anemic patients do not survive unless transfused.[1,2] Where should the priority be?

The shockwave of the human immunodeficiency virus (HIV) epidemics put overwhelming emphasis on blood safety, but now the supply of blood should take back its legitimate place as a priority. An adequate and sustainable blood supply would go a long way to reducing mortality in developing countries, especially among women and children.

The World Health Organization (WHO) has identified 4 key objectives for blood services to ensure that blood is safe for transfusion:

- Establish a coordinated national blood transfusion service that can provide adequate and timely supplies of safe blood for all patients in need.
- Collect blood only from voluntary nonremunerated blood donors from low-risk populations, and use stringent donor selection procedures.
- Screen all blood for transfusion-transmissible infections, and have standardized procedures in place for grouping and compatibility testing.
- Reduce unnecessary transfusions through the appropriate clinical use of blood, including the use of intravenous replacement fluids and other simple alternatives to transfusion, wherever possible.

The WHO also emphasizes that effective quality assurance should be in place for all aspects of the transfusion process, from donor recruitment and selection through to infection screening, blood grouping and blood storage to administration to patients and clinical monitoring for adverse events.[3]

BLOOD-BORNE INFECTIONS

Local blood transfusion services encounter many problems, including lack of funding, insufficient training, poor management, frequent failure in supply of reagents and consumables, and breakdown of the cold chain (mostly related to frequent power cuts). Since 2000, a lot of investment has gone into providing HIV, hepatitis

B surface antigen (HBsAg), and to some extent, hepatitis C virus (HCV) tests in Africa. In particular, there have been enormous efforts to ensure that blood collected in Africa is tested for HIV.

Blood-Borne Viral Infections

The overall prevalence of HIV antibody in sub-Saharan Africa ranges between 0.5% and 16.0%. In donors, it tends to remain less than 5% in West Africa, less than 10% in East and Central Africa and more than 10% in southern Africa.[4–7]

Chronic hepatitis B prevalence, as indicated by the presence of circulating HBsAg, ranges between 5% and 25% of the population, including blood donors. This high prevalence is due to (vertical) transmission at birth or (horizontal) infection in infancy and limited national vaccination programs, indeed infection after 10 years of age is uncommon. HBsAg is more prevalent in West Africa (10%–25%) than in East or Central Africa (5%–10%), whereas the lowest prevalence is found in southern Africa (5% or less).

Antibody to HCV is not routinely screened for in many parts of Africa, but the prevalence of this infection ranges between 0.5% and 3.0% and reaches 10% to 15% in Egypt. There is evidence of geographically limited pockets of high prevalence, suggesting the importance of specific factors, such as various types of injections and past diagnostic or vaccination campaigns, contributing to the spread of infection.

Other Infections

Most countries in sub-Saharan Africa do not screen for human T-lymphotropic virus 1 (HTLV-1) because the prevalence is low (<2%). However, in other areas of the world, more than 10% of chronically transfused patients have evidence of exposure to HTLV-1.[8] Although the risk of acquiring syphilis from infected blood is low, most blood banks in sub-Saharan Africa do screen for *Treponema pallidum*. Fresh blood is potentially infectious for syphilis, but storage at 4°C can inactivate the bacterium.

Malaria is not only the leading cause of anemia requiring transfusion across Africa[9–12] but can also be transmitted by transfusion. In North America and Europe, transmission of malaria from donors who have visited malaria-endemic areas and have a subclinical patent blood stage infection can transmit the parasite, often with fatal results.[13,14]

In areas of low or no malaria transmission, screening for the parasite is important, as recipients are likely to have no immunity. In countries where malaria is highly endemic, the prevalence of *Plasmodium* spp in donor blood is often very high (16%–55%).[15] Excluding donors with low-grade parasitemia would reduce the supply of blood; in any event, the current methods of screening donors by blood film or rapid diagnostic tests may be insufficiently sensitive to prevent transmission of malaria.[16] Preemptive treatment of recipients of red cells with antimalarial drugs may be a viable alternative.[17,18]

Bacterial contamination of blood components is poorly recognized, although some surveys suggest bacterial infection may be present in 10% of products at the time of issue.[19,20] The most common bacterial infections were due to gram-negative organisms, and the most likely source of contamination was the blood bank and not donors.[20] More widely, the testing of components is limited by the expense of facilities for rapid detection of bacterial contamination. Assessing the scale of the problems and factors behind bacterial contamination of blood would be a priority for future hemovigilance and quality-assurance programs.

TESTING BLOOD PRODUCTS

Test sensitivity and coverage is critical in the face of high prevalence rates for HIV, hepatitis B virus (HBV) and HCV.[4,6,7,21] Some 15 years ago, a survey of blood collection services across India showed that 87% of the donor units were screened for HBV, 95% for HIV, 94% for syphilis, 67% for malaria, and 6% for HCV. Only 13% of blood banks used enzyme-linked immunosorbent assay (ELISA) kits for HBsAg. Notification of the occurrence of transfusion-associated hepatitis was provided less than 40% of the time.[22] There have been substantial efforts to improve the coverage and quality of testing for these viruses over the last decade.

Even with good coverage, the residual risk of all viral infections is high because of the window period of patent infection before detectable antibody, antigen or viral nucleic acid. The residual risk of HBV has always been substantial because of donations containing undetected low levels of HBsAg or occult HBV DNA. Estimates of the residual risk of HIV transmission in the preseroconversion window period were 1:2600 to 6000, hepatitis C 1:400 to 1500, and hepatitis B 1:300 to 500, when using enzyme immunoassay (EIA) screening.[23,24]

In spite of these substantial problems, the considerable international effort to improve the blood safety led by PEPFAR and the Global Fund seems now to be showing significant improvements in the number of units donated and the number of countries screening at least 95% of donations for HBV and HCV, whereas the median of national prevalence for HBV and HCV markers reactive blood donations has declined between 2004 and 2011.[25–28]

The fruits of this work can be seen in the reduction in HCV prevalence over time in cohorts of chronically transfused patients across Africa.[29,30] Some more recent estimates for the residual risk for HIV for Zimbabwe are 1:7500 units for first-time donors and 1:5500 for repeat donors.[30,31] In Gabon, the current residual risks are HIV 1:16,000, HCV 1: 4800 and HBV 1:2000, again showing a broad improvement when compared with previous estimates from Africa.[32]

Across the world there is increasing concern over the transmission of West Nile virus and in Asia and Latin America concern about infection with dengue and chikungunya viruses through blood products.[33,34] These mosquito-borne infections (or arboviruses) are of wide concern for global transfusion practice as asymptomatic, but viremic donors, may transmit infection through blood products. Furthermore, the diseases may spread to areas with suitable mosquito vectors in tropical and subtropical zones and by travelers to nonendemic countries.

Since 2003, all donations in the United States are tested for West Nile virus by nucleic acid testing.[33] There is less certainty over what measures should be used to prevent arboviral transfusion-transmitted infection in epidemics.[35] During epidemics of dengue, screening for donors at risk, donor tracing, and a 7-day quarantine of blood components at risk were undertaken to reduce the risk of viral transmission.[36] In Reunion during the chikungunya epidemic in 2006, the French Blood Service interrupted blood donations on the island, except donations for platelets, whereby they implemented systematic screening for the virus by nucleic acid testing (NAT).[37]

SUPPLY AND USAGE
Blood Donors

Recruiting voluntary donors from the community is complex and expensive and depends on regular education programs, collection teams, vehicles and cold storage. It is proving problematic to expand the number of volunteer donors.[38] Some difficulties remain in persuading donors to donate in the light of HIV testing. There are also cultural beliefs surrounding blood donation that inhibit donors coming forward. Some of these seem to be misinformation about donating blood (eg, men will become impotent if they donate blood; HIV can be caught from the blood bag needle). There are, however, other cultural beliefs related to understanding the value of blood to the individual and to society, for example, blood is related to kinship or personal health. Understanding local beliefs surrounding blood and blood donation is likely to be important in developing effective services. It is worth noting that similar problems were a barrier to widespread acceptance of blood donation in London more than 70 years ago.[39]

As volunteer donors are in short supply, family members are frequently used to provide blood for their relatives in hospital. In 2002, in Africa as a whole, WHO estimated that more than 60% of blood originated from replacement/family donors. In sub-Saharan Africa, the proportion of blood derived from replacement donors is certainly higher. Most viral infections, such as HIV, HBV, and HCV, have similar prevalence in age-matched replacement and volunteer donors.[40] Nevertheless, in Brazil, one-third of donors who were seropositive for syphilis came to the blood bank to help a friend or a relative who needed blood. Although they reported and recognized some high-risk behavior, most were motivated by direct appeal to donate blood.[41] The ultimate aim should be to maximize conversion of voluntary and replacement donors into regular donors because those who are successful repeat donors have the best safety profile.

Notwithstanding the problems in recruiting donors from the community, there is still an argument that a centralized community-based blood service is a necessity to ensure that there is an adequate blood supply to meet clinical demand. Reliance on family replacement donors does not yield sufficient blood units; therefore, there needs to be a dedicated effort to collect from voluntary nonremunerated donors in the community.

Use of Blood Products

In contrast to higher-income countries, most transfusions in sub-Saharan Africa are given for life-threatening emergencies. Transfusions are administered to children predominantly for malaria-related anemia. Many clinical guidelines suggest that transfusions for children are indicated if hemoglobin (Hb) less than 40 or 50 g/L with symptoms of decompensation (**Table 1**).[1,42] The evidence is that children with severe anemia (Hb <50 g/L) who are not transfused have a high chance of dying, often soon after admission. In a recent study in East Africa, 52% (54 of 103) of severely anemic children who were not transfused died within 8 hours, and 90% of these deaths occurred within 2.5 hours of admission. Anemia is an independent risk factor for death during admission; by 24 hours, 128 of 1002 (13%) severely anemic children had died, compared with 36 of 501 (7%) and 71 of 843 (8%) of those with moderate and mild anemia, respectively.[43]

Pregnant women are the second most common recipients of blood, particularly for hemorrhagic emergencies. Hemorrhage during pregnancy or at the time of delivery may contribute to a significant proportion of maternal deaths. In Botswana, a review of the causes of maternal deaths suggested that hemorrhage contributed to 40% of deaths, and overall two-thirds of the women who died were HIV positive.[44] Risk factors for transfusion in pregnancy include not only hemorrhage but also prenatal anemia, lack of prenatal care, gestational age of less than 34 weeks at delivery and HIV infection.[45]

Although improved transfusion services would be an important component of strategies to reduce maternal mortality, they are not sufficient on their own. In many

Table 1
Blood transfusion guidelines for children in Africa

| | Indications for Transfusion | | Volume and Speed |
	Hb Level (g/L)	Clinical Symptoms	of Transfusion
WHO Pocket Book of Hospital Care for Children (2005)	40 or less OR 60 or less PLUS 1 or more	Not required Deep and labored breathing Cardiac failure Clinical dehydration or shock Impaired concentration Malaria parasitaemia >10%	20 mL/kg whole blood or 10 mL/kg packed cells over 3–4 h
Kenya Guidelines for Appropriate Use of Blood and Blood Products (2004)	<40 OR <50 PLUS	Not required Respiratory distress	20 mL/kg whole blood over 3–4 h
Ugandan National Guidelines (2010)	40 or less OR 60 or less PLUS 1 or more	Not required Hypoxia Cardiac decompensation Acidosis Impaired consciousness or cerebral malaria Septicaemia Meningitis Malaria parasitaemia >20%	20 mL/kg whole blood or 10 mL/kg packed cells over 3–4 h
Tanzania National Malaria Guidelines (2006)	40 or less OR 60 or less PLUS	Not required Cardiac failure	20 mL/kg whole blood or 10 mL/kg packed cells over 3–4 h

Adapted from Kiguli S, Maitland K, George EC, et al. Anemia and blood transfusion in African children presenting to hospital with severe febrile illness. BMC Med 2015;13:21.

countries, a comprehensive emergency obstetric and neonatal care, that provides a continuous service, is still only available in a minority of regional and district hospitals.[46] The picture of current care suggests that there is a real need to integrate hematology and blood transfusion, HIV management and antenatal care if substantial progress is to be made in reducing the terrible burden of maternal mortality in low- and middle-income countries (LMICs).

Significant quantities of blood are also used in trauma, often related to motor vehicle accidents, surgery and general medicine. There are neither systematic reviews nor international guidelines covering the use of blood and blood products in these specific contexts and few audits of blood use. The scope for improving clinical practice and reducing unnecessary transfusion is probably substantial.

The success of chronic blood transfusion in the primary and secondary prevention of stroke in sickle cell disease has significantly improved the outcome for severe sickle cell disease in Europe and North America. However, implementing these life-enhancing regimes in Africa faces substantial challenges, including costs, unreliable and insufficient supply of blood for elective procedures, cultural beliefs, and the high frequency of transfusion reactions.[47] Hydroxyurea may offer a more viable route not only for the management of severe sickle cell disease[48–50] but also to reduce transfusion requirements in thalassemia intermedia.[51]

As LMICs improve their public and primary health care, chronic medical illnesses, such as cardiac disease, diabetes and cancer, become more of a priority for health care needs.[52,53] To be able to provide therapies for these disorders, especially for cancer, transfusions are needed to support patients through bone marrow suppression. Unfortunately, in some instances, the unreliability of the supply of whole blood and blood components to support elective blood transfusion may force treating physicians to choose less rigorous chemotherapeutic regimens, which can affect long-term outcomes. Initiatives to improve cancer care and cardiac surgery in LMICs must also include attention to blood supply and safety to support patients through intensive treatments.

Systems

Taken together, small numbers of volunteer blood donors, a frequently fragile cold chain, and difficulties with pathogen testing, lead to low stocks of blood and blood products that ultimately affect patient care and outcomes. Patients in poorer countries usually present late in the course of their disease, and the need for urgent transfusion coupled with shortages of blood, mean that patients may die before a blood transfusion can be organized. In situations where blood must be donated by relatives before a patient can be transfused, several hours or even days can elapse. The process can be speeded up if relatives are asked to donate after patients have been transfused with blood from the hospital's stocks. In this way a combination of voluntary donations to maintain some emergency stocks, combined with posttransfusion donations from patients' relatives, may provide a practical solution to blood shortages.

Even in tertiary centers, many patients with anemia die within a few hours of admission before they can be transfused. Ten years ago, one clinical research center reported the average wait for blood transfusion in children with severe anemia to be 6 hours.[54] Last year, a recent survey of clinical practice during trial of fluid replacement showed that 82% of children with severe anemia were transfused within 8 hours.[43]

Focus on Sub-Saharan Africa

It is axiomatic that transfusion medicine should be incorporated into national health plans. The WHO has provided a recommended structure of national blood transfusion services.[3] They suggest that at the national level the transfusion service should have a medical director, an advisory committee, and clear national transfusion policies and strategies with the appropriate statutory instruments to ensure the national co-ordination and standardization of blood testing, processing and distribution.[55] Notwithstanding these recommendations, transfusion activities must be integrated with other services at local and national levels.

There has been some progress to realize the WHO's recommendations for a national blood program. In Africa in 2002, the WHO estimated that among the 46 member states in the African continent, only 14 had a national blood policy and just 6 had a policy to specifically encourage and develop a system of voluntary nonremunerated donation. In the most recent survey in 2007, 40 out of 41 of the African states surveyed had a national blood policy; but only 56% (23 out of 41) countries were able to implement their policies.

It is worthwhile reflecting on why the development of national transfusion services has not been achieved. A key reason is that it is expensive and logistically complex.

Management skills to run such services are insufficient and the cost of blood transfusion is high in relation to disposable income and health care budgets.

When a transfusion service is provided by individual hospitals, it places an enormous burden on laboratory resources. One survey showed that in a typical district hospital in southern Africa, the overall cost of the transfusion service, including consumables, proportional amounts for capital equipment, staff time, and overheads, was 36% of total laboratory costs. In hospital-based systems that depend on replacement donations, it is the patients' family that bears the cost of donor recruitment.

The cost of a national service is even greater because of the additional costs of quality assurance, local education programs, dedicated collection teams, vehicles, and cold storage. In addition, a national service has to solve the very real practical problems of maintaining regular distributions of blood to remote facilities. A unit of blood in a centralized service costs around 4 times as much as one from a hospital-based system that uses family replacement donors (this cost does not include capital costs). Blood is, therefore, an expensive commodity in relation to the annual per capita budget for health care in these countries; it remains to be seen if blood costing more than $50 per unit when produced in centralized, externally funded units is sustainable. Precise cost-benefit analyses for the use of blood have not been done.

A perennial problem in health care systems is the availability of skilled technical staff; this may be compounded by internal migration of technical staff from hospitals to national or regional centers. There is a severe lack of training and career advancement opportunities for technical and clinical blood service staff. Training programs to increase capacity for the processing, testing, and issue of blood are, therefore, an integral part of service development.

IMPROVEMENTS
Putting the World Health Organization Objectives into Practice

In middle-income countries in Asia, many countries have established national blood services. For example, the Iranian Blood Transfusion Organization was established in 1974 as a national centralized organization to supply blood products free of charge to both public and private hospitals.[56] With external assistance from Germany, Pakistan has moved to establish national and provincial blood transfusion programs.[57]

In sub-Saharan Africa some countries have used external funds to establish an integrated national service; but few have been able to make the transition to a sustainable, national transfusion service in the absence of external funding, and even fewer have been able to reach an adequate blood supply.[58] However, some recent success has been achieved in developing a transfusion service in several centers in Nigeria (see later discussion). The alternative is that transfusion services have to be optimized within the existing general hospital budget. Whatever sums are available, the problems surrounding the supply, safety, cost, and use of blood must be addressed. There has to be a balance between providing an ideal, integrated national service and the more pragmatic solutions afforded by local services.

Development of a National Transfusion Service in Nigeria

In 2004, Nigeria, a country of more than 140 million people, had a highly fragmented hospital-based transfusion system, with little co-ordination from the central government. Most donated blood collected was from replacement and paid donors. Testing for transmissible disease markers was inconsistent and poorly controlled. The practice of family replacement donors in a hospital-based blood service was, at that time, the most economical option; but in the face of high child and maternal mortality rates, the blood supply was insufficient. There was, therefore, the need to change practice.

The Safe Blood for Africa Foundation with a grant from US Agency for International Development and later the President's Emergency Plan for AIDS Relief (PEPFAR) established a demonstration blood service in the capital, Abuja. This service collected blood from voluntary unremunerated donors in the local community. The blood was tested for HIV, hepatitis B and C, and syphilis and distributed to the local hospitals. A simple, but effective, quality management system was established with standard operating procedures written and followed. The objective of this project was to be the model for other centers throughout the country.

Subsequently, the Federal Ministry of Health established 6 zonal transfusion centers under the umbrella of the National Blood Transfusion Service. In addition, 10 states opened transfusion centers; there is one that serves the needs of the military forces. The Federal Ministry of Health also established an expert committee, which drafted a national blood policy and national guidelines for the standards for the practice of transfusion in Nigeria. The Safe Blood for Africa Foundation has, to date, provided technical assistance for the establishment of these centers and provided training to the staff in all elements of transfusion.[59]

The major problem was to recruit blood donors. The youth were encouraged to donate with the establishment of a Club 25 program for donors less than 25 years of age. There was active promotion through the media, and it was highlighted by a televised donation by the president on the occasion of the official opening of the Abuja center. A problem encountered was the high number of donors presenting with Hb levels less than the required standard of 125 g/L. This problem is probably a reflection of the poor health status within the community.

Improving the Blood Supply

Careful donor selection is crucial not only to improve the supply of blood but also to reduce transfusion-transmitted infection risk. The selection of volunteer donors from lower-risk populations is considered the most effective approach, and considerable effort has been devoted to promoting voluntary, repeat donations. In practice, these are often secondary school students with median age ranging between 16 and 20 years. They are younger and have a greater proportion of females than replacement donors; but there are some concerns that, although these younger donors have a lower prevalence of transfusion-transmitted infections than older donors, they may have a higher incidence of new infections. Experience has shown that, although recruiting volunteer donors in schools can be relatively straightforward, making them into repeat donors is difficult and expensive. Encouraging both volunteer nonremunerated and family replacement donors to donate blood repeatedly is the challenge for sub-Saharan African blood services in order to provide safer blood.[40,60,61]

Several strategies have been devised to encourage repeat donors and, thus, reduce the risk of virus carriage. In Zimbabwe, the Pledge 25 Club, a program using education and incentives to attract school students to give blood 25 times, has been successful. Similar, less ambitious schemes, for example, a Club 5, could also be effective. The WHO slogan of "Safe Blood Starts with Me" has also resulted in educational programs around the world. These schemes can be complemented by strategies to recruit donors from faith-based organizations or collaborating with radio stations to organize and promote blood donations. Specific strategies intending to encourage family replacement donors to become repeat donors are being developed.

The best use of fluid replacement, pressure devices, and pharmaceuticals, such as tranexamic acid for severe hemorrhage, are under study. The landmark CRASH-2 study (Clinical Randomisation of an Antifibrinolytic in Significant Haemorrhage-2) showed that after major trauma the antifibrinolytic tranexamic acid, given within 3 hours of the initial trauma as a loading dose 1 g over 10 minutes then infusion of 1 g over 8 hours, reduced all-cause mortality by 10%.[62]

Several studies have shown the use of placental blood to prevent neonatal anemia, particularly in malarious areas. The high hematocrit from the placental blood and easy availability may make it suitable for small-volume emergency transfusions.[63] However, the logistics and infrastructure needed to collect placental blood free of bacterial contamination, to obtain consent from women in labor and test and distribute these small volumes of blood, should not be underestimated.[64]

Improving Screening for Blood-Transmitted Infections

New approaches to blood donor testing for transfusion-transmitted diseases have been adapted to local situations. Rapid immunochemical tests are being developed for blood-borne pathogens and may cut the cost of predonation and postdonation testing to a tenth of present costs. Many rapid diagnostic tests (RDTs) for anti-HIV and HBsAg are available, although fewer for anti-HCV; but sensitivity and specificity, ease of use, and cost vary greatly. The WHO has established systematic evaluations of both EIA and rapid tests to guide developing countries in their choice of tests. The current reviews of rapid diagnostic tests using immunochromatography have shown the limitations of these tests for screening for HIV, HBV, and HCV.[65,66] Operator errors may be improved through training; but many rapid diagnostics tests (RDTs), especially hepatitis B rapid assays, are less sensitive than the respective EIAs; this must question the suitability of rapid diagnostic test as the sole test, particularly where the prevalence of these viral infections is high.[66–68]

Nucleic acid testing (NAT) is highly effective and has been introduced in South East Asia, South Africa, Brazil, and a few centers elsewhere.[69–71] The efficiency of individual-donation and mini-pool NAT is driven by the size of pool of samples treated.[70,72,73] Widespread use of NAT is out of reach for most countries; cheaper, simpler methods to perform NAT testing would be useful.[74] However, a recent rapid amplification method for quantization of HIV load has produced equivalent results to the current gold standard methods.[75] Large-scale evaluation of these and similar tests is now planned.

Another approach to improve the sensitivity of HIV ELISA testing in the absence of NAT screening has been to use 2 HIV ELISA tests in parallel. This approach has prevented a substantial number of HIV-infected donations from entering the Chinese blood supply, at the cost of discarding many false-positive donations.[76] Test performances of all tests may be improved by the development of an external quality-assurance scheme.[68]

Blood safety has often focused on the risk of viral infection in donors, but bacterial contamination of units is also a substantial problem. Two studies have highlighted the considerable risk of bacterial infection in nearly 10% of whole blood units.[19,20] Contamination seems to be of environmental, rather than of donor, origin and reducing these hazards will be an important challenge in the future.

Meeting the Financial Requirements of Transfusion Services

The challenge for poorer countries is that enough safe blood should be available for health services and individuals even when resources are extremely limited. The high cost of providing blood makes it impossible to recoup the cost of blood by user fees alone, and blood services will require internal or external public funding for the foreseeable future.[77] Developing systems that rely more on local resources means that in the long term they may be more flexible, productive and sustainable.

Improving the Clinical Use of Blood

Monitoring and improving the appropriate use of blood is crucial to preserve the supply of blood and to improve patient care. The scope for improvement in clinical practice is great. For example, strict enforcement of a transfusion protocol in a Malawian hospital reduced the number of transfusions by 75% without any adverse effect on mortality. Even in a trial setting, the WHO's or local guidelines for the transfusion of acute anemia in children (see **Table 1**) are frequently breached.[43] As the scope of transfusion in LMICs expands into nonemergency settings, there is perhaps not surprisingly emerging evidence of inappropriate use of platelets[78] or of neonatal transfusions.[79]

Reduction in blood use has been achieved in Africa by improved or modified surgical techniques[80] or cell salvage.[81] In other circumstances, transfusion procedures can be adapted to local circumstance, for example, the use of exchange transfusion when leukapheresis or plasmapheresis is not available.[82]

The use of guidelines can reduce unnecessary transfusions, and many institutions in sub-Saharan Africa and Asia have developed guidelines to promote rational use of blood transfusions and blood components.[23] The principles underlying most transfusion guidelines are similar and combine a clinical assessment of whether patients are developing complications of inadequate oxygenation, with measurement of their Hb (as a marker of intracellular oxygen concentration). In the United States, anesthetists suggest that transfusions are almost always indicated when the Hb concentration is less than 60 g/L, whereas in many sub-Saharan African countries transfusions are recommended for children at Hb concentrations less than 40 g/L, provided there are no other clinical complications. Moreover, the lack of fractionated blood products and the reliance on whole blood should be considered in context. Using whole blood for many of the common emergent indications for transfusion in Africa may be advantageous, as it supplies critical coagulation factors for patients facing hemostatic challenge, such as in the setting of postpartum hemorrhage and following a significant trauma.

Ensuring that the transfusion guidelines are implemented is extremely difficult without formal monitoring and auditing systems. This issue is particularly problematic if the quality of Hb measurements is not assured as clinicians may rely entirely on clinical judgment to guide transfusion practice with an inevitably high proportion of inappropriate transfusions. As the cost of providing a unit of blood is approximately 40 times the cost of a quality-assured Hb test, investment in improving the Hb testing is likely to not only improve practice but also reduce transfusion costs.

Hospital transfusion committees have been an important part of improving transfusion practice in higher-income countries;[83] now such committees have begun to spread in LMICs and started to develop policy and guidelines in tertiary centers in Kumasi, Ghana and elsewhere.[84] One important function of these committees is to review and prevent adverse events, although they are grossly underreported in passive hemovigilance schemes.[84] However, prospective studies suggest that adverse events are more common in resource-poor settings.[85,86] National hemovigilance schemes are exceptional, but have been established in Namibia and Burkina Faso.[87,88]

Within the hospital blood bank, the ability to supply blood rapidly is a priority given the high proportion of blood required for medical and obstetric emergencies. There are encouraging reports of the rapid provision of blood for emergency use in district hospitals with a time of 1 hour from requisition to supply, which would be a worthwhile and achievable target for supply of blood.[26]

There are many developments in improving the supply and safety of blood, and the serologic side of transfusion has often been benignly neglected. Alloimmunization rates have been reported to be between 5% and 30% in multi-transfused patients.[89–91] In some settings, the clinical significance of regional differences in the frequency of minor alleles of the major blood group systems is now being explored.

The complex blood group antigen genotypes and phenotypes in Africa, particularly of the Rh system,[92,93] suggest that more detailed typing of variants of the *RHCE* gene in patients (5.5% prevalence of variants across Africa) and in donors, RH54 (DAK) (frequency of 8.1%) may be valuable when more detailed, large-scale blood group phenotyping is possible.

In China, a careful study of 140 women with the partial DEL has shown that they are at risk of alloimmunization to the D antigen and that they require RhD immunoglobulin prophylaxis. Women expressing the partial DEL should receive only RhD-negative red blood cells (RBCs), whereas patients with DEL with complete expression of antigen can safely receive RhD-positive RBCs.[94]

The technical infrastructure and skills needed to screen patients for alloantibodies and to provide antigen-negative blood is frequently absent in many countries and regional centers in sub-Saharan Africa. Developing reliable panels of screening cells and reagents locally and providing the requisite training and establishing quality-assurance schemes may be feasible developments with external support.[95,96]

The Ebola Pandemic in West Africa

The outbreak of the Ebola virus in 3 West African countries caused loss of life to many thousands of people. At the time of the outbreak, there was no proven therapy for the disease; however, 40% to 65% of patients made a full recovery. Those who survived have a developed immunity, and it has been hypothesized that antibody-containing plasma recovered from these individuals could be used as a passive therapy for Ebola-infected patents.[97,98] The epidemic has highlighted the needed for well-organized hospital services. It may be that blood centers could play a significant role in providing treatment if it is proven that plasma, harvested from convalescent patients, is efficacious in the treatment of acutely ill patients; trials to test this were set up during the recent epidemic.[99]

Research Directions in Transfusion Medicine

International policies and guidelines for blood transfusion, including blood donation, screening, clinical practice, and service organization, are based on experience from, and evidence generated in, high-income countries. Consequently, they are not necessarily appropriate for poorer countries. To improve the effectiveness of their internal operations, blood services need to be constantly conducting their own research, for example, to validate new kits or equipment or to change donor recruitment strategies. However, blood services invest very little in developing research skills among their staff and even less in conducting research that is of international quality and that could be shared across different services.

Most published transfusion-related research has been heavily biased toward transfusion-transmitted infections, particularly HIV. However, the major problem facing many blood services in poorer countries is blood shortages; but good-quality research exploring strategies for innovative donor recruitment and improving the effectiveness of clinical use of blood and economic aspects of transfusion is extremely limited.

There is increasing interest in research, audit, and collaboration in Africa[95,100] and Latin America[101] in addition to well-established postgraduate teaching in South Africa,[102,103] Nigeria[104] and Tanzania,[105] to name but a few examples. Both the Anglophone and Francophone Transfusion Research Groups have multinational research programs.[68,106]

Some key research needs of transfusion services identified at a workshop in Africa in 2015, which are likely to be relevant for other resource-limited settings, were an in-depth understanding of pragmatic and culturally sensitive approaches to blood donor recruitment; good evidence of the costs and effectiveness of different blood service models; and the critical need for appropriate information technology systems to manage and optimize blood stocks and blood donor recruitment and tracking.[107] Transfusion research into the complex issues of systems, costs and models of sustainable funding is virtually nonexistent but is essential to guide the design and operation of cost-effective and feasible blood services in poorer countries.

For all of these, research needs to be addressed; not only does research capacity within blood services need to be improved but also the national and international societies for blood transfusion and the blood transfusion leadership in the WHO need to be strengthened to facilitate coordination, knowledge exchange, and evidence-based policy making.

SUMMARY

Fulfilling the first WHO objective of establishing "a national blood system with well-organized and co-ordinated blood transfusion services, effective evidence-based and ethical national blood policies ... that can provide sufficient and timely supplies of safe blood and blood products to meet the transfusion needs of all patients" has proved to be very difficult in many countries, even given the substantial external funding. Nevertheless, some countries have made progress and have recently established national transfusion services. On the other hand, progress has been made by developing local services; there has to be a balance between providing an ideal integrated national service and the more pragmatic solutions afforded by local services. There remains considerable scope to optimize fluid management and other ancillary treatments and to reduce unnecessary transfusions through the appropriate clinical use of blood and products.

Increased blood supply depends on the recruitment of all types of nonremunerated donors, whether volunteer nonremunerated donors or family replacement donors, and the development of innovative strategies to encourage both groups of donors to give blood regularly.

Resources must be made available by governments to ensure that the essential supplies are available, such as blood bags, grouping reagents and test kits. Laboratory and blood bank management systems also need to be improved to ensure effective testing and processing and the maintenance of the cold chain. Hospitals and other health facilities could co-operate to directly purchase cheap, high-quality tests adapted to their needs. Significant efforts need to be made to ensure that blood services in poorer countries are underpinned by feasible and sustainable internal financing mechanisms, so they can operate independently of external donors.

There is currently a feeling of guarded optimism about the future of blood supply and safety in developing countries. The recent increase in the allocation of resources for the prevention of HIV across the world, including the investment by governments of wealthy countries and contributions from international and private agencies, have begun to recognize the importance of reducing HIV transmission through blood, but run the risk of neglecting other basic laboratory services, for example, blood grouping and Hb measurements. Parallel to the price reduction for antiviral drugs, the cost of screening tests supplied to developing countries has also decreased. The high cost of anti-HCV testing should now be reduced as the patent has expired in Europe. More effective and efficient methods for testing blood are to be welcomed, and pathogen-reduction methods applicable to whole blood would be an enormous relief if affordable. The real challenge will be to integrate improvements in the supply and safety of blood in sustainable, co-ordinated national transfusion services.

REFERENCES

1. Lackritz EM, Campbell CC, Ruebush TK 2nd, et al. Effect of blood transfusion on survival among children in a Kenyan hospital. Lancet 1992;340(8818): 524–8.
2. Bates I, Chapotera GK, McKew S, et al. Maternal mortality in sub-Saharan Africa: the contribution of ineffective blood transfusion services. BJOG 2008; 115(11):1331–9.
3. World Health Organization. Developing a national blood system. 2015. Available at: http://www.who.int/bloodsafety/clinical_use/en/. Accessed November 1, 2015.
4. Tapko JB, Sam O. Diarra-Nama A. Report on the status of blood safety in the WHO African region for 2004. Geneva, Switzerland: World Health Organization; 2007.
5. Cunha L, Plouzeau C, Ingrand P, et al. Use of replacement blood donors to study the epidemiology of major blood-borne viruses in the general population of Maputo, Mozambique. J Med Virol 2007;79(12):1832–40.
6. Tagny CT, Diarra A, Yahaya R, et al. Characteristics of blood donors and donated blood in sub-Saharan Francophone Africa. Transfusion 2009;49(8): 1592–9.
7. Tagny CT, Owusu-Ofori S, Mbanya D, et al. The blood donor in sub-Saharan Africa: a review. Transfus Med 2010;20(1):1–10.
8. Keshvari M, Hajibeigi B, Azarkeivan A, et al. Seroepidemiology of human T-cell lymphotropic virus among Iranian adult thalassemic patients. Transfus Med 2014;24(4):227–32.
9. Kiggundu VL, O'Meara WP, Musoke R, et al. High prevalence of malaria parasitemia and anemia among hospitalized children in Rakai, Uganda. PLoS One 2013;8(12):e82455.
10. Bugge HF, Karlsen NC, Oydna E, et al. A study of blood transfusion services at a district hospital in Malawi. Vox Sang 2013;104(1):37–45.
11. Comfort AB, van Dijk JH, Mharakurwa S, et al. Association between malaria control and paediatric blood transfusions in rural Zambia: an interrupted time-series analysis. Malar J 2014;13:383.
12. Austin N, Adikaibe E, Ethelbert O, et al. Prevalence and severity of malaria parasitemia among children requiring emergency blood transfusion in a tertiary hospital in Imo State, Nigeria. Ann Med Health Sci Res 2014;4(4):619–23.
13. Mungai M, Tegtmeier G, Chamberland M, et al. Transfusion-transmitted malaria in the United States from 1963 through 1999. N Engl J Med 2001;344(26): 1973–8.
14. O'Brien SF, Delage G, Seed CR, et al. The epidemiology of imported malaria and transfusion policy in 5 nonendemic countries. Transfus Med Rev 2015; 29(3):162–71.
15. Owusu-Ofori AK, Parry C, Bates I. Transfusion-transmitted malaria in countries where malaria is endemic: a review of the literature from sub-Saharan Africa. Clin Infect Dis 2010;51(10):1192–8.

16. Owusu-Ofori AK, Betson M, Parry CM, et al. Transfusion-transmitted malaria in Ghana. Clin Infect Dis 2013;56(12):1735–41.
17. Rajab JA, Waithaka PM, Orinda DA, et al. Analysis of cost and effectiveness of pre-transfusion screening of donor blood and anti-malarial prophylaxis for recipients. East Afr Med J 2005;82(11):565–71.
18. Owusu-Ofori AK, Bates I. Impact of inconsistent policies for transfusion-transmitted malaria on clinical practice in Ghana. PLoS One 2012;7(3): e34201.
19. Adjei AA, Kuma GK, Tettey Y, et al. Bacterial contamination of blood and blood components in three major blood transfusion centers, Accra, Ghana. Jpn J Infect Dis 2009;62(4):265–9.
20. Hassall O, Maitland K, Pole L, et al. Bacterial contamination of pediatric whole blood transfusions in a Kenyan hospital. Transfusion 2009;49(12):2594–8.
21. Keshvari M, Alavian SM, Aghaee B, et al. Seroepidemiology and clinical features of hepatitis delta among HBsAg carriers: a study from hepatitis clinic of Iranian Blood Transfusion Organization. Transfus Med 2014;24(6):411–7.
22. Kapoor D, Saxena R, Sood B, et al. Blood transfusion practices in India: results of a national survey. Indian J Gastroenterol 2000;19:64–7.
23. Chaudhuri V, Nanu A, Panda SK, et al. Evaluation of serologic screening of blood donors in India reveals a lack of correlation between anti-HBc titer and PCR-amplified HBV DNA. Transfusion 2003;43(10):1442–8.
24. Basavaraju SV, Mwangi J, Nyamongo J, et al. Reduced risk of transfusion-transmitted HIV in Kenya through centrally coordinated blood centres, stringent donor selection and effective p24 antigen-HIV antibody screening. Vox Sang 2010;99(3):212–9.
25. Adouani B, Alami R, Laouina A, et al. Hepatitis B in Moroccan blood donors: a decade trend of the HBsAg prevalence in a resources limited country. Transfus Med 2013;23(6):432–7.
26. Alvarado-Mora MV, Pinho JR. Epidemiological update of hepatitis B, C and delta in Latin America. Antivir Ther 2013;18(3 Pt B):429–33.
27. Apata IW, Averhoff F, Pitman J, et al. Progress toward prevention of transfusion-transmitted hepatitis B and hepatitis C infection–sub-Saharan Africa, 2000-2011. MMWR Morb Mortal Wkly Rep 2014;63(29):613–9.
28. WHO. Global database on blood safety. Available at: http://www.who.int/bloodsafety/global_database/en/. Accessed November 1, 2015.
29. Mansour AK, Aly RM, Abdelrazek SY, et al. Prevalence of HBV and HCV infection among multi-transfused Egyptian thalassemic patients. Hematol Oncol Stem Cell Ther 2012;5(1):54–9.
30. Seck SM, Dahaba M, Gueye S, et al. Trends in hepatitis C infection among hemodialysis patients in Senegal: results of a decade of prevention. Saudi J Kidney Dis Transpl 2014;25(6):1341–5.
31. Mapako T, Mvere DA, Chitiyo ME, et al. Human immunodeficiency virus prevalence, incidence, and residual transmission risk in first-time and repeat blood donations in Zimbabwe: implications on blood safety. Transfusion 2013;53(10 Pt 2):2413–21.
32. Rerambiah LK, Rerambiah LE, Djoba Siawaya JF, et al. The risk of transfusion-transmitted viral infections at the Gabonese National Blood Transfusion Centre. Blood Transfus 2014;12(3):330–3.
33. Dodd RY, Foster GA, Stramer SL. Keeping blood transfusion safe from West Nile virus: American red cross experience, 2003 to 2012. Transfus Med Rev 2015; 29(3):153–61.

34. Arellanos-Soto D, B-d I Cruz V, Mendoza-Tavera N, et al. Constant risk of dengue virus infection by blood transfusion in an endemic area in Mexico. Transfus Med 2015;25(2):122–4.

35. Lanteri MC, Busch MP. Dengue in the context of "safe blood" and global epidemiology: to screen or not to screen? Transfusion 2012;52(8):1634–9.

36. Gan VC, Leo YS. Current epidemiology and clinical practice in arboviral infections - implications on blood supply in South-East Asia. ISBT Sci Ser 2014; 9(1):262–7.

37. Brouard C, Bernillon P, Quatresous I, et al. Estimated risk of chikungunya viremic blood donation during an epidemic on Reunion Island in the Indian Ocean, 2005 to 2007. Transfusion 2008;48(7):1333–41.

38. Bates I, Manyasi G, Medina Lara A. Reducing replacement donors in Sub-Saharan Africa: challenges and affordability. Transfus Med 2007;17(6): 434–42.

39. Starr D. Blood: an epic history of medicine and commerce. New York: Harper Collins; 2002.

40. Allain JP. Moving on from voluntary non-remunerated donors: who is the best blood donor? Br J Haematol 2011;154(6):763–9.

41. Ferreira SC, de Almeida-Neto C, Nishiya AS, et al. Demographic, risk factors and motivations among blood donors with reactive serologic tests for syphilis in São Paulo, Brazil. Transfus Med 2014;24(3):169–75.

42. Akech SO, Hassall O, Pamba A, et al. Survival and haematological recovery of children with severe malaria transfused in accordance to WHO guidelines in Kilifi, Kenya. Malar J 2008;7:256.

43. Kiguli S, Maitland K, George EC, et al. Anaemia and blood transfusion in African children presenting to hospital with severe febrile illness. BMC Med 2015; 13:21.

44. Ray S, Madzimbamuto FD, Ramagola-Masire D, et al. Review of causes of maternal deaths in Botswana in 2010. S Afr Med J 2013;103(8):537–42.

45. Bloch EM, Crookes RL, Hull J, et al. The impact of human immunodeficiency virus infection on obstetric hemorrhage and blood transfusion in South Africa. Transfusion 2015;55(7):1675–84.

46. Compaore GD, Sombié I, Ganaba R, et al. Readiness of district and regional hospitals in Burkina Faso to provide caesarean section and blood transfusion services: a cross-sectional study. BMC Pregnancy Childbirth 2014;14:158.

47. Lagunju IA, Brown BJ, Sodeinde OO. Chronic blood transfusion for primary and secondary stroke prevention in Nigerian children with sickle cell disease: a 5-year appraisal. Pediatr Blood Cancer 2013;60(12):1940–5.

48. Lagunju IA, Brown BJ, Sodeinde OO. Stroke recurrence in Nigerian children with sickle cell disease treated with hydroxyurea. Niger Postgrad Med J 2013;20(3): 181–7.

49. Galadanci NA, Abdullahi SU, Tabari MA, et al. Primary stroke prevention in Nigerian children with sickle cell disease (SPIN): challenges of conducting a feasibility trial. Pediatr Blood Cancer 2015;62(3):395–401.

50. Lagunju I, Brown BJ, Sodeinde O. Hydroxyurea lowers transcranial Doppler flow velocities in children with sickle cell anaemia in a Nigerian cohort. Pediatr Blood Cancer 2015;62(9):1587–91.

51. El-Beshlawy A, El-Ghamrawy M, EL-Ela MA, et al. Response to hydroxycarbamide in pediatric beta-thalassemia intermedia: 8 years' follow-up in Egypt. Ann Hematol 2014;93(12):2045–50.

52. Javadzadeh Shahshahani H, Hatami H, Meraat N, et al. Epidemiology of blood component recipients in hospitals of Yazd, Iran. Transfus Med 2015; 25(1):2–7.
53. Butler EK, Hume H, Birungi I, et al. Blood utilization at a national referral hospital in sub-Saharan Africa. Transfusion 2015;55(5):1058–66.
54. English M, Ahmed M, Ngando C, et al. Blood transfusion for severe anaemia in children in a Kenyan hospital. Lancet 2002;359(9305):494–5.
55. Organization, W.H. Universal access to safe blood transfusion. 2015. Available at: http://www.who.int/bloodsafety/universalbts/en/. Accessed November 1, 2015.
56. Pourfathollah AA, Hosseini Divkolaye NS, Seighali F. Four decades of National Blood Service in Iran: outreach, prospect and challenges. Transfus Med 2015; 25(3):138–43.
57. Zaheer HA, Waheed U. Legislative reforms of the blood transfusion system in Pakistan. Transfus Med 2014;24(2):117–9.
58. Ala F, Allain JP, Bates I, et al. External financial aid to blood transfusion services in sub-Saharan Africa: a need for reflection. PLoS Med 2012;9(9):e1001309.
59. Africa, S.B.f. Safe Blood for Africa Foundation 2015. Available at: http://www.safebloodforafrica.org/index.php?option=com_content&view=article&id=344&Itemid=516. Accessed November 11, 2015.
60. Allain JP, Sarkodie F, Boateng P, et al. A pool of repeat blood donors can be generated with little expense to the blood center in sub-Saharan Africa. Transfusion 2008;48(4):735–41.
61. Muthivhi TN, Olmsted MG, Park H, et al. Motivators and deterrents to blood donation among Black South Africans: a qualitative analysis of focus group data. Transfus Med 2015;25(4):249–58.
62. CRASH-2 Trial Collaborators, Shakur H, Roberts I, et al. Effects of tranexamic acid on death, vascular occlusive events, and blood transfusion in trauma patients with significant haemorrhage (CRASH-2): a randomised, placebo-controlled trial. Lancet 2010;376(9734):23–32.
63. Hassall O, Bedu-Addo G, Adarkwa M, et al. Umbilical-cord blood for transfusion in children with severe anaemia in under-resourced countries. Lancet 2003; 361(9358):678–9.
64. Hassall OW, Thitiri J, Fegan G, et al. The microbiologic safety of umbilical cord blood transfusion for children with severe anemia in Mombasa, Kenya. Transfusion 2012;52(7):1542–51.
65. Laperche S, Francophone African Group for Research in Blood Transfusion. Multinational assessment of blood-borne virus testing and transfusion safety on the African continent. Transfusion 2013;53(4):816–26.
66. Pruett CR, Vermeulen M, Zacharias P, et al. The use of rapid diagnostic tests for transfusion infectious screening in Africa: a literature review. Transfus Med Rev 2015;29(1):35–44.
67. Orkuma JA, Egesie JO, Banwat EB, et al. HIV screening in blood donors: rapid diagnostic test versus enhanced ELISA. Niger J Med 2014;23(3):192–200.
68. Bloch EM, Shah A, Kaidarova Z, et al. A pilot external quality assurance study of transfusion screening for HIV, HCV and HBsAG in 12 African countries. Vox Sang 2014;107(4):333–42.
69. Vermeulen M, Lelie N, Sykes W, et al. Impact of individual-donation nucleic acid testing on risk of human immunodeficiency virus, hepatitis B virus, and hepatitis C virus transmission by blood transfusion in South Africa. Transfusion 2009; 49(6):1115–25.

70. Bruhn R, Lelie N, Custer B, et al. Prevalence of human immunodeficiency virus RNA and antibody in first-time, lapsed, and repeat blood donations across five international regions and relative efficacy of alternative screening scenarios. Transfusion 2013;53(10 Pt 2):2399–412.

71. Andrea P, Kupek E, Genovez G, et al. NAT yield for human immunodeficiency and hepatitis C viruses in Brazilian blood donors: preliminary results. Transfus Med 2015;25(2):125–7.

72. Vermeulen M, Coleman C, Mitchel J, et al. Sensitivity of individual-donation and minipool nucleic acid amplification test options in detecting window period and occult hepatitis B virus infections. Transfusion 2013;53(10 Pt 2):2459–66.

73. Cable R, Lelie N, Bird A. Reduction of the risk of transfusion-transmitted viral infection by nucleic acid amplification testing in the Western Cape of South Africa: a 5-year review. Vox Sang 2013;104(2):93–9.

74. Shyamala V. Transfusion transmitted infections in thalassaemics: need for reappraisal of blood screening strategy in India. Transfus Med 2014;24(2):79–88.

75. Ritchie AV, Ushiro-Lumb I, Edemaga D, et al. SAMBA HIV semiquantitative test, a new point-of-care viral-load-monitoring assay for resource-limited settings. J Clin Microbiol 2014;52(9):3377–83.

76. Zeng P, Liu J, Wang J, et al. Parallel enzyme-linked immunosorbent assay screening for human immunodeficiency virus among blood donors in five Chinese blood centres: a retrospective analysis. Transfus Med 2015;25(4):259–64.

77. Hensher M, Jefferys E. Financing blood transfusion services in sub-Saharan Africa: a role for user fees? Health Policy Plan 2000;15:287–95.

78. Sonnekus PH, Louw VJ, Ackermann AM, et al. An audit of the use of platelet transfusions at Universitas Academic Hospital, Bloemfontein, South Africa. Transfus Apher Sci 2014;51(3):44–52.

79. Harrison MC, Pillay S, Joolay Y, et al. Resource implications of adopting a restrictive neonatal blood transfusion policy. S Afr Med J 2013;103(12):916–7.

80. Adeleye AO. Targeting a zero blood transfusion rate in the repair of craniospinal dysraphism: outcome of a surgical technique for developing countries. Neurol Res 2015;37(2):125–30.

81. Solomon L, von Rahden RP, Allorto NL. Intra-operative cell salvage in South Africa: feasible, beneficial and economical. S Afr Med J 2013;103(10):754–7.

82. Barrett CL, Louw VJ, Webb MJ. Exchange transfusion as a life-saving intervention in three patients with different haematological malignancies with severe hyperleukocytosis where leukapheresis was not available. Transfus Apher Sci 2013;49(3):397–402.

83. Murphy MF. The Choosing Wisely campaign to reduce harmful medical overuse: its close association with Patient Blood Management initiatives. Transfus Med 2015;25(5):287–92.

84. Opare-Sem O, Bedu-Addo G, Karikari P, et al. Fourteen-year experience of a tertiary hospital transfusion committee in West Africa. Transfusion 2014;54(11):2852–62.

85. Ibrahim NU, Garba N, Tilde IM. Acute blood transfusion reactions in pregnancy, an observational study from North Eastern Nigeria. J Blood Disord Transfus 2013;4:145. http://dx.doi.org/10.4172/2155-9864.1000145.

86. Meza BP, Lohrke B, Wilkinson R, et al. Estimation of the prevalence and rate of acute transfusion reactions occurring in Windhoek, Namibia. Blood Transfus 2014;12(3):352–61.

87. Dahourou H, Tapko JB, Nébié Y, et al. Implementation of hemovigilance in Sub-Saharan Africa. Transfus Clin Biol 2012;19(1):39–45 [in French].

88. Basavaraju SV, Lohrke B, Pitman JP, et al. Knowledge and barriers related to reporting of acute transfusion reactions among healthcare workers in Namibia. Transfus Med 2013;23(5):367–9.
89. Diarra AB, Guindo A, Kouriba B, et al. Sickle cell anemia and transfusion safety in Bamako, Mali. Seroprevalence of HIV, HBV and HCV infections and alloimmunization belonged to Rh and Kell systems in sickle cell anemia patients. Transfus Clin Biol 2013;20(5–6):476–81 [in French].
90. Hussein E, Desooky N, Rihan A, et al. Predictors of red cell alloimmunization in multitransfused Egyptian patients with beta-thalassemia. Arch Pathol Lab Med 2014;138(5):684–8.
91. Zaidi U, Borhany M, Ansari S, et al. Red cell alloimmunisation in regularly transfused beta thalassemia patients in Pakistan. Transfus Med 2015;25(2):106–10.
92. Granier T, Beley S, Chiaroni J, et al. A comprehensive survey of both RHD and RHCE allele frequencies in sub-Saharan Africa. Transfusion 2013;53(11 Suppl 2):3009–17.
93. Kappler-Gratias S, Auxerre C, Dubeaux I, et al. Systematic RH genotyping and variant identification in French donors of African origin. Blood Transfus 2014; 12(Suppl 1):s264–72.
94. Wang M, Wang BL, Xu W, et al. Anti-D alloimmunisation in pregnant women with DEL phenotype in China. Transfus Med 2015;25(3):163–9.
95. Dzik WS, Kyeyune D, Otekat G, et al. Transfusion Medicine in Sub-Saharan Africa: conference summary. Transfus Med Rev 2015;29(3):195–204.
96. Waiswa MK, Moses A, Seremba E, et al. Acute transfusion reactions at a national referral hospital in Uganda: a prospective study. Transfusion 2014;54(11):2804–10.
97. Gulland A. Clinical trials of Ebola therapies to begin in December. BMJ 2014; 349:g6827.
98. Gutfraind A, Meyers LA. Evaluating large-scale blood transfusion therapy for the current Ebola epidemic in Liberia. J Infect Dis 2015;211(8):1262–7.
99. Burnouf T, Emmanuel J, Mbanya D, et al. Ebola: a call for blood transfusion strategy in sub-Saharan Africa. Lancet 2014;384(9951):1347–8.
100. Eichbaum Q, Shan H, Goncalez TT, et al. Global health and transfusion medicine: education and training in developing countries. Transfusion 2014;54(7):1893–8.
101. Damulak OD, Jatau E, Akinga E, et al. The prevalence of syphilis among blood donors in a centralized Nigerian Blood Transfusion Service Centre. Niger J Med 2013;22(2):113–6.
102. Louw VJ. Determining the outcomes for clinicians completing a postgraduate diploma in transfusion medicine. Transfus Apher Sci 2014;51(3):38–43.
103. Louw VJ. Transfusion education and practice in South Africa. Transfus Apher Sci 2014;51(3):6–7.
104. Olaleye DO, Odaibo GN, Carney P, et al. Enhancement of health research capacity in Nigeria through north-south and in-country partnerships. Acad Med 2014;89(8 Suppl):S93–7.
105. MUHAS. Muhimbili Wellcome Programme. Training and Capacity Building - MMed in Haematology and Blood Transfusion. Available at: http://www.muhimbili-wellcome.org/training. Accessed November 11, 2015.
106. Tagny CT, Murphy EL, Lefrère JJ, et al. The Francophone Africa Blood Transfusion Research Network: a five-year report. Transfus Clin Biol 2014;21(1):37–42 [in French].
107. Bates I, Hassall O. Workshop on blood transfusion research in sub-Saharan Africa. 2015. Available at: http://www.t-rec.eu/highlights/documents/Workshoponbloodtransfusionresearchinsub-SaharanAfricaexternal.pdf. Accessed November 1, 2015.

Improving Laboratory and Clinical Hematology Services in Resource Limited Settings

Angela Allen, PhD[a,b,]*, Stephen Allen, MD[b],
Nancy Olivieri, MD, FRCP[c,d,e,f]

KEYWORDS

- Laboratory hematology • Clinical hematology • Thalassemia • Quality improvement
- Resource limited

KEY POINTS

- Every step in the sample journey, from initial request to timely delivery of results, needs to be considered to improve services.
- Quality improvement approaches offer opportunities to improve service delivery even within existing resources.
- Approaches to improve clinical services should benefit from focus on establishing continuity of care.
- National patient registries may serve to inform governments about the demands for increased resources for management.

BACKGROUND

The recommendations of this article are based in part upon work in the thalassemias, inherited disorders of hemoglobin that are widely prevalent in Asia, which may serve as a model that is applicable to other common, chronic disorders in resource-poor

Disclosure Statement: The authors have nothing to disclose.
[a] Molecular Haematology, Weatherall Institute of Molecular Medicine, John Radcliffe Hospital, Headington, Oxford, UK; [b] Department of Clinical Sciences, Liverpool School of Tropical Medicine, Pembroke Place, Liverpool L3 5QA, UK; [c] Pediatrics, Toronto General Hospital, University of Toronto, 200 Elizabeth Street, Eaton Wing North, EN12-238, Toronto, Ontario M5G 2C4, Canada; [d] Medicine, Toronto General Hospital, University of Toronto, 200 Elizabeth Street, Eaton Wing North, EN12-238, Toronto, Ontario M5G 2C4, Canada; [e] Public Health Sciences, Toronto General Hospital, University of Toronto, 200 Elizabeth Street, Eaton Wing North, EN12-238, Toronto, Ontario M5G 2C4, Canada; [f] Hemoglobal®, 75 Indian Grove, Toronto, Ontario M6R 2Y5, Canada
* Corresponding author. Liverpool School of Tropical Medicine, Pembroke Place, Liverpool L3 5QA, UK.
E-mail address: aallengm@yahoo.co.uk

Hematol Oncol Clin N Am 30 (2016) 497–512
http://dx.doi.org/10.1016/j.hoc.2015.11.012
0889-8588/16/$ – see front matter © 2016 Elsevier Inc. All rights reserved.

settings. The decline in childhood mortality rates in Asian countries over the past four decades has resulted in substantial proportions of many countries' health-care budgets now being consumed in the management of surviving patients. We had previously estimated that in Sri Lanka, the management of thalassemia could shortly require about 5% of the country's health budget.[1] Therefore, even in Sri Lanka where care has reached a commendable standard,[2] it remains critical to continue to plan not only for programs for screening and counseling in thalassemia, but for improvements in clinical and laboratory services in patients whose lengthening survival is often associated with increasingly complex care.

IMPROVING CLINICAL SERVICES IN RESOURCE-POOR SETTINGS

The approaches suggested here to improve clinical services include *education* to increase the knowledge base about thalassemia, including approaches to long-distance education. Improvements in the *delivery of care* will include those in clinical facilities as well as in the organization of health care, with emphases on continuity of care and on accountability. Meticulous approaches to history and physical examination and to record keeping in local clinics may assist development of national programs of data management. Extending the *access to essential medicines* is a critical issue in almost all Asian countries. As well, there is a view – not usually overtly expressed – in many countries that thalassemia is a hopeless disease in which a substantial investment is wasted. This requires efforts to *change attitudes* within health care systems and governments who may not provide many basic health services to their citizens. South-South partnerships may be critical in many of these approaches (See Fucharoen S, Weatherall DJ: Progress towards the control and management of the thalassemias, in this issue).

Expansion of Medical Education

Early investment to increase the knowledge base in the thalassemias, beginning in medical school and including training in pediatrics and hematology, would represent a long term positive investment in improving clinical management of these complex disorders. Examples are illustrated from Sri Lanka.

Medical school

In Sri Lanka exposure to thalassemia in medical school includes a few lectures on hematologic disorders, including thalassaemia, two practical laboratories including one during the later clinical rotation and, during clinical clerkship, opportunities to manage patients.

Pediatrics

As in many other countries in Asia, in Sri Lanka thalassemia patients are generally managed by pediatricians, many of whom may have received limited exposure to thalassemia following medical school. Over 4 years of pediatric training, including one as a registrar, a week-long, largely laboratory-based, rotation in hematology is provided. During a mandatory subsequent year of training overseas, there may be opportunities to manage patients with thalassemia (Professor Sanath Lamabadusuriya, personal communication, 2015).

Hematology

Thalassemia patients in Sri Lanka are not managed by hematologists, whose training, as per the traditional British model, focuses primarily on laboratory experience with less extensive clinical training. During 4 years of formal laboratory training and a relatively shorter period of clinical training, there may be no experience in thalassaemia, although there may be clinical exposure during years as a registrar, or overseas (Dr Senani Williams, personal communication, 2015).

The upshot of all this is that a newly-qualified pediatrician may be charged with responsibility of hundreds of patients in a rural setting, despite limited expertise and experience in either laboratory or clinical problems of thalassaemia; in parallel, individuals who have extensive hematology training in thalassemia may possess limited understanding of clinical issues. Similar situations exist in other emerging countries, but may be evolving, as they are in Sri Lanka. In Sri Lanka at present approximately ten pediatricians and a few consultant hematologists are trained annually. The doctor-patient ratio in 2010 in Sri Lanka was 0.7/1000 population (compared to 2.7 in the UK, 2.4 in the United States, and 2.1 in Canada); in many emerging countries, this ratio is much lower.[3] Yet even in countries where chronic understaffing may be accepted as inevitable, the optimal arrangement and one that would improve care without additional extensive financial outlay is a network of dedicated clinicians, working with designated laboratories, in a few expert centers.

Possible approaches to change
Expansion of the medical school curriculum to include exposure to the evidence for current practices in thalassemia, with emphasis on independent guidelines of management, may stimulate early scientific interest in this fascinating disease. Following medical school, more comprehensive laboratory training for pediatric trainees and extended clinical rotations for those in hematology might usher in a new era of cooperative care. Some of the country's prominent pediatricians have suggested that in future, defined periods spent in dedicated thalassemia units be mandated as part of pediatric training. These units need to be expanded to more centers, given that in many emerging countries many patients live hours from the closest center of excellence with a potential inaccessibility to expert care. Efforts to expand the expertise that is often concentrated in urban centers have been assisted over the last decade with advances in communication technology, including the potential for telemedicine to play a potential role.[4–6]

Improved Delivery of Care

Organization of clinical facilities
In many emerging countries, in the absence of hemoglobin screening programs, thalassemia patients are often first diagnosed during an admission to an emergency department, where a variable range of understanding of thalassemia care may be encountered. In Sri Lanka, if admission is required, a patient aged older than 13 years (the age after which a child is registered as an "adult") will be admitted to an adult ward. If a pediatrician trained in thalassemia management (or if expert "on call" advice was available), a child could be reviewed and if necessary admitted to a pediatric ward, improving continuity of care. With respect to thalassemia *outpatient* management, a separate facility need not be a freestanding structure. Two or three dedicated rooms, including a transfusion and treatment area, a (private) patient consultation area and, if possible a waiting area, are sufficient.

Re-organization of the structure of the health care team
Arguably the most effective approach to improve clinical services for this disorder would be to ensure *continuity of care*. Efforts to establish dedicated expert centers in which interested, motivated pediatricians and hematologists act as Thalassemia Center Directors with extended terms of appointment, who supervise all care and mentor junior staff, would improve a common arrangement by which senior staff relocate every few years. Prior to taking up a post as a Thalassemia Center Director,

dedicated short courses could be provided to consultants interested in thalassemia management, who would then be assigned ultimate responsibility for all patients, if not permanently, for extended periods.

Management guidelines providing evidence-based recommendations for clinical assessment, medication use, and patient monitoring that is tailored to the center can be provided. Regular review of all clinical and laboratory data on each patient, at not longer than 3-month intervals, and seminars and meetings focusing on evidence-based management, will maintain compliance with management guidelines. Interest can thereby be promoted in trainees, for whom a process should be established for regular attendance at each center. Because ongoing assessment of complications including those in the cardiac, hepatic and endocrine systems is critical in thalassaemia care, relationships with consultants in the relevant sub-specialities should be established, and may help to expand sub-networks of interested and expert care. Related to continuity is *accountability* in care. The concept of a minimum standard of care, even in rural settings, is of critical importance. Regular mortality/morbidity rounds to document causes of death, complications, and parameters of iron control can evaluate the compliance with management guidelines, and direct optimization of care. The use of quality assessments by impartial independent reviewers can help guide physicians in appropriate practices.

In parallel, it is equally important that staff morale be maintained. Efforts toward academic work should be encouraged and promoted. Not only Center Directors, but others including nursing staff, should be provided with opportunities for continuing medical education, both locally and abroad.

Emphasis on clinical skills and 'low tech' approaches to care

Clinical care may be facilitated by encouraging what could be termed "low tech" approaches with a targeted meticulous approach to history and physical examination and careful record keeping. **Boxes 1** and **2** highlight some important points from the history and physical examination, using the example of thalassemia, which when documented over time allow substantial understanding of the patient's status.

Box 1
Important points to be obtained in the history

Date of diagnosis

Presenting symptoms and signs at diagnosis

Hemoglobin prior to first transfusion

Date of first transfusion

Date of initiation of regular transfusions (8 or more transfusions/year)

Reasons for initiation of regular transfusions, if applicable

Transfusion history including regular update of number of transfusions received to date

Year of initiation of iron-chelating therapy if applicable

Initial clinical parameters at initiation of iron-chelating therapy

Year of, and indication for, splenectomy if applicable

Compliance with medication

Age at menarche (and mother's age at menarche if available)

Box 2
Physical and laboratory findings

Documented meticulously in the clinical record on each visit, the following allows substantial understanding of the patient's status.

- In children, height and weight and comparison with healthy siblings to identify potential growth attenuation commonly observed in thalassaemia; in adults, comparison to parental height;

- Spleen size to permit evaluation of extramedullary activity, indications for increased intensity of transfusions, and/or consideration of splenectomy;

- In older patients, Tanner staging to permit identification of pubertal delay and failure and interpretation of growth pattern;

- In all patients, hematocrit and date of each unit of packed cells administered, to estimate annual iron accumulation and the cumulative body iron burden;

- In all, pre-transfusion hemoglobin (by automated counters) including to identify early hypersplenism, evaluate growth difficulties, interpret marrow expansion;

- In children greater than 4 years, bone age to interpret potential delays of linear growth;

- In all patients annual facial photography to record potential bony expansion.

Data management

In our experience at the National Thalassemia Center in Sri Lanka, the presence of an efficient, dedicated, multi-tasking clinic manager with broad responsibility but above all that for organizing data and charts, has been extremely valuable. Data does not have to be recorded electronically; indeed, this is often not practical in many settings. Where sufficient staff are available there is value in developing a local data base which among other goals, permits tracking of numbers and of local statistics; a uniform country-wide system of recording clinical and laboratory data assists in evaluation of national trends. It is a common but, in our view, inadvisable practice to have the patient keep even limited medical records at home as these may often be misplaced. Finally, as identified in other chronic disorders[6] maintenance of a national registry by a trusted source may assist the understanding by the government of the necessity to increase resources for care.

Increased access to essential medicines

In many cases high drug prices, often the result of intellectual property "protection", are a serious barrier to access to essential medicines. Efforts to reduce drug prices are opposed by many industrialized countries and the pharmaceutical industry. The potential solutions to this are complex, including alliances with Health Directors and ministries, education and organization of parents' groups, and continued resistance from humanitarian organizations.[7]

Changes in attitude

Changes in the perception of thalassemia is critical to the success of the initiatives outlined above. There remains a contrast between the expectations of care in richer countries for thalassemia and many other once predictably-fatal disorders which have evolved to a chronic disease, and emerging countries, in which many patients remain under-diagnosed and under-treated. However, even in countries lacking the public health system of Sri Lanka, survival in thalassemia has almost doubled over the past four decades, due primarily to the wider availability of iron-chelating therapy.[8]

Given recent initiatives in India, the previously discouraging general lack of access to chelation therapy[9] may be changing.

Governments, companies interested in corporate social responsibility, and interested charities may be accessed to provide resources with varying success. As an example, our charity, Hemoglobal in cooperation with a private health facility in Sri Lanka, recently was able to begin quantitative testing to evaluate iron overload *in vivo*.[10] Following this effort, the Sri Lankan Director General of Health reinforced the commitment to make such monitoring available annually for a cohort of patients. Similar approaches may be feasible in other countries.

Of course, as long as governments do not support basic health priorities including sanitation and immunization, thalassaemia – whatever its prevalence – will not be conceived as a high national priority. But there is no doubt that continued lack of attention leading to poor physical, psychological and social functioning, as these patients survive but develop irreversible complications, is increasingly costly in social and economic terms.[11] Furthermore, experience in other diseases also shows that governments respond to pressure and that individual efforts to improve care and awareness may have long-lasting impact. Our own experience in Sri Lanka emphasizes that even one dedicated individual, over years of effort, can increase the involvement of a government willing to listen. One example includes the observed doubling over the past 20 years, in Sri Lanka, of the use of iron-chelating therapy. Still another is the initiation of a screening, education and prevention program in Sri Lanka, where the government has recognized that such approaches are key to reducing the burden of disease.

IMPROVING LABORATORY SERVICES IN RESOURCE-POOR SETTINGS

Gaps in access to essential laboratory testing are costly to excellent patient care. An early example from our work in Sri Lanka was the (former) limited availability of the measurement of serum ferritin as a measure of the common complication of iron overload in thalassemia. This prevented the reliable interpretation of clinical status and, therefore, the provision of safe and effective care. Expanded access to this testing has helped to encourage evidence-based management.

The difficulties in establishing and delivering reliable clinical diagnostic laboratory services in resource-limited settings are well recognised.[12–16] Limited equipment, consumables, reagents, standards and quality control materials coupled with intermittent water and electricity supplies, make day to day work quite a challenge. Although these difficulties are faced in the large city hospital and reference laboratories, they are often more pronounced in the smaller district hospitals and village health centers, which are often last in the chain to receive what already limited resources are available. Unfortunately, health burdens are usually greatest in the very places where resources for health care are the most limited.[17]

The problems of limited resources are compounded by difficulties in providing adequate training so that laboratory staff lack the skills necessary to deliver reliable results that are essential for effective health care. This can lead to clinical staff mistrusting laboratory results, which in turn leads to low staff morale. Morale can be further undermined by inadequate supervision and also career progression opportunities.

Degree and diploma courses in Biomedical Sciences and laboratory technology are often only available in the larger cities, in neighboring countries or overseas. Limited laboratory staff and funding means that these courses are often not easily accessible, particularly to those based in the more remote laboratories where they may be the sole provider of the laboratory services. Furthermore, laboratory personnel may lack the necessary qualifications for enrollment. Therefore, it is often necessary to provide meaningful training for laboratory personnel, that is appropriate for their capabilities, relevant to the laboratory in which they work and the population they serve and delivered within existing resources. We will focus on what can be achieved through locally-led initiatives and without formal external training courses as these may not be available for the majority of staff.

Investments in training are justified if they result in improved practice. Therefore, to ensure that training is relevant to the local service, it is best delivered as part of broader quality improvement (QI). Simple, generic tools for improving the quality of services are readily available and can be applied to a laboratory setting.

Implementing Quality Improvement

"Everyone in healthcare really has two jobs when they come to work every day: to do their work and to improve it"[18] applies equally to laboratory staff. The World Medical Association guidelines on continuous QI in health care are targeted at physicians and health institutions but are relevant to all healthcare professionals.[19]

Locally driven QI initiatives can engage all members of the laboratory team and provide a broad range of training and capacity development opportunities including leadership, team working, problem solving and communication.

QI has been defined as "the combined and unceasing efforts of everyone—healthcare professionals, patients and their families, researchers, payers, planners and educators—to make the changes that will lead to better patient outcomes (health), better system performance (care) and better professional development (learning)".[19] This definition highlights that the critical outcome is the whole service delivered to the patient, of which individual laboratory procedures are only a part. Therefore, laboratory staff need to lead or join QI initiatives that take a patient-centred and comprehensive approach and engage a broad range of stakeholders. **Table 1** presents the key elements of QI and how these can be applied to laboratory services.

Improvement in services requires a sequence of activities to be undertaken (**Box 3**). It is important to note that, rather than "task and finish", QI is an on-going, cyclical process so that continual improvements in services occur. Where laboratory technicians are working in isolation, local networks can be formed to deliver QI addressing basic procedures across several laboratory facilities.

Step 1 of Quality Improvement Cycle: Benchmarking

The QI cycle starts by identifying universally accepted standards of laboratory practice that can provide benchmarks for the development of services. This is also critical in advocating for additional resources to enable practice to improve toward these standards. All clinical diagnostic laboratories in resource limited settings should strive to work in accordance with nationally agreed standards and, where possible, to International Organization for Standardization (ISO) standard ISO 15189. This ensures an excellent laboratory quality management system, technical competence and the ability to provide reliable and accurate results.

In South East Asia, laboratory accreditation programs are well established in India, Indonesia and Thailand.[20] Following a WHO South East Asian inter-country laboratory accreditation workshop held in Thailand in 2006, a laboratory accreditation program was started in Sri Lanka adopting ISO 15189 as the standard. To date, many private hospital laboratories have been accredited.

Table 1
Five foundation stones for quality improvement applied to laboratory practice

1. Focus on the client	• View the service that you provide from the patient's perspective • Engage patient representatives as key members of your QI team
2. Focus on team work	• Efficient and effective services require team work • What can each member of your existing staff contribute? • Who might require additional in-service training? • Could staff be better organized to improve the service delivered?
3. Focus on data	• Rather than anecdotal reports, what information is available about your service? • Undertake audit to obtain data about specific aspects of the service • Qualitative information from service-users (patients, clinical staff) is essential
4. Focus on systems and processes	• Take a comprehensive view of the whole service from the patient's perspective • Consider systems such as patient waiting times, the environment where samples are collected and the reporting of results as well as processes such as laboratory protocols
5. Communication and feedback	• Critically important throughout • Starts with engaging key stakeholders to identify areas for service improvement • Regular feedback of performance should encourage staff and identify areas for further improvement

Adapted from Quality Improvement Guide. Quality improvement - the key to providing improved quality of care. Republic of South Africa: Department of Health; 2012. Available at: www.rudasa.org.za. Accessed July 13, 2015.

In the Government sector, the National blood transfusion service laboratory is accredited and there are plans to extend the program to include all other Government hospital laboratories. With this in mind, National External Quality Assurance (NEQAs) programs have been established since 2012, and workshops for technical officers and provincial training programs are conducted regularly by the Ministry of Health, Sri Lanka College of Haematologists and the Sri Lanka Accreditation Board (Dr Chandana Wickremaratne, personal communication, 2015).

Box 3
The quality improvement cycle

1. Use core standards as a benchmark to assess current services, and to provide a baseline to compare future changes

2. Engage in QI starting by identifying gaps or deficiencies in current provision

3. Understand the whole system to uncover barriers; analyze causes, and explore alternative ways to improve

4. Develop a plan to address the gaps or deficiencies and improve provision

5. Test and monitor the changes; implement successful changes

6. Sustain changes; continuous quality improvement

Adapted from Quality Improvement Guide. Quality improvement - the key to providing improved quality of care. Republic of South Africa: Department of Health; 2012. Available at: www.rudasa.org.za. Accessed July 13, 2015.

In Africa, the Maputo Declaration[21] and Joint WHO-CDC Conference on Health Laboratory Quality Systems,[22] both in 2008, aimed to strengthen and support laboratory systems in resource-limited settings to achieve national or the ISO 15189 international standards. In 2009, the Stepwise Laboratory Improvement Process Toward Accreditation (SLIPTA) and the Strengthen Laboratory Management Toward Accreditation (SLMTA) initiatives were established under WHO-Afro.[23,24] At the same time, a training tool kit developed by WHO, US Center for Disease Control and Prevention and the Clinical Laboratory Standards Institute was launched to assist laboratory trainers to educate and train laboratory staff in best practice.[25] This includes a Clinical Laboratory Standards Institute library of bench aids and guidance documents. These guidelines and resources are comprehensive and are most appropriate for the larger hospital and reference laboratories, but also provide a useful template and resource for all laboratory facilities.

Findings from a recent survey conducted in 49 countries in sub Saharan Africa showed that 380 laboratories have been accredited to international standards, and 91% of these laboratories are in South Africa. However, there were no accredited laboratories in 37/49 countries surveyed.[26]

Step 2 of Quality Improvement Cycle: Identify Gaps or Deficiencies in Current Provision

Based on a project in a clinical laboratory in West Africa, a requirement for patients to return the following day to collect hemoglobin (Hb) results was observed to delay clinical management (eg, blood transfusion), incur avoidable patient expenses and increase defaulting (patients often failed to return). A multi-stakeholder QI team, including two patient representatives, analyzed the likely causes and represented them in a fishbone diagram (**Fig. 1.**)

Step 3 of Quality Improvement Cycle: Consider the Whole System - the Sample Journey

It is critical to take a whole system approach as road blocks can occur at any step. Careful attention to quality control and standardizing sample testing is important as a laboratory may use instruments and reagents from several manufacturers to measure the same parameter.

The reliability of results can be evaluated according to:

- Accuracy – degree of closeness to the true value (eg, validated using a standard)
- Repeatability – the same result is obtained when the same parameter is measured multiple times in a single sample by the same technician using the same method
- Reproducibility – the same result is obtained from a single sample when different methods or instruments are used to measure the same parameter

Regular calibration and maintenance of equipment are essential to ensure reliability of tests, and where possible service contracts should be established at the time of purchase. External quality assurance programs such as NEQAS, tend to operate in the larger hospital laboratories in cities. However, it is also important to establish local laboratory networks that can facilitate the appropriate storage and distribution of control blood samples from a central hospital to neighboring peripheral laboratories. Control samples should be tested each morning to check instrument accuracy before testing patient samples. Control samples should also be included in subsequent batches of samples to monitor accuracy and test repeatability over the course of

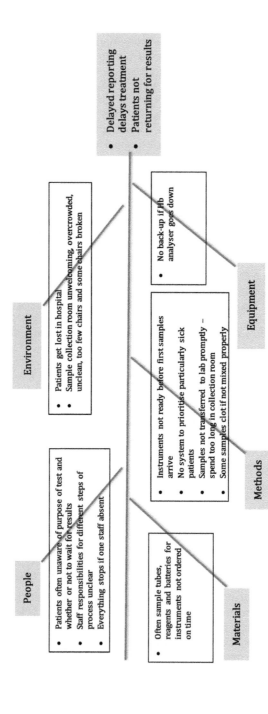

Fig. 1. Analysis of causes and effects: fishbone diagram.

Box 4
The "sample journey"

Laboratory request slip to request investigations

- Improves communication between clinical and laboratory staff

- Must be readily available in all departments where sample collection takes place

- Limited only to tests that the laboratory does, rather than aspires to do, to avoid frustration to clinicians!

- An adaptable template showing essential information is available.[27]

Sample collection

- Sample collection area should be clean, well lit, quiet and screened off from the laboratory and patient waiting area

- Acknowledge local greetings and put the patient and parent/carer at ease by speaking to them in a professional and pleasant manner; especially in children who are often frightened and upset

- Always explain what you are going to do and why you are doing it

- Ensure that everything needed is to hand

- Following collection, briefly review the patient and ensure that the puncture site has stopped bleeding

- Transfer the blood samples to the laboratory immediately

Reception in laboratory and sample log

- Ensure samples are in good condition, clearly labeled and have an accompanying laboratory request form with matching patient information

- Reject samples that are leaking, clotted or where patient information is inadequate and request a repeat sample immediately

- Record patient details (full name, date of birth, hospital or clinic number, ward), laboratory tests requested and the time and date of receipt in log book

Analyses

- Follow standard operating procedure (SOP) for each assay to ensure that equipment is operated correctly, safely and efficiently and procedures are carried out consistently by different members of staff

- Refer to trouble-shooting advice in the SOP for common problems that arise

- Make SOPs readily available especially where staff turnover is high

- Perform all measurements in duplicate or, where reagents are scarce, repeat measurements in every nth sample

- Templates for laboratory SOPs are readily available.[28]

Step 4: Reporting of results

- Check that results are presented clearly and correspond with the patient details

- Use the correct units and include normal reference ranges

- Confirm any abnormal results before reporting to the clinician or ward staff

- Be alert to results that are not in keeping with the clinical information provided on the laboratory form as these need particularly careful review

- Reporting must be timely to ensure that the patient receives prompt treatment

- Keep a separate record of all tests that can not be completed immediately and notify the clinician that the missing result will follow on

- Follow up on any outstanding results

Data from Laboratory quality stepwise implementation tool. Develop a request form for laboratory testing. Available at: https://extranet.who.int/lqsi/content/develop-request-form-laboratory-testing. Accessed June 29, 2015; and Laboratory quality stepwise implementation tool. Make SOPS for all tests performed by the laboratory. Available at: https://extranet.who.int/lqsi/content/make-sops-all-tests-performed-laboratory. Accessed June 29, 2015.

each day. Control results from each laboratory can be reviewed by the distributing laboratory to monitor performance across the network and identify if any remedial action is needed.

Where a regular supply of external control material is not achievable, it is still possible to establish internal quality control procedures:

- Repeat measurements in previously tested samples with normal, high and low values and known positive and negative samples when testing for hemoglobinopathies.
- Perform all measurements in duplicate when possible. However, where reagents are scarce, repeat measurements in every nth sample.

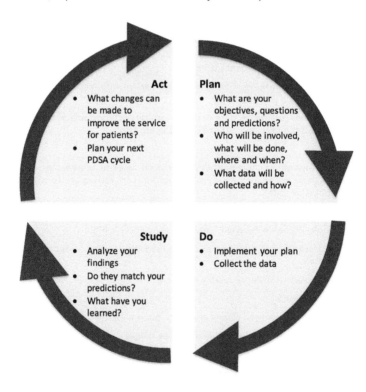

Fig. 2. The plan, do, study, act (PDSA) cycle. (*Adapted from* NHS Institute for Innovation and Improvement 2008. Available at: http://www.institute.nhs.uk/quality_and_service_improvement_tools/quality_and_service_improvement_tools/plan_do_study_act.html. Accessed July 13, 2015.)

Box 5
PDSA cycle to achieve timely clinical management through prompt reporting of hemoglobin values

Plan	• Question: Why can we not report Hb values promptly?
	• Aim: Report Hb value within one hour of sample collection
	• Prediction: All results can be reported within 1 h of sample collection
	Establish a QI team comprising: two patient representatives, phlebotomist, lab staff, clinician, store man, hospital manager
	Complete QI initiative within 6 mo including evaluation of impact
Do	Baseline audit of time from sample request (recorded on the investigation request form) to providing the result to the patient (recorded in a ledger in the lab reception area)
Study	Review findings from baseline audit
	Undertake analysis of barriers and causes of delays; present findings in a fishbone diagram (see **Fig. 1**)
Act	Main elements of QI implementation

	People	• Ward/clinic staff explain reasons for measuring Hb
		• Phlebotomist advises patient to return for result to lab reception area in 30 min
		• Individual lab staff allocated responsibility for sample transport, recording and Hb measurement
		• Deputy identified if staff member absent
	Environment	• Colored signs to sample collection room put-up in hospital
		• Room, cleaned, painted, provided with benches
		• Only one parent/guardian per patient allowed in to sample collection room
	Materials	• Daily check on supply of basic reagents and sample tubes
		• When to re-order from stores clarified
	Methods	• SOP for daily lab set-up; start at 07.30 h, instrument warm-up and running quality control samples
		• Tick box on investigation request form to prioritise sick patients (eg, may need urgent transfusion)
		• 15 min schedule for sample transfer; designated staff members
		• Training to ensure all samples awaiting analysis placed on roller mixer
	Equipment	• PCV measured and reported immediately if Hb value not available within 30 min

Re-audit at 6 months. Feedback findings in a hospital meeting. Identify on-going problems to further improve the service.

• Ensure that all blood films are read twice, preferably by two independent microscopists, save every nth blood film and send to an expert microscopist at the regional hospital laboratory on a monthly basis to check the quality of the blood film preparation and staining and the accuracy of reading.

Box 4 outlines the key steps in the sample journey which may need attention to ensure that the whole process is performed to the desired standard.

Step 4 of the Quality Improvement Cycle - Developing a Plan for Service Improvement

The "Plan, Do, Study, Act" (PDSA) cycle provides a useful structure for developing a plan and can be adapted to laboratory settings (**Fig. 2**). Again using the West Africa project as an example, the main elements of the cycle for this project are shown in **Box 5**.

Steps 5 and 6 of the Quality Improvement Cycle: Test, Monitor, Implement and Sustain Successful Changes

Although clearly critical to improving services over the longer term, these are often the most difficult elements of QI to achieve. The initial enthusiasm often wanes as improvements are achieved and key staff move on. Establishing a continuous QI ethos amongst all laboratory staff takes time and this overall aim should be explicit in all projects. Integrating meaningful training activities to QI initiatives is a key element in engaging staff and ensuring that service improvement is a routine part of everyone's day.

SUMMARY

Over the last few years, a number of resource-poor countries, obtaining support from appropriate governmental sources, have assessed the gaps in care and improved clinical services for patients with thalassemia. Despite limited resources, much can be achieved through a concerted QI approach. Attention to systems and processes quickly identifies opportunities for staff training that directly improves the service. A home grown quality improvement ethos within clinical and laboratory departments is also essential to maximize the impact of any additional resources and external training that can be secured. Assisting federal or state governments to understand the many complex demands of clinical care in thalassaemia and other chronic and common disorders is a critical element in improving patient outcomes.

REFERENCES

1. De Silva S, Fisher CA, Premawardhena A, et al. Thalassaemia in Sri Lanka: implications for the future health burden of Asian populations. Lancet 2000;355(9206): 786–91.
2. Olivieri NF, Muraca GM, O'Donnell A, et al. Studies in hemoglobin E beta-thalassaemia. Br J Haematol 2008;141:388–97.
3. The World Bank data. Physicians (per 1000 people). Available at: http://data.worldbank.org/indicator/SH.MED.PHYS.ZS. Accessed June 29, 2015.
4. Graham LE, Zimmerman M, Vassallo DJ, et al. Telemedicine: the way ahead for medicine in the developing world. Trop Doct 2003;33:36–8.
5. Pal A, Mbarika VWA, Cobb-Payton F, et al. Telemedicine diffusion in a developing country: the case of India (March 2004). IEEE Trans Inf Technol Biomed 2005;9: 59–65.
6. O'Mahony B, Black C. Expanding hemophilia care in developing countries. Semin Thromb Hemost 2005;31:561–8.
7. MSF Launches Global Campaign Urging India to Protect Access to Affordable Medicines. Available at: http://www.msfaccess.org/about-us/media-room/press-releases/msf-launches-global-campaign-urging-india-protect-access. Accessed June 29, 2015.

8. Chakrabarti P, Bohara V, Ray S, et al. Can the availability of unrestricted financial support improve the quality of care of thalassemics in a center with limited resources? A single center study from India. Thalassemia Reports 2013;3:e2, 6–10.

9. Modell B, Darlison M. Global epidemiology of hemoglobin disorders and derived service indicators. Bull World Health Organ 2008;86:480–7.

10. St. Pierre TG, Clark PR, Chua-anusorn W, et al. Non-invasive measurement and imaging of liver iron concentrations using proton magnetic resonance. Blood 2005;105:855–61.

11. Merchant RH, Shirodkar A, Ahmed J. Evaluation of growth, puberty and endocrine dysfunctions in relation to iron overload in multi transfused Indian thalassemia patients. Indian J Pediatr 2011;78:679–83.

12. Petti CA, Polage CR, Quinn TC, et al. Laboratory medicine in Africa: a barrier to effective health care. Clin Infect Dis 2006;42(3):377–82.

13. Bates I, Maitland K. Are laboratory services coming of age in sub-Saharan Africa? Clin Infect Dis 2006;42(3):383–4.

14. Okeke IN. Diagnostic insufficiency in Africa. Clin Infect Dis 2006;42(10):1501–3.

15. Muula AS, Maseko FC. Medical laboratory services in Africa deserve more. Clin Infect Dis 2006;42(10):1503.

16. Nkengasong JN, Nsubuga P, Nwanyanwu O, et al. Laboratory systems and services are critical in global health. Time to end the neglect. Am J Clin Pathol 2010; 134:368–73.

17. Bates I, Carter J. Haematology in under resourced laboratories. In: Bain BJ, Bates I, Laffan M, et al, editors. Dacie and lewis practical haematology. 11th edition. London: Elsevier Churchill Livingstone; 2012. p. 607.

18. Batalden PB, Davidoff F. What is "quality improvement" and how can it transform healthcare? Qual Saf Health Care 2007;16:2–3.

19. WMA declaration on guidelines for continuous quality improvement in health care. Available at: http://www.wma.net/en/30publications/10policies/g10/. Accessed June 29, 2015.

20. WHO Report of Inter country workshop in Thailand Oct 9-13th 2006. Establishment of quality systems and accreditation in health laboratories. Available at: http://www.apps.searo.who.int/PDS_DOCS/B0405.pdf. Accessed June 29, 2015.

21. The Maputo declaration-World Health Organization. Available at: www.who.int/diagnostics_laboratory/Maputo-Declaration_2008.pdf. Accessed June 29, 2015.

22. Joint WHO-CDC conference on health laboratory quality systems. Lyon (France), 2008. Available at: http://www.who.int/ihr/lyon/report20080409.pdf. Accessed June 29, 2015.

23. WHO Guide for the Stepwise Laboratory Improvement Process Towards Accreditation in the African Region (with checklist) - WHO Regional Office for Africa. Accessed June 29, 2015. Available at: http://www.afro.who.int. Accessed December 16, 2015.

24. SLMTA Strengthening Laboratory Management Toward Accreditation. Accessed June 29, 2015. Available at: http://www.slmta.org. Accessed December 16, 2015.

25. Laboratory quality management systems training kit. Available at: http://www.who.int/ihr/training/laboratory_quality/doc/en. Accessed June 29, 2015.

26. Schroeder LF, Amukele T. Medical Laboratories in sub-Saharan Africa that meet international quality standards. Am J Clin Pathol 2014;141:791–5.

27. Laboratory quality stepwise implementation tool. Develop a request form for laboratory testing. Available at: https://extranet.who.int/lqsi/content/develop-request-form-laboratory-testing. Accessed June 29, 2015.

28. Laboratory quality stepwise implementation tool. Make SOPS for all tests performed by the laboratory. Available at: https://extranet.who.int/lqsi/content/make-sops-all-tests-performed-laboratory. Accessed June 29, 2015.

FURTHER READINGS

Bain BJ, Bates I, Laffan M, et al, editors. Dacie and lewis practical haematology. 11th edition. London: Elsevier Churchill Livingstone; 2012. ISBN 9780702034077.

Cheesbrough M, editor. District laboratory practice in tropical countries, part 1. 2nd edition update. Cambridge (UK): Cambridge University Press; 2006. ISBN. 978-0-521-67632-8.

Cheesbrough M, editor. District laboratory practice in tropical countries, part 2. 2nd edition update. Cambridge (UK): Cambridge University Press; 2006. ISBN. 978-0-521-67633-5.

Cheesbrough M. Tropical medicine microscopy. Norwich (United Kingdom): Swallowtail Print; 2014. Distributed by Teaching Aids at Low Cost (TALC), St Albans (United Kingdom).

Index

Note: Page numbers of article titles are in **boldface** type.

Hematol Oncol Clin N Am 30 (2016) 513–527
http://dx.doi.org/10.1016/S0889-8588(16)30009-0
0889-8588/16/$ – see front matter © 2016 Elsevier Inc. All rights reserved.

hemonc.theclinics.com

Moving?

Make sure your subscription moves with you!

To notify us of your new address, find your **Clinics Account Number** (located on your mailing label above your name), and contact customer service at:

Email: journalscustomerservice-usa@elsevier.com

800-654-2452 (subscribers in the U.S. & Canada)
314-447-8871 (subscribers outside of the U.S. & Canada)

Fax number: 314-447-8029

Elsevier Health Sciences Division
Subscription Customer Service
3251 Riverport Lane
Maryland Heights, MO 63043

*To ensure uninterrupted delivery of your subscription, please notify us at least 4 weeks in advance of move.

Printed and bound by CPI Group (UK) Ltd, Croydon, CR0 4YY

07/10/2024

01040505-0007